The Middleboro Casebook

Second Edition

The Middleboro Casebook

Healthcare Strategy and Operations

Lee F. Seidel
James B. Lewis

AUPHA

Health Administration Press, Chicago, Illinois

Association of University Programs in Health Administration, Washington, DC

Acquisitions editor: Janet Davis; Project manager: Jane Calayag; Cover designer: James Slate; Layout: Virginia Byrne

Found an error or a typo? We want to know! Please e-mail it to hapbooks@ache.org, mentioning the book's title and putting "Book Error" in the subject line.

For photocopying and copyright information, please contact Copyright Clearance Center at www.copyright.com or at (978) 750-8400.

Health Administration Press
A division of the Foundation of the American
   College of Healthcare Executives
One North Franklin Street, Suite 1700
Chicago, IL 60606-3529
(312) 424-2800

Association of University Programs
   in Health Administration
1730 M Street, NW
Suite 407
Washington, DC 20036
(202) 763-7283

Dedicated to Dr. Mary Fox Arnold (1920–2005), a dynamic professor and healthcare professional. She inspired the early works that led to this book.

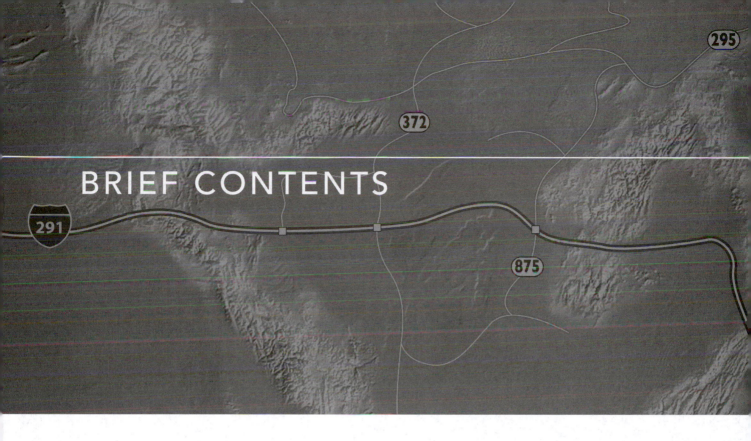

BRIEF CONTENTS

DETAILED CONTENTS

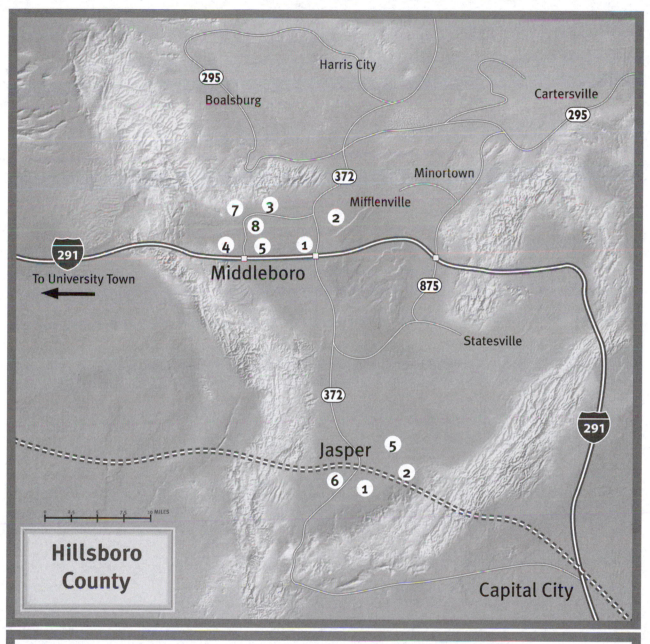

Map Legend

Mountains

County and State Roads

Interstate Highway

Interstate Highway
(Under Construction)

❶ Hillsboro Health (HH)–Middleboro and Jasper
❷ Physician Care Services (PCS)–Mifflenville and Jasper
❸ Middleboro Medical Center (MIDCARE)–Middleboro
❹ Webster Health System (WHS)–Middleboro
❺ Medical Associates (MA)–Middleboro and Jasper
❻ Jasper Gardens (JG)–Jasper
❼ Hillsboro County Health Department (HCHD)–Middleboro
❽ Middleboro Community Mental Health Center (MCMHC)–Middleboro

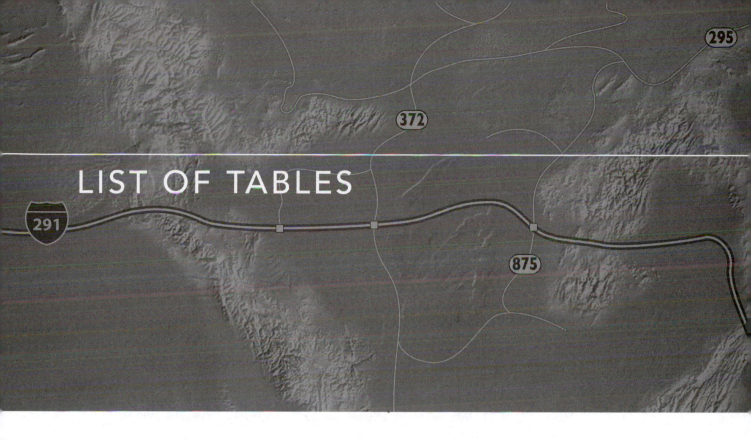

LIST OF TABLES

An asterisk (*) indicates that an Excel version of the table is available on the web at *ache.org/books/Middleboro2.*

Case 1

Case 5

Case 6

Case 7

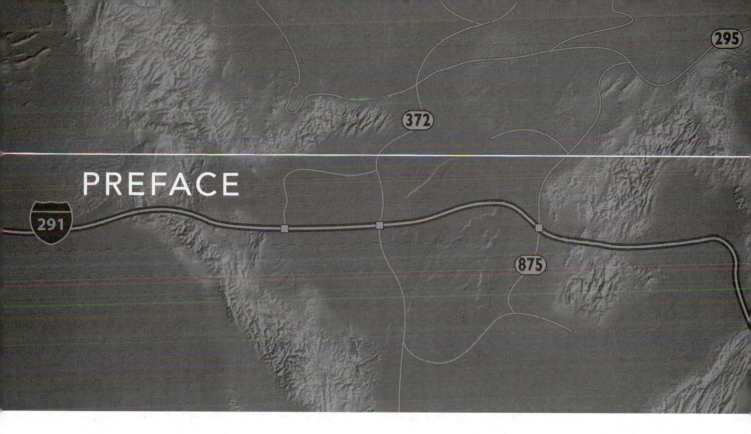

PREFACE

The *Middleboro Casebook* is a flexible and integrated case study that focuses on the strategy and operations of eight healthcare organizations—two hospitals, a long-term care facility, a home health agency, two physician group practices, a community mental health center, and a local health department—located in and around the community of Middleboro. The book introduces students to the community as well as its demographic, socioeconomic, political, economic, epidemiological, and environmental characteristics. Data presented in the tables enable students to analyze the community in detail, focusing on those factors that drive the need for and use of healthcare services as well as framing the strategic decisions made by healthcare organizations. The cases provide information about the primary healthcare organizations in Middleboro and the surrounding area. Each case includes the organization's history, governance, organizational structure, programs and services, finances, and particular issues and challenges.

CONCEPT OF THE BOOK

We developed *The Middleboro Casebook* to bring authentic management and policy issues into the classroom and to assist students and faculty with integrating an academic curriculum in health administration. It provides the basis for identifying many types of problems and issues and for formulating management plans and strategies. Since its inception, it has assisted faculty with providing a robust integrating seminar between traditional academic study and professional practice.

This is a unique casebook. It is designed specifically for the field of health administration. The cases and the setting—Hillsboro County—are totally fictitious, removing "what really happened" scenarios from the solutions and strategies provided by students. Also, each healthcare organization featured here is described in detail in the context of its common community. Each case requires understanding from many fields and disciplines, not just one. The cases blend together the national forces and issues that influence the management of healthcare organizations today with the local forces and issues that make health services management unique. Sensitivity to local events, circumstances, and issues is essential; just as in professional practice, the local dimension is impossible to exclude from the management of health services.

This is a unique academic text as well. It provides student and faculty users with the freedom and flexibility to achieve many different types of learning outcomes. For example, students can be asked to define a comprehensive strategy for a specific business unit or to complete a focused analysis on a specific aspect of an organization (e.g., financial, marketing). Each case presents a detailed picture of the structure and operation of a different type of healthcare organization. Notice that no specific student assignments have been included. The reason for that is to allow the instructor to define how the book is used and decide what assignments—and, if needed, additional information—to give. The Instructor Resources include field-tested assignments for many types of graduate- and baccalaureate-level courses and select companion texts. For example, in our class, we hand out one- or two-page "Assignment Letters" that include questions and often additional information to support specific assignments.

THE SECOND EDITION

The first edition of this book—published in 2014—found its niche in many academic settings, including baccalaureate and graduate programs, schools of business, and public health and human services. It was used to support traditional study as well as executive education and online instruction. It met our original goal of helping students assess and develop their professional repertoire via practice and application.

This second edition includes all of the original cases, each of which has been revised and expanded to reflect contemporary trends and issues, and a new case about a community mental health center (case 4). *Note that the data in the second edition have no relationship with the data in the first edition. Each edition is independent.* We appreciate

Health Administration Press's understanding that this type of book must be refreshed and updated regularly if it is to continue as an authentic instructional resource for health administration education.

As was true of the first edition, this edition can be used in many ways. First, it can be the stand-alone text for an integrating course or a course in strategic planning or management. Second, as some faculty members have done, it can be the course in a graduate program that introduces students to the "real world" issues in health services management and familiarizes them with the structure and function of a regional healthcare system. Third, it can be the basis for a model—such as the one developed by Dr. Gary Filerman at Georgetown University—whereby the cases are used in multiple foundation courses in which students develop strategic analyses and business plans for a specific organization featured in the casebook. This model approach, which we call "Middleboro Across the Curriculum," provides depth, breadth, and integration to many courses. Other universities have reported using the book with a similar approach.

Helping students integrate and apply their learning is an essential component of any academic curriculum intended to prepare professionals. This casebook serves as an alternative to approaches such as directed field-based consulting and projects, which by their very nature are limited by the particular project and may not be truly integrative.

The cases reflect contemporary, plausible reality—a reality influenced by many events and forces. Since the 2010 passage of the Affordable Care Act (Public Law 111–148), health services providers in the United States have been facing new and ever-evolving requirements and issues. The suggested assignments in the Instructor Resources are intended to ensure that students are dealing with current issues and reality.

CONCLUSION

Middleboro, Hillsboro County, and all the organizations and people described in the book are, again, totally fictitious. Any similarity to real people, places, or events is merely an unintended consequence. (For the record, Middleboro, Jasper, and Hillsboro County are not in New Hampshire.) Also, there are no preconceived outcomes here. Management is both an art and a science. We hope health administration students use both to define and address problems, improve access and quality, and lower costs.

Remember that every case is layered, so students—and other users of the book—should peel it like an onion. Read it over—numerous times. Look for connections. Explore it. Think about it. Understand that the cases are related and integrated. For example, some of the physicians affiliated with Medical Associates (case 7) are on the medical staff of MIDCARE, Inc. (case 6). Even though an assignment may focus on one organization, relevant information can be gathered from the other cases.

The book requires students to apply their managerial repertoires to sort through the facts and issues. They must decide what is important and what is trivial. They may use the cases to integrate and broaden—as well as sharpen—their analytical and intuitive abilities as a professional manager of health services. They may "connect the dots" they deem important. For example, in Hillsboro County, the same last name may suggest people are related by birth or marriage.

One cannot become an accomplished musician merely by studying music theory. The same can be said of health administration students who merely learn management skills, insights, and principles but do not apply and test them. This book helps students mature beyond the silos of learning that characterize higher education. Remember that truly integrating learning is the student's responsibility; faculty can only provide the opportunity, support, and general direction. Most students, regardless of their background, both love and hate this book. Some think it has too much information, while others think it offers not enough. Over many years, however, most students have agreed that—on their way to becoming proficient managers of organized health services—the book validated, changed, and sharpened their professional skills, values, and insights.

Health services management requires both educational and experiential preparation. We hope this book provides some of each. Welcome to Middleboro and Hillsboro County. It is midnight January 1, 2020. The year 2019 has just ended and 2020 has just begun.

Lee F. Seidel, PhD
James B. Lewis, ScD

ACKNOWLEDGMENTS

To ensure that all cases are realistic, we asked senior healthcare executives to review and comment on each case. Cathy, Dan, Dennis, Ellen, Eugene, Fritz, Jay, Mike, Steve, Tim, Tom, and Yousef have read these cases and given us their perspectives as successful managers in different sectors of our industry. Many others have volunteered their advice, as we continue to strive to provide our students with an effective foundation. Over the years, the cases also have benefited from the insights and suggestions by faculty members, senior healthcare executives, and students—especially the students and faculty in the Executive MBA program at the University of Colorado, Denver. Professor Errol Biggs, director of the Executive MBA in Health Administration at CU Denver, deserves our special recognition and appreciation. Errors in the many tables of data, however, are solely our responsibility.

INSTRUCTOR RESOURCES

This book's Instructor Resources include the following:

- *Using Middleboro* presents many issues and suggestions related to problem-based learning and case-method teaching applied to this case. This section includes using Assignment Letters and Case Assignments to create the "problems" for student attention.
- *Teaching Notes* provides short essays that describe what the instructor needs to know to use these cases effectively.
- *Suggested Assignments* recommends assignments in three categories: (1) assignments for each individual case (e.g., Webster Hospital); (2) assignments by subject (e.g., marketing); and (3) assignments for specific companion texts, including the following:

    Dunn, R. T. 2016. *Dunn & Haimann's Healthcare Management*, 10th edition. Chicago: Health Administration Press.

    Gapenski, L. C. 2013. *Fundamentals of Healthcare Finance*. Chicago: Health Administration Press.

    Gapenski, L. C., and K. L. Reiter. 2016. *Healthcare Finance: An Introduction to Accounting and Financial Management*, 6th edition. Chicago: Health Administration Press.

    Olden, P. C. 2015. *Management of Healthcare Organizations: An Introduction*, 2nd edition. Chicago: Health Administration Press.

    Thomas, R. K. 2015. *Marketing Health Services*, 3rd edition. Chicago: Health Administration Press.

    Walston, S.L. 2014. *Strategic Healthcare Management: Planning and Execution*. Chicago: Health Administration Press.

    White, K. R., and J. R. Griffith. 2015. *The Well-Managed Healthcare Organization*, 8th edition. Chicago: Health Administration Press.

    Zuckerman, A. M. 2012. *Healthcare Strategic Management*, 3rd edition. Chicago: Health Administration Press.

- *Other Materials* includes references and suggested URLs for instructors and students, including references related to oral presentations and business plans.

For the most up-to-date information about this book and its Instructor Resources, go to ache.org/HAP and browse for the book's title or author names.

This book's Instructor Resources are available to instructors who adopt this book for use in their course. For access information, please e-mail hapbooks@ache.org.

STUDENT RESOURCES

Excel versions of select tables are available online. In the book, tables that are posted online are indicated with a 🖥 and this line: On the web at *ache.org/books/Middleboro2*. The tables themselves and the List of Tables are marked by these indicators.

CASE 1

THE COMMUNITY

Many people regard Hillsboro County as a comfortable place to raise a family. It is an area known for its social and economic stability. While the residents are generally aware of national and world events, the local media coverage is dominated by news about the area's youth teams, social and fraternal organizations, church outings, and high school sports. Multiple generations of families live in Middleboro and the surrounding towns that make up Hillsboro County.

DEMOGRAPHIC CHARACTERISTICS

Middleboro and Hillsboro County are classified as non–metropolitan areas. Middleboro has been the economic, political, and social hub for Hillsboro County. The average family size is 2.57 people. Basic demographic data are given in tables 1.1 through 1.3 at the end of this case. (Note that the entire casebook is set at the start of 2020, so all tables are dated for the preceding years.)

On the web at ache.org/books/Middleboro2

    The other major town in Hillsboro County is Jasper, located 23 miles southeast of Middleboro. Jasper is a growing community that benefits from being close to Capital City, the state capital. Jasper is becoming a bedroom community for Capital City and is continuing to develop as an economy that is independent from Middleboro.

Geographic Characteristics

Surrounded on two sides by relatively high mountains, Middleboro is 45 miles northwest of Capital City and 70 miles east of University Town, the location of State University. Access to Middleboro is limited to rail (freight), bus, automobile, and truck. The majority of private and commercial travel is done on the auxiliary four-lane, east–west interstate highway, which is typically closed an average of three days per year because of weather conditions. Commercial air travel is available in Capital City. The mountains on the east and west make winter travel outside Middleboro especially difficult. The fertile valleys on the north and south are known for agricultural activities.

Outside of Middleboro and Jasper, the population lives in small, scattered villages. The only transportation linkages to Middleboro from these scattered communities are the rural county and state highways. Limited bus service is available throughout Hillsboro County. Middleboro serves as the regional transportation hub, and the bus station in Middleboro offers connections to major population centers in the state. Jasper is also served by this bus system. Recently, a commuter bus system began linking Jasper with Capital City.

Hillsboro County stretches 45 miles to the north, 15 miles to the west, 28 miles to the east, and 37 miles to the south of Middleboro. Seventy-one percent of the total area is developed, and the remainder is taken up by forest, the state park, and rivers. This area experiences four distinct seasons, but tourists find it especially attractive during the fall and spring. Sports of all types play an important role in the life of its communities. Table 1.4 indicates the miles between the communities located in Hillsboro County.

Middleboro is located along Swift River, which was instrumental in the commercial development of the city in the early 1800s. Before the turn of the century, Swift River and the commercial barges that traversed it were the city's primary linkage with the rest of the state. Now the river is used for recreational purposes, and some limited redevelopment of the riverside property has begun.

Swift River divides Middleboro into two almost equal parts. The north side of the river is the site of the central business district, large manufacturing plants, the railroad station, older residential neighborhoods, and the county government. During the 1970s, federal funds were used to develop low-income housing on the north side. The south side of the river, which is closer to the interstate highway, is the site of newer residential neighborhoods, the new Middleboro High School, and small shopping centers. To date, the City of Middleboro has not approved any significant development—residential or commercial—in the vacant 150-acre land adjacent to the interstate highway.

SOCIAL AND EDUCATIONAL CHARACTERISTICS

The population of Hillsboro County is predominantly of German, Irish, and English extraction. Racial minority groups compose about 13 percent of the population. Most of the African Americans arrived in the 1960s, and most of the other racial groups arrived in the late 1970s. The number of households headed by a female is 10.6 percent.

The median education level of the population older than 25 years is 10.7 years. Approximately 13.5 percent of the population has completed college, and 89.3 percent has completed high school. The current dropout rate from area high schools is 3 percent, an improvement over the 17 percent rate experienced 20 years ago.

Middleboro is the site of numerous elementary schools (K–6), a regional middle school (7–8), and a high school (9–12) that serve students from all over the city. Other communities in the county can send their children to Middleboro schools, using tuition arrangements on a space-available basis. Although all the schools are owned and operated by the City of Middleboro, a separately elected Middleboro School Board makes educational policy. One-third of the nine-member school board is elected each year in a special school-district election held in Middleboro. Each year, the school board submits a recommended budget for consideration by the Middleboro City Council. The city council approves the school budget before it is submitted, as part of the town's total budget, for voter approval. All employees of the Middleboro School Department—except the school superintendent Dr. Sam Drucker—are unionized. Abby O'Hara is currently the chair of the school board, a position she has held for the past ten years. The new $28.5 million high school located in Middleboro opened last year after being considered by the city council for about eight years. The town is heavily involved in high school sports. Middleboro Memorial Stadium is a landmark in regional high school football.

Jasper is the site of numerous elementary schools, a regional middle school (5–8), and a high school (9–12). A state-supported junior college is scheduled to open. A five-member elected school board that is independent of the town governs the Jasper Regional Educational Cooperative. Each year, this school board submits a recommended budget directly to the voters. Once approved, the funds are collected by the Town of Jasper from local taxes. The Jasper Regional Education Cooperative has expressed interest in working with the state to develop a regional vocational high school to complement the new Hillsboro County Junior College.

State University (SU) in University Town is the land-grant university within the state. It has a nursing, public health, and allied health school connected to its relatively large liberal arts and agricultural schools. Its 39,000 students make SU the largest public university in the state. A private liberal arts college of 1,000 students is also located in Capital City. SU maintains a small branch campus in Capital City as well.

Church membership remains strong in Hillsboro County. Aside from their religious influence, churches sponsor many of the youth sports leagues and are the site of many social gatherings.

Local chapters of Rotary International meet monthly in Middleboro and Jasper. AARP—formerly called the American Association of Retired Persons—maintains a chapter in Middleboro. The local chapter of American Red Cross, located in Middleboro, sponsors monthly blood drives throughout the county.

When statistics are adjusted for demographic characteristics, crime rates in the county are 10 percent below the national averages for non–metropolitan areas.

POLITICAL CHARACTERISTICS

Middleboro and its surrounding communities are politically conservative. Unlike other areas in the state, the same political party has dominated Middleboro for the past 45 years, except in presidential elections. Its politicians have gained statewide political power by consistently being reelected to office. The city is especially proud that the area's representative to the US Congress, James Giles, is a Middleboro native who retains his law practice in town.

Middleboro is governed by a six-member city council whose members are elected every two years. By tradition, the council member who receives the largest number of popular votes is appointed by the council to serve as mayor. Although the office's powers are mostly ceremonial, the mayor has the ability to influence decisions by presiding over council meetings and by making appointments to boards and commissions. Keith Edwards, a local retailer, has held the position of mayor for 17 years. Other members of the Middleboro City Council are Frederick Washburn, Diana Story, David Alley, Patricia Hood, and Michael York. The city's largest department is the school department, and the second largest is public works. York is the council member who has lead responsibilities for all healthcare-related issues and programs.

The City of Middleboro has recently begun legal action to block the licensing of three group homes for the developmentally disabled population. Middleboro Community Mental Health Center currently owns and operates Justin Place, a four-bed group home in Middleboro. Group Homes Inc., a national corporation, has a contract with the state to own and operate these homes. According to Mayor Edwards, the Hillsboro County Health Department has failed to take into consideration the serious implications these homes will create for Middleboro. Mayor Edwards recommends that the application for licensure be turned down on grounds related to negative community impact. Stephanie Jervis-Washburn, the executive director of Middleboro Community Mental Health Center, has also questioned the need for additional group homes, although at the same time indicating that her organization would be willing to assess the need for such services and possibly develop them should a need be identified.

Middleboro is the county seat for Hillsboro County. Three county commissioners elected by the population at large govern Hillsboro County. While the county level of government is not a powerful political subdivision in this region, it does control the court system, the penal system, and the registry of motor vehicles; it also provides some human service programs. Hillsboro County owns and operates a nursing home located in Middleboro. It is a major county employer in Middleboro. The current Hillsboro County Commissioners are Janet Ruseski, Bill Nelligan, and Mary Harrison.

Jasper is governed by a 12-member town council and a mayor. All are elected for four-year terms. William Hines is the mayor, a position he has held for the past nine years. The town council employs a professional city manager, Susan Giles-Harrison. The Jasper Industrial Development Authority (JIDA)—authorized by the voters 15 years ago—is a subunit of the town council and has the authority to issue bonds to support industrial development in Jasper. State law allows a municipal government to use tax-increment financing for purposes of economic development. Giles-Harrison also serves as the executive director of JIDA. Two years ago, JIDA formed a special committee to consider the feasibility of a hospital located on its property that was to be owned and operated by the town. This committee is chaired by Sharon Lee, who is the spouse of a Jasper physician, a member of the town council, and a former consultant for a national consulting firm that specializes in healthcare. Other members of this committee include Mayor Hines and town councilor Ed Hicks. Giles-Harrison provides staff support for the committee.

Under a program supported by the federal Department of Homeland Security, the mayors of all the communities located in Hillsboro County and their fire and police officials have created a task force to estimate surge capacity in an emergency or mass casualty situation. Officials from the two Middleboro hospitals—MIDCARE and Webster Health System—have attended task force meetings. The task force continues to update its estimate of potential evacuation or triage locations and beds that could be used. The Office of the Governor supports this project by funding a countywide assessment of surge capacity conducted by State University.

Initial findings and results from the surge capacity study indicate the following:

- At least 385 hotel or motel rooms are available in Hillsboro County.

- Public schools are able to hold 4,500 citizens, although none has provisions for emergencies.

- The disaster plans for both hospitals have not been coordinated. Each has its own plan and has estimated that it can accommodate at least 150 percent to 180 percent of its inpatient capacity for one week.

◆ No countywide, centralized communication system or command-and-control system exists that is able to direct resources and responses in the face of a significant disaster.

A more comprehensive assessment and plan is expected in six months.

Since 2009, Hillsboro County has sponsored a Community Emergency Response Team program to educate residents about disaster preparedness for hazards that may arise such as fires, floods, and weather-related disasters. Classes are held three times a year; to date, approximately 120 residents have completed training. Program instructors have been drawn from local police and fire departments, both local hospitals, and the Hillsboro County Health Department.

For the past five years, the state legislature has attempted to make the state a right-to-work state. Although the bill was not passed, it did secure 52 percent approval in the state senate last year. The current governor has indicated that, if the legislation passes in both houses, he would veto it. His political opponents have indicated their support for the right-to-work legislation.

ECONOMIC CHARACTERISTICS

Middleboro's tax profile reflects the conservative nature of the community. Increases in property taxes have just barely kept pace with inflation. The state has both a graduated income tax and a sales tax. By state law, any incorporated city is allowed to add a 0.5 percent local sales tax to the state sales tax. The Middleboro City Council has repeatedly rejected all proposals to do this.

Middleboro is the site of important wholesale and retail trade in Hillsboro County. Its major industries include manufacturing, finance, and service. Jasper is also establishing itself as a manufacturing center. Agriculture, which once dominated, now accounts for 20 percent of income and 16 percent of all employment in the county. Manufacturing accounts for 32 percent of income and 30 percent of employment. Per capita income is 5 percent below the national average. Fourteen percent of the county's population falls below the federal poverty standard. In Capital City, 18 percent of the population is under the federal poverty level.

Local banks estimate that approximately 8 percent of the single homes in the county have outstanding mortgages greater than the homes' current market value. The regional foreclosure rate is 1 percent greater than the national rate.

Three of Middleboro's manufacturing companies employ nearly 15 percent of the community's workforce, down 7 percent from five years ago:

1. Carlstead Rayon, a privately controlled textile corporation, employs 5.1 percent of the workforce.

2. River Industries, a division of National Auto Technology, manufactures rubber products for automobiles. For the past three years, it has reduced its workforce by 9 percent but still accounts for 4.5 percent of the workforce.

3. Master Tractor, formerly a division of United Agricultural Supply, was recently sold to a Japanese firm, which indicated that some parts for tractors will be imported from offshore and South American suppliers. A leader in the market for small tractors, Master Tractor employs 4.6 percent of the workforce.

The manufacturing plants of Carlstead Rayon, River Industries, and Master Tractor are all adjacent to Middleboro's rail service.

Following are employment opportunities in Jasper:

◆ Blue Bear Ale is a popular, locally owned, statewide microbrewery. Its sites are located in Middleboro and Mifflenville. The company plans to open a new site in Jasper in 2017.

◆ U.S. Parts, a division of a national corporation that manufactures components for large air conditioning units, relocated to Jasper three years ago. Today, it employs 2.2 percent of Jasper's workforce.

◆ National Yearbooks, a corporation headquartered in a major western city, established a modern printing and manufacturing plant in Jasper last year, using resources provided by JIDA. The company specializes in manufacturing yearbooks for colleges and high schools. Although currently it employs only 81 workers, it estimates that employment will increase 10 percent for each of the next ten years as it reduces its existing regional manufacturing sites and concentrates its entire North American manufacturing at the Jasper plant. National Yearbooks is not unionized and offers a full range of health insurance options to its full-time workers.

◆ Office Pro, a retail and wholesale provider of office supplies and office furniture, operates its regional warehouse in the Jasper Industrial Park, located on the western boundary of Jasper.

Agriculture and construction companies in the rest of Hillsboro County are primarily small, family-owned businesses. Chicken Farms, Inc., located in Harris City, is a national corporation that specializes in raising chickens for fast-food restaurants. It recently began to acquire family farms in the area and has announced plans to locate a processing plant somewhere in the county.

Countywide, housing construction permits have steadily declined over the past seven years. The housing stock is considered old—except in Jasper—by both national and state standards. The recent real-estate exception is the area between Jasper and Capital City.

Hillsboro County has one state-chartered commercial bank—Middleboro Trust Company—that has offices in Middleboro, Mifflenville, Statesville, Harris City, and Jasper. The county also has four small savings-and-loans (S&L) institutions, which were started principally to provide capital to the agricultural sector. To avoid insolvency 12 years ago, the Merchants Bank of Capital City acquired the Carterville Bank (S&L). Harry Carter, Carterville Bank's president, was a prominent politician at that time and was subsequently convicted of investor fraud.

Major capital financing is available through Middleboro Trust Company, a correspondent bank of a major national financial institution, or through a commercial bank located in Capital City. Bankers' Cooperative, a multistate commercial bank headquartered in another state, has recently announced plans to expand into Jasper.

MEDIA RESOURCES

The major newspaper in the county is the *Middleboro Sentinel*. It has a daily as well as a Sunday edition, and it maintains a comprehensive website. Its circulation is 22,000 for the daily edition and 8,200 for the Sunday edition. Three years ago, National News Stands, Inc., a national owner and operator of local newspapers, acquired the *Middleboro Sentinel*. Jack Donnelly has been its editor for 16 years. In Jasper, *The Capital City News* reaches approximately 25 percent of all households in town. Its rates are similar to those of the *Middleboro Sentinel*.

Middleboro has three local radio stations—AM-75, AM-1220, and FM-89.7— that cover local news and current events. TV Channel 32 is an independent station located in Middleboro. It provides network and independent programs. Affiliates of national television networks are located in Capital City, and their broadcast reaches most residents in the county. Cable TV and high-speed Internet from national and local providers are available throughout the county as well.

MEDICAL RESOURCES

HILLSBORO HEALTH

This tax-exempt, Medicare-certified home health agency provides a broad range of home-based services throughout the county. Two years ago, the agency was formed after a merger and expanded its mission and focus. It established a Medicare-certified hospice service and curtailed a number of community health programs. It uses funds provided by the towns and cities in the area, Hillsboro County, and United Way to support indigent care associated with Medicare-certified services. It transferred maternal and child health programs, funded by a grant from the state's Department of Health and Human Services, to voluntary health agencies. Martha Washington is Hillsboro Health's CEO, and Janet Myer is president of its board of directors.

PHYSICIAN CARE SERVICES, INC.

Physician Care Services (PCS), Inc. is a private, tax-paying corporation that owns and operates two urgent care/occupational health centers—one located in Mifflenville and the other in Jasper. PCS employs physicians and other professionals to provide walk-in ambulatory care, a full range of diagnostic services, and an occupational health program. Currently, PCS is considering opening a third center in the Jasper Industrial Park. Dr. Stephen Tobias is the president/CEO and medical director of PCS.

MIDDLEBORO COMMUNITY MENTAL HEALTH CENTER

In 1964, Middleboro Community Mental Health Center (MCMHC) was established as a tax-exempt 501(c)(3) corporation; it is one of two such designated centers in Hillsboro County. MCMHC provides a range of services and programs, including adult, child and family, emergency, and education. In addition, it owns and operates a central office called Gardner Place as well as a four-bed group home called Justin Place; both facilities are located in northwest Middleboro. Stephanie Jervis-Washburn serves as MCMHC's executive director.

WEBSTER HEALTH SYSTEM

Webster Health System owns and operates a fully accredited, tax-exempt, 85-bed osteopathic hospital located in Middleboro adjacent to the interstate highway. Named after its founder Dr. Edward W. Webster, this system was founded as Webster Hospital in 1930. Currently, the hospital has an active medical staff and makes use of many other physicians with consulting privileges from Osteopathic Medical Center (OMC) in Capital City. Ten years ago, Webster Hospital changed its name to Webster Health System and became an affiliate corporation of Osteopathic Hospitals of America, Inc. (OHA). Under this affiliation, OMC and OHA support the management of the system, provide joint-purchasing and supply-chain opportunities, and provide capital. In return, OMC and OHA have an exclusive contract to receive all medically appropriate referrals. Since executing the agreement, Webster Health System has established Quick Med, a walk-in ambulatory care clinic adjacent to its emergency department; recruited physicians; and expanded all services related to birthing. The system and members of its medical staff jointly own Webster Health, Inc., a tax-paying corporation, to support joint ventures. In 2015, the system appointed Steve Swisher as president and CEO.

MIDCARE, Inc.

Middleboro Medical Center, or MIDCARE, is a health system established on January 1, 2015, to "meet the needs of Hillsboro County." The system grew out of Middleboro Community Hospital, a fully licensed, tax-exempt acute care hospital founded in 1890 on the north side of Middleboro. Most of MIDCARE's current beds are located in wings originally constructed in 1962 and 1966 with the assistance of federal Hill-Burton funds; these wings have now been modernized. In 2014, this modernization involved converting a significant number of semiprivate rooms into private rooms and updating the birthing facilities. MIDCARE provides a full range of diagnostic, outpatient, therapeutic, and emergency medical services, including a cancer center. Adjacent to the hospital is the Middleboro Medical Office Building; ample parking is available for both facilities. Although licensed for 272 beds, the hospital had to reduce its inpatient capacity to lower costs and adjust to new hospital utilization patterns.

In 2015, the system signed a ten-year agreement to become an affiliate member of Treeline Health Systems, Inc. Under this affiliation, MIDCARE pays dues to be part of Treeline; in return, Treeline provides medical oversight and direction for MIDCARE's cancer center, access to its national supply chain management system, and technical assistance and support for MIDCARE's clinical data systems. In addition, both parties agreed to develop a clinical residency program for primary care practitioners. In 2012, a physician–hospital organization was created to facilitate the development of joint and other collaborative ventures involving the medical staff. James Higgens is the president of MIDCARE.

Medical Associates

Medical Associates is a multispecialty physician group with offices in downtown Middleboro and in Jasper. Founded in 1951, it is a tax-paying private corporation organized as a professional partnership. Physicians in the group provide specialty and subspecialty care on an ambulatory basis, and in the Jasper location, they also offer ambulatory surgical services. All of its physicians are board certified and maintain active medical staff privileges at area hospitals. Over the past three years, to facilitate the expansion of its primary services, the group has added more physicians in its Jasper office as well as advanced registered nurse practitioners in both locations. In 2017, it introduced Medical Associates Express, a 24/7 walk-in clinic, to its Jasper office. The group contracts with Wythe Laboratories in Capital City for all medical tests and with Radiology Partners for all diagnostic images. Cynthia Worley is the executive manager at Medical Associates.

JASPER GARDENS

Jasper Gardens is a private, tax-paying, 110-bed long-term care facility located in Jasper. It qualifies for Medicare, Medicaid, all private insurance plans, and self-pay. Its owners—Jefferson Partners, LLC of Capital City—recently announced plans to expand its inpatient and outpatient rehabilitation services. Also, Jefferson Partners recently submitted to the Town of Jasper an application to build an 88-bed assisted living facility as well as 50 adult single-family homes on the same campus as Jasper Gardens. At the news conference, Jefferson Partners indicated that this "continuing care retirement community" will be operational within three years. Jayne Winters is the licensed administrator of Jasper Gardens.

HILLSBORO COUNTY HEALTH DEPARTMENT

Located in Middleboro, this department is responsible for the distribution of state health agency funds to local health agencies, immunizations, environmental health, the long-term care facility Manorhaven, and the implementation of county health priorities using county tax revenues. Using a statewide data system, the department gathers vital and mortality statistics and provides the data to the state as part of its annual report to the Hillsboro County Commissioners. John Snow is the director of the health department, and Dr. Doris Felix is the current chair of the Hillsboro County Board of Health, which oversees the department. The board comprises 12 members, each of whom is appointed for an overlapping five-year term by the Hillsboro County Commissioners. Other professionals the department employs include registered nurses, public health assistants, and experts in public health.

OTHER HEALTH SERVICES

Aside from Medical Associates, many small, single-specialty and solo medical practices operate out of Hillsboro County.

The Carter Home—located north of Middleboro and Jasper near Mifflenville—is a tax-paying, 110-bed long-term care facility that qualifies for both Medicare (as a skilled nursing facility) and Medicaid (as an intermediate care facility). Jack H. Carter has been president of the Carter Home Corporation, Inc. for the past 20 years and is currently the administrator of the Carter Home. Recently, the corporation opened Carter Village, an assisted living facility comprising 50 two-bedroom apartments with a congregate meal facility, 24-hour access to nursing services, access to physical and occupational therapists, and van service to shopping areas in Middleboro.

Manorhaven—located in Middleboro—is a 110-bed long-term care facility that is owned and operated by Hillsboro County. It also operates a limited adult day care program for residents of Middleboro. Services at the facility qualify for both Medicare and Medicaid reimbursement. Jennifer Jones has been Manorhaven's administrator for the past eight years.

Rock Creek—located north of Mifflenville near Harris City—is a private, 126-bed nursing home and 84-bed assisted living facility. It qualifies for Medicaid insurance, but it serves no Medicare patients. Five years ago, a statewide proprietary chain purchased Rock Creek. Its current administrator is John Lipman.

Senior Living of Mifflenville—located between Middleboro and Mifflenville—is an assisted living facility that offers two types of living arrangements. In the 45-unit assisted living facility, residents rent a private, one- or two-bedroom apartment with a small kitchen. Amenities include congregate meals, transportation services, and a full recreational program. In the adult home, 125 residents are provided either private or semi-private room accommodation. A 24-hour nursing staff provides supervision. Senior Living of Mifflenville opened four years ago and is owned and operated by a national corporation. Its adult home is not a licensed nursing home.

Sockalexis Center—located in Jasper—has the contract to provide behavioral health and counseling services to the Jasper schools and is moving aggressively into the corporate substance abuse and employee assistance program market. The center is staffed by four doctorally trained clinical psychologists, three master's-level social workers, and three substance abuse counselors.

Greenwood Group—located just east of Jasper—is a provider of substance abuse therapy known for its "upscale" setting. It is staffed by psychiatrists, clinical psychologists, a social worker, substance abuse counselors, and health-and-wellness personnel. The organization has targeted commercially insured clients.

Royman Oaks, LLC, offers employment counseling and job placement for clients with a history of behavioral disorders.

Grosvenor Arms—located in Jasper—is a seven-bed adult group home. Its staff includes residential counselors, a clinical psychologist, a social worker, and a marriage-and-family therapist.

A state-supported, 154-bed inpatient psychiatric institution is located nearly 150 miles northeast of Middleboro.

Churches throughout Hillsboro County coordinate and provide Meals on Wheels, a program that delivers hot lunches to homebound elderly and disabled populations.

In Middleboro, the Fire Department provides emergency services staffed with emergency medical technicians (EMTs). In Jasper, the Fire Department uses paramedics to provide emergency services. Other communities rely on volunteer firefighters and emergency responders, some of whom require basic EMT certification. This year, the county launched a countywide 911 emergency dispatch system.

Statewide Blue Cross and Blue Shield is headquartered in Capital City, along with the state chapters of the following organizations:

◆ AARP

◆ Alzheimer's Association

◆ American Cancer Society

◆ American Diabetes Association

◆ American Heart Association

◆ American Lung Association

◆ Brain Injury Association of America

◆ Epilepsy Foundation

◆ Mental Health America (formerly National Mental Health Association)

◆ Muscular Dystrophy Association

◆ Planned Parenthood Federation of America

◆ United Cerebral Palsy

The statewide Alzheimer's Association has publicly expressed its priority to establish a membership office in Middleboro and throughout Hillsboro County.

The state has two medical schools. One is public and located on the eastern boundary, and the other one is private with an osteopathic focus and located on the northern boundary. Both are located in major cities and are more than 250 miles away from Capital City. Over the past 30 years, the hospitals in Capital City have become major referral centers for the community hospitals located within a 100- to 150-mile geographic circle. Capital City General Hospital and Osteopathic Medical Center—the two largest hospitals in the city—maintain teaching affiliations with the two medical schools in the state.

In Hillsboro County, there are this many healthcare professionals per 100,000 people:

◆ 42.0 dentists, most of whom are independent practitioners with private offices;

◆ 20.3 veterinarians;

◆ 811.4 registered nurses; and

◆ 27.0 physicians.

Six licensed mortuaries work in the county—four in Middleboro and two in Jasper.

STATE REGULATIONS

The state continues to maintain a certificate-of-need (CON) law for all acute and specialty hospitals and long-term care facilities that receive Medicaid and/or Medicare. Home health agencies were exempted from the law 12 years ago. Also specifically excluded from the law are private physician offices, clinics, and dispensaries for employees and health maintenance organizations. The thresholds for application of CON are $4 million for major medical equipment, $10 million for new construction, any transfer of ownership, and any increase in the number of licensed bed size equal to or greater than 15 beds or 20 percent of the facility (whichever is less). CON proposals are evaluated on the basis of the proposal's ability to better address the needs of the service area, immediate and long-term financial viability, cost control, and quality-of-care implications.

CON applications are forwarded to the State Commissioner of Health and Welfare and then analyzed by the State Bureau of Healthcare Services. The state's CON Board renders the final decision. The governor, following the recommendation of the state legislature, appoints the seven-member board. Jack Carter, the only local representative on this board, owns a nursing home in Hillsboro County. Working with a committee in the state legislature, the governor will be issuing recommendations on whether CON should be reauthorized, changed, or allowed to lapse as a state statute.

COMMUNITY CONCERNS AND ISSUES

Local political leaders have long recognized that Middleboro is economically stagnant. They have discussed the need to build a major industrial park adjacent to the interstate highway. Local business leaders, however, have resisted this venture, arguing that the funds designated for an industrial park be invested instead in improving the central business district to bolster the city's existing retail trade business. As a result of these competing views, Middleboro has not invested in either development.

The entire city has been affected by the national downturn in the traditional industrial and manufacturing sector. The current unemployment rate in Hillsboro County is 3.4 percentage points higher than the state's overall rate. Most of this unemployment is in the Middleboro area.

Twenty-five years ago, a flood hit Middleboro, heavily damaging Carlstead Rayon's plant. While some of this damage has been repaired, the corporation did not return to full production. It elected to use the insurance settlement to open a new production facility in another state with a right-to-work law and to switch some of its production to an overseas location. In an emergency settlement one month before Carlstead Rayon was about to completely close its Middleboro plant, it agreed to maintain a scaled-down manufacturing operation—as long as the city waived in perpetuity all of the company's real estate taxes and the state provided it with industrial-development bonds for capital acquisition.

Although this settlement did save a significant number of jobs, local and state political leaders continue to be criticized for the terms of the agreement. Earlier this year, the *Middleboro Sentinel* ran a series of stories on the environmental hazards caused by Carlstead Rayon's questionable handling of waste materials through the years. Finally, about one month ago, the Hillsboro County Health Department requested a Health Consultation of the Carlstead site by the Agency for Toxic Substances and Disease Registry of the US Department of Health and Human Services, Public Health Service. The consultation report is due to be released within the next two months, and the expected conclusion is that portions of Carlstead will be designated as hazardous waste sites and thus subject to remediation requirements.

Meanwhile, the company has recently informed the city that it wants a 25 percent reduction in the price it pays for water. The Middleboro City Council has repeatedly asked all tax-exempt healthcare providers to make a payment in lieu of taxes to cover municipal services costs. Last year, Steven Local ran for city council with one campaign promise: He would convince nonprofit hospitals and other healthcare "free riders" to "pay their fair share" or face consequences from the city, including court action. He lost the election by 21 votes but vowed to return next year with an even stronger campaign. For the past five years, Hillsboro County has received an annual payment of $28,000 under the federal Payment in Lieu of Taxes program (Public Law 113–79).

For the past five years, Middleboro politics has been dominated by three issues: (1) the increases in property taxes, (2) the cost of schools, and (3) the use of funds included in Medicaid to pay for abortions. Planned Parenthood continues to attract demonstrations and protests. Generally, economic development issues do not characterize the local political campaigns.

Over the past three years, major industrial development has occurred in Jasper. U.S. Parts arrived in town, and today the company occupies almost 60 percent of the Jasper Industrial Park, a campus established five years ago. National Yearbooks is expected to fill the remaining capacity in the Jasper Industrial Park within five years. Plans are also underway to expand the park or to construct another one next to the new interstate highway between Jasper and Capital City. City officials in Middleboro are still being criticized for letting Jasper "beat out" Middleboro in attracting these major employers.

In 18 months, the state will open a moderate-security prison as part of the plan to develop regional prison facilities. The prison will have a capacity of 600 inmates and will be located 30 miles south and west of Jasper. It is expected to become another major employer in town. Seven years ago, Floyd Donovan, a state senator from Jasper, began the community's effort to secure the prison for Jasper.

Issues involving growth continue to dominate the politics in Jasper. While the entire community seems very satisfied with the success of JIDA, many are dissatisfied with the impact the developments have had on municipal services and the local education system. Responsible Growth, a four-year-old group comprising 100 Jasper residents who voice community concerns, succeeded in electing two of its members—Jennifer Kip and Alan Simpson—to the Jasper Town Council. Both expressed concern that Jasper was too quickly becoming a bedroom community to Capital City.

It is common knowledge that Kip and Simpson have approached the governor about opening a hospital in Jasper. "Residents in Jasper need access to a hospital, especially an emergency room," Kip stated. "Too many of our residents have to travel too many miles when they most need these types of services." The governor has recommended the two work with the State Commissioner of Health and Welfare to determine whether a small hospital in Jasper is a viable venture. The governor has promised his support to ensure the residents "of this growing community have access to the type of health services they need and can support." Kip and Simpson have told the press they will ask the Jasper Town Council to authorize the hiring of a consulting firm to study this issue.

National Development Corp. has recently presented to the Jasper Planning Board a proposal to construct an 800-unit subdivision of moderately priced housing on land adjacent to the new interstate highway. The proposal holds the developer responsible for all infrastructures.

NEW INTERSTATE HIGHWAY

Three years ago, Representative Giles announced with the governor that a new four-lane interstate highway would be built from Jasper to Capital City and University Town. This road would shorten the travel distance from downtown Jasper to downtown Capital City (currently, 32 miles) to 16 miles and from Jasper to University Town (currently, 93 miles) to 70 miles. Representative Giles acknowledged that this project would inject numerous new jobs into the local economy and would provide Jasper with the transportation link it has needed for 15 years. The road from Jasper to Capital City should be completed in the next 12 months, while the road from Jasper to University Town will be finished in 18 months.

Over the past three years, the south of Jasper and land between Jasper and Capital City have experienced significant attention and a number of development proposals. For example, the Jasper Town Council, including Kip and Simpson, recently approved the zoning application for a major shopping mall complex, which will be located adjacent to the new highway and at the edge of Jasper—approximately six miles from downtown Jasper and ten miles from the boundary of Capital City and Capital County.

When contacted by Mayor Edwards of Middleboro, Representative Giles indicated that the new interstate is unlikely to be extended from Jasper to Middleboro. Long-term plans have this new highway intersecting the existing east–west highway in University Town. Representative Giles did say, however, that he would ask the governor whether state funds exist to upgrade the existing road between Jasper and Middleboro to a limited-access highway.

Under recent federal legislation, the State Department of Transportation issued a feasibility study for a commuter rail link between Jasper and Capital City. The study indicates that such a rail system may be feasible if Jasper continues to grow at its current rate over the next five to seven years.

Tables 1.5 through 1.12 show the health insurance profile, hospital data, and mortality rates in Hillsboro County.

On the web at ache.org/books/ Middleboro2

COUNTYWIDE GRIEVANCES

Citizens Against Abortions is a small but vocal political force in Jasper. On three occasions, the group has picketed in front of the offices of physicians known to have performed abortions at hospitals in either Middleboro or Capital City and a Planned Parenthood clinic. TV Action 12, the largest TV station in Capital City, broadcasted on the evening news two of these demonstrations in Jasper. This group has announced plans to picket area hospitals. The *Middleboro Sentinel* has estimated that this organization has 35 to 40 members.

Leaders from other communities in Hillsboro County—Harris City, Boalsburg, Minortown, and Carterville—have begun to meet monthly to discuss common concerns. The group recently issued a statement directed at the Hillsboro County Commissioners. The statement indicated that too many county resources are being devoted to develop the southern part at the expense of the northern, smaller communities.

Philanthropy has declined in the county. As a condition of receiving funds from United Way, a nonprofit agency must forgo any independent fund-raising, although it can accept individual gifts. The rate of giving throughout the county has declined 30 percent, and the amount disbursed by United Way has also shrunk by 16 percent. Even though all large industries and many small employers in the county cooperate with United Way, measures suggest that philanthropy has significantly decreased over the past ten years.

Five years ago, a state law was passed prohibiting health insurers doing business in the state from excluding people from coverage because of their preexisting conditions. This action was taken independently of the same provisions in the federal Affordable Care Act (ACA). In addition, debate about a small-group health insurance reform bill is ongoing in the statehouse. If passed, the law will allow small employers—those with fewer than ten employees—to participate in health insurance purchasing pools, which offer more coverage options at a lower rate than available from the employers' previous arrangements. The state decided not to participate in the insurance exchange originally stipulated by the ACA.

All employers in the state are required to obtain workers' compensation insurance. Currently, employees injured on the job are free to choose which healthcare provider would treat them. A new workers' comp law has been recently enacted, however. In 18 months, the responsibility for choosing the medical provider to care for an injured worker will be, by law, the employer's—not the employee's. This legislation also changes the workers' comp appeal process. Appeals will continue to flow through the circuit court and the State Supreme Court, and employees will still have 30 days from the time of the injury to initiate an appeal. However, questions reviewed under the new appeals process will pertain to law only and will not permit a jury trial. The old process permitted reviews of law and fact as well as a jury trial. In addition, the new law will increase competition for workers' comp business among healthcare providers. Most residents and observers feel that the changes amount to a tightening up of the workers' comp system, at the expense of employees. By all indications, the new law and its yet-to-be-seen impacts will be watched carefully. For example, a recent article in *The Capital City News* reported that a study by the Teamsters and Service Workers Unions found that, under the current system, the state's rejection rate of workers' comp claims was extremely high and had been rising for at least the past four years. According to the study, rejected claims are not paid by the state but by the employees' regular health insurance plans, which often include deductibles and copayments. The unions identified the shift of insurance coverage from the state workers' comp system to the employees and employers as a major way of increasing health insurance expenses.

At a recent annual meeting, the State Medical Society endorsed statewide tort reform, similar to the reform adopted in Texas in 2003. The group recommends limiting awards for noneconomic damages to $750,000. Policy action committees have been established in each county to work with state representatives to implement this revision to the tort system.

Capital City Medical Center has purchased a five-year land option in Jasper (near the new interstate) and indicated that it is considering constructing a medical office with select ancillary services for its physicians. The medical center is expected to announce a formal plan in 18 to 24 months.

City/Town	1994	1999	2004	2009	2014	2019
Jasper	31,560	39,871	42,657	46,902	49,247	51,230
Middleboro	45,460	45,861	46,995	47,364	47,590	48,502
Statesville	11,788	11,750	11,790	12,750	14,350	14,780
Harris City	12,009	12,203	12,953	12,951	12,904	12,835
Mifflenville	10,325	10,623	10,945	10,952	11,240	11,253
Carterville	2,356	2,367	2,145	2,378	2,066	2,198
Minortown	2,160	2,163	2,190	2,056	2,103	2,005
Boalsburg	1,790	1,885	1,893	1,891	1,935	1,965
Total	**117,448**	**126,723**	**131,568**	**137,244**	**141,435**	**144,768**
Outside Hillsboro County						
Capital City	110,450	120,450	155,340	160,230	163,440	177,560
University Town	78,990	81,044	81,370	83,560	84,500	85,840

Table 1.1
Hillsboro
County
Population

*On the web at
ache.org/books/
Middleboro2*

Table 1.2
Hillsboro
County
Population by
Race

City/Town	Population	White	Black	Other
Jasper				
2019	51,230	47,162	1,534	2,534
2014	49,247	46,879	1,367	1,001
Middleboro				
2019	48,502	35,440	9,095	3,967
2014	47,590	34,891	9,234	3,465
Statesville				
2019	14,780	14,371	42	367
2014	14,350	14,078	16	256
Harris City				
2019	12,835	12,130	145	560
2014	12,904	12,256	130	518
Mifflenville				
2019	11,253	10,859	314	80
2014	11,240	10,855	301	84
Carterville				
2019	2,198	2,104	16	78
2014	2,066	1,958	7	101
Minortown				
2019	2,005	1,989	9	7
2014	2,103	2,099	0	4
Boalsburg				
2019	1,965	1,942	14	9
2014	1,935	1,924	6	5
Total				
2019	**144,768**	**125,997**	**11,169**	**7,602**
2014	**141,435**	**124,940**	**11,061**	**5,434**

City/Town	Total	Ages						
		Under 5	5–14	15–24	25–44	45–64	65–74	75+
Jasper	51,230	3,942	7,647	7,533	15,726	11,487	3,083	1,812
Male	25,796	2,010	3,910	3,810	7,977	5,740	1,537	812
Female	25,434	1,932	3,737	3,723	7,749	5,747	1,546	1,000
Middleboro	48,502	3,203	7,060	6,725	13,904	10,661	3,522	3,427
Male	24,341	1,625	3,610	3,456	7,052	5,320	1,745	1,533
Female	24,161	1,578	3,450	3,269	6,852	5,341	1,777	1,894
Statesville	14,780	1,022	2,151	1,920	4,516	3,282	903	986
Male	7,287	521	1,107	996	2,273	1,651	441	298
Female	7,493	501	1,044	924	2,243	1,631	462	688
Harris City	12,835	805	1,868	1,780	3,629	2,850	848	1,055
Male	6,429	407	943	900	1,827	1,428	413	511
Female	6,406	398	925	880	1,802	1,422	435	544
Mifflenville	11,253	712	1,448	1,259	3,655	2,499	743	937
Male	5,617	362	730	643	1,837	1,239	358	448
Female	5,636	350	718	616	1,818	1,260	385	489
Carterville	2,198	102	320	305	655	488	156	172
Male	1,064	52	162	156	320	238	70	66
Female	1,134	50	158	149	335	250	86	106
Minortown	2,005	109	292	278	497	445	163	221
Male	1,011	55	152	140	266	222	77	99
Female	994	54	140	138	231	223	86	122
Boalsburg	1,964	114	286	272	586	436	143	128
Male	958	60	140	133	292	210	68	55
Female	1,007	54	146	139	294	226	75	73
Total	144,768	10,009	21,072	20,072	43,168	32,148	9,561	8,738
Male	72,503	5,092	10,754	10,234	21,844	16,048	4,709	3,822
Female	72,265	4,917	10,318	9,838	21,324	16,100	4,852	4,916

Table 1.3
Hillsboro County Age Profile by Sex

On the web at ache.org/books/ Middleboro2

Table 1.4
Distance (Miles) Between Hillsboro County Communities

City/Town	Boalsburg	Carterville	Harris City	Jasper	Middleboro	Mifflenville	Minortown	Statesville
Boalsburg	0	23	9	37	20	16	18	35
Carterville		0	18	28	11	7	13	15
Harris City			0	32	15	11	17	30
Jasper				0	23	21	27	3
Middleboro					0	4	10	23
Mifflenville						0	6	19
Minortown							0	25
Statesville								0
Outside Hillsboro County								
Capital City	61	52	60	32	45	49	55	25
University Town	90	81	85	93	70	74	80	93

	Percentage of Coverage					
	Not Covered Any Time During the Year	Covered by Employment-Based Insurance	Covered by Self-Employment Insurance	Covered by Medicaid	Covered by Medicare	Covered by Medicare and Medicaid
All Residents	14.1	47.8	6.0	21.0	17.0	3.1
Employer Size, Workers Aged 18–64						
Fewer than 25 Employees	26.8	34.7	14.6	1.0	0.2	0.2
25–99 Employees	23.5	64.3	7.4	1.5	0.1	0.0
100–499 Employees	14.9	76.6	4.7	1.5	0.2	0.3
500–999 Employees	13.6	78.8	0.0	0.7	0.2	0.3
1,000+ Employees	0.0	0.0	0.0	0.0	0.0	0.0
Household Income						
Less than $25,000	28.3	13.9	8.2	43.50	8.1	0.00
$25,000–$49,999	22.8	35.4	23.6	12.20	7.9	0.00
$50,000–$74,999	13.2	66.3	30.5	0.00	7.5	0.00
$75,000 or More	9.3	72.4	39.4	0.00	5.7	0.00

Table 1.5
Hillsboro County Health Insurance Profile

Note: Percentages may exceed 100%, depending on changes during the year of study and multiple coverage.

Table 1.6
Health
Insurance
Benefits
of Major
Employers
in Hillsboro
County

Employer	Fee-for-Service		Managed Care	
	Deductible ($)	Coinsurance (%)	Deductible ($)	Coinsurance per MD Visit (%)
Carlstead Rayon	3,200	80/20		
PPO			6,400	80/20
HMO			4,000	70/30
HD	12,900	70/30		
River Industries				
LD	2,500	70/30		
HD	12,900	60/40		
Master Tractor				
PPO			7,500	60/40
HMO			7,500	70/30
HD	12,900	60/40		
U.S. Parts				
PPO			7,500	60/40
HMO			7,500	70/30
National Yearbooks				
PPO			1,000	70/30
HMO			800	80/20
HD	10,500	70/30		
POS	400	80/20		
Office Pro	2,500	60/40		
Chicken Farms, Inc.	12,900	50/50	300	85/15
Middleboro Trust Company				
PPO			2,000	70/30
HMO			1,500	80/20
HD	12,900	60/40		

Notes: (1) Deductibles shown are for family coverage. (2) State law mandates mental health coverage in any insurance plan with more than 25 participants. The plan must include 30 hours coverage for outpatient visits and 20 days for inpatient. (3) HD: high deductible; HMO: health maintenance organization; LD: low deductible; POS: point of service; PPO: preferred provider organization

Coverage	1994	1999	2004	2009	2014	2019
No Insurance	12.5	12.9	14.5	19.1	19.3	15.5
Medicaid	12.7	15.1	15.2	16.3	19.2	19.7
Any Private Plan	63.6	59.6	58.4	56.3	55.1	49.3
Medicare	14.3	13.7	14.1	14.9	15.0	16.1
Military Healthcare	2.0	2.5	2.8	2.4	2.4	2.6

Table 1.7
Hillsboro County Estimated Health Insurance Coverage

Note: Numbers are a percentage of total. Total insured and totals may exceed 100% due to multiple coverages.

City/Town	Population	Hospital Discharges	Patient Days			
			Total	Webster Health System (WHS)	MIDCARE	Other
Jasper						
2019	51,230	4,771	25,859	4,668	12,000	9,191
2014	49,247	5,352	24,084	3,013	17,100	3,971
2009	46,902	4,878	22,926	3,078	17,664	2,184
2004	42,657	4,795	24,453	3,105	19,825	1,523
Middleboro						
2019	48,502	6,023	32,343	5,037	27,002	304
2014	47,590	6,201	35,346	7,076	27,830	440
2009	47,364	6,394	33,889	4,850	28,185	854
2004	46,995	7,364	43,448	4,445	38,143	860
Statesville						
2019	14,780	1,528	8,918	2,490	6,356	72
2014	14,350	1,530	7,191	3,020	4,056	115
2009	12,750	1,469	7,938	3,175	4,673	90
2004	11,790	1,455	8,293	3,375	4,846	72
Harris City						
2019	12,835	1,581	8,468	6,590	1,720	158
2014	12,904	1,730	8,996	6,743	2,020	233
2009	12,951	1,756	12,117	9,866	2,006	245
2004	12,953	1,886	12,447	7,856	4,360	231
Mifflenville						
2019	11,253	1,324	7,378	2,291	4,938	149
2014	11,240	1,456	7,280	2,839	4,288	153
2009	10,952	1,687	8,939	3,320	5,475	144
2004	10,945	1,795	10,411	2,003	8,230	178

Table 1.8
Hillsboro County Hospital Discharges and Patient Days

On the web at ache.org/books/ Middleboro2

continued

Table 1.8
Hillsboro
County Hospital
Discharges and
Patient Days
(continued)

*On the web at
ache.org/books/
Middleboro2*

City/Town	Population	Hospital Discharges	Patient Days			
			Total	Webster Health System (WHS)	MIDCARE	Other
Carterville						
2019	2,198	275	1,442	390	1,000	52
2014	2,066	194	1,716	596	1,077	43
2009	2,378	338	1,891	702	1,177	12
2004	2,145	332	2,095	723	1,283	89
Minortown						
2019	2,005	194	1,127	94	1,001	32
2014	2,103	420	2,408	601	1,796	11
2009	2,056	317	1,963	508	1,448	7
2004	2,190	382	2,446	468	1,962	16
Boalsburg						
2019	1,965	229	1,326	528	798	0
2014	1,935	220	1,217	681	513	23
2009	1,891	236	1,395	747	608	40
2004	1,893	254	1,547	707	761	79
Hillsboro County Totals						
2019	**144,768**	**15,925**	**86,861**	**20,288**	**56,815**	**9,758**
2014	**141,435**	**17,103**	**88,238**	**24,569**	**58,680**	**4,989**
2009	**137,244**	**17,075**	**91,058**	**26,246**	**61,236**	**3,576**
2004	**131,568**	**18,263**	**105,140**	**22,682**	**79,410**	**3,048**
Noncounty Residents						
2019		26	126	71	55	
2014		32	176	86	90	
2009		24	128	45	83	
2004		21	124	44	80	
Total						
2019			**86,987**	**20,359**	**56,870**	**9,758**
2014			**88,414**	**24,655**	**58,770**	**4,989**
2009			**91,186**	**26,291**	**61,319**	**3,576**
2004			**105,264**	**22,726**	**79,490**	**3,048**

continued

2019 Hospital Discharges by Town and Hospital				
City/Town	Total Discharges	WHS	MIDCARE	Other
Jasper	4,771	802	2,202	1,767
Middleboro	6,023	967	5,000	56
Statesville	1,528	450	1,064	14
Harris City	1,581	1,228	325	28
Mifflenville	1,324	503	801	20
Carterville	275	71	195	9
Minortown	194	20	170	4
Boalsburg	229	94	135	0
Total Discharges	**15,925**	**4,135**	**9,892**	**1,898**

Table 1.8
Hillsboro County Hospital Discharges and Patient Days *(continued)*

On the web at ache.org/books/ Middleboro2

Specialty	Total	MIDCARE	WHS	Other
Family Practice	**41**	**5**	**27**	**9**
Middleboro	9	0	9	0
Jasper	14	0	6	8
Harris City	3	0	3	0
Statesville	3	1	1	1
Mifflenville	6	1	5	0
Carterville	2	1	1	0
Minortown	2	1	1	0
Boalsburg	2	1	1	0
Internal Medicine	**47**	**33**	**2**	**12**
Middleboro	12	10	2	0
Jasper	22	10	0	12
Harris City	2	2	0	0
Statesville	2	2	0	0
Mifflenville	4	4	0	0
Carterville	2	2	0	0
Minortown	2	2	0	0
Boalsburg	1	1	0	0
Pediatrics	**28**	**16**	**4**	**8**
Middleboro	14	10	4	0
Jasper	14	6	0	8

Table 1.9
Hillsboro County Physicians by Specialty, City/Town, and Hospital Affiliation

continued

Specialty	Total	MIDCARE	WHS	Other
Allergy Immunology	5	3	0	2
Middleboro	2	2	0	0
Jasper	3	1	0	2
Cardiology	8	5	1	2
Middleboro	5	5	0	0
Jasper	3	0	1	2
Gastroenterology	6	6	0	0
Middleboro	4	4	0	0
Jasper	2	2	0	0
Psychiatry	8	8	0	0
Middleboro	6	6	0	0
Jasper	2	2	0	0
Other Medical*	17	12	3	2
Middleboro	15	10	3	2
Jasper	2	2	0	0
Orthopedic	13	8	3	2
Middleboro	11	8	3	0
Jasper	2	0	0	2
General Surgery	18	12	4	2
Middleboro	14	10	4	0
Jasper	4	2	0	2
OB/GYN	22	12	8	2
Middleboro	14	8	6	0
Jasper	8	4	2	2
Other Surgical**	17	16	1	0
Middleboro	17	16	1	0
Jasper	0	0	0	0

continued

Specialty	Total	MIDCARE	WHS	Other
Hospital-Based	**61**	**43**	**18**	**0**
Emergency	20	12	8	0
Anesthesiology	14	10	4	0
Radiology	16	13	3	0
Pathology	11	8	3	0
Total	**291**	**179**	**71**	**41**

Table 1.9
Hillsboro County Physicians by Specialty, City/Town, and Hospital Affiliation *(continued)*

Notes: (1) Table includes only physicians who have active medical staff privileges or are employed by an accredited hospital. (2) * includes dermatology, pulmonology, endocrinology, otolaryngology, pulmonary medicine, ear/nose/throat, oncology, and hematology; ** includes vascular surgery, bariatric surgery, ophthalmology, plastic surgery, thoracic surgery, urology, and neurosurgery; (3) WHS is Webster Health System, and Other is a hospital not located in Hillsboro County.

Coverage	1989	1994	1999	2004	2009	2014	2019
Live Births	1,282	1,746	1,945	2,205	2,678	2,935	2,254
Deaths (Except Fetal)	833	890	967	1,085	1,210	1,236	1,193
Infant Deaths	16	13	21	14	14	17	15
Neonatal Deaths*	10	12	13	10	8	6	7
Postneonatal Deaths**	6	1	8	4	6	11	8
Maternal Deaths	2	1	1	2	1	2	3
Out-of-Wedlock Births	140	167	175	216	299	355	256
Marriages	1,053	977	923	901	1,051	981	995

Table 1.10
Hillsboro County Vital Statistics

On the web at ache.org/books/ Middleboro2

Note: * fewer than 28 days after birth; ** within 28–365 days of birth.

Table 1.11
Hillsboro
County Resident
Deaths by
Cause of Death

Cause of Death	ICD-10 Codes	1989	1994	1999	2004	2009	2014	2019
Diseases of the Heart	Ioo–Io9, I11, I13, 120–151	302	325	361	390	418	401	367
Malignant Neoplasms	Coo–C97	212	221	234	240	245	256	262
Chronic Lower Respiratory Diseases	J40–J47	32	32	34	34	36	40	60
All Accidents	Vo1–X59, Y85–Y86	44	45	49	59	70	64	62
Cerebrovascular Diseases	I60–I69	57	60	67	73	86	93	78
Alzheimer's Disease	G30	0	10	16	20	26	34	38
Diabetes Mellitus	E10–E14	25	22	30	30	33	33	32
Influenza and Pneumonia	Jo9–J18	31	27	31	40	34	30	37
Nephritis, Nephrotic Syndrome, and Nephrosis	Noo–No7, N17–N19, N25–N27	16	23	20	18	21	22	20
Intentional Self-Harm	Uo3, X60–X84, Y87.0	14	21	18	20	26	24	17
Total Deaths from Leading Causes		**733**	**786**	**860**	**924**	**995**	**997**	**973**
All Deaths		**833**	**890**	**967**	**1,085**	**1,210**	**1,236**	**1,193**

Cause of Death	Total	Age Group							
		Under 1	1–4	5–14	15–24	25–44	45–64	65–75	75+
Diseases of the Heart									
2019	367	1	0	0	3	18	62	120	163
2014	401	2	0	0	2	14	58	124	201
2009	418	0	0	0	0	11	50	139	218
2004	390	0	0	0	0	9	40	120	221
Malignant Neoplasms									
2019	262	2	0	2	3	20	34	67	134
2014	256	1	0	1	1	24	38	79	112
2009	245	0	0	2	4	19	24	75	121
2004	240	0	0	0	0	14	31	77	118
Chronic Lower Respiratory Diseases									
2019	60	0	0	0	0	0	15	20	25
2014	40	0	0	0	0	0	13	13	14
2009	36	0	0	0	0	0	11	9	16
2004	34	0	0	0	0	0	12	8	14
All Accidents									
2019	62	3	5	10	10	5	7	9	13
2014	64	5	2	9	8	6	7	8	19
2009	70	3	4	4	18	15	12	5	9
2004	59	5	1	2	13	16	8	3	11
Cerebrovascular Diseases									
2019	78	0	0	0	0	2	12	28	36
2014	93	0	0	0	1	3	10	26	53
2009	86	0	0	0	0	2	14	23	47
2004	73	0	0	0	0	5	17	16	35
Alzheimer's Disease									
2019	38	0	0	0	0	0	0	12	26
2014	34	0	0	0	0	0	2	3	29
2009	26	0	0	0	0	0	1	0	25
2004	20	0	0	0	0	0	1	2	17
Diabetes Mellitus									
2019	32	0	0	0	0	0	3	14	15
2014	33	0	0	0	0	0	5	12	16
2009	33	0	0	0	0	2	10	12	9
2004	30	0	0	0	0	1	12	12	5

Table 1.12
Hillsboro County Causes of Resident Death by Age Group

continued

Table 1.12
Hillsboro
County Causes
of Resident
Death by
Age Group
(continued)

Cause of Death	Total	Age Group							
		Under 1	1–4	5–14	15–24	25–44	45–64	65–75	75+
Influenza and Pneumonia									
2019	37	1	1	0	0	0	2	14	19
2014	30	1	0	0	0	0	1	12	16
2009	34	1	2	0	0	0	2	8	21
2004	40	0	1	0	0	4	4	9	22
Nephritis, Nephrotic Syndrome, and Nephrosis									
2019	20	0	1	0	1	3	3	4	8
2014	22	0	1	0	1	2	4	5	9
2009	21	0	0	1	2	4	6	2	6
2004	18	0	1	3	3	1	2	2	6
Intentional Self-Harm									
2019	17	0	0	1	6	2	3	2	3
2014	24	0	0	0	2	2	9	5	6
2009	26	0	0	4	6	6	4	2	4
2004	20	0	0	3	2	3	6	4	2
Septicemia									
2019	16	1	2	0	0	0	3	1	9
2014	14	1	0	0	0	0	2	2	9
2009	13	0	0	0	0	0	1	4	8
2004	14	1	0	0	0	0	3	3	7
Chronic Liver Disease and Cirrhosis									
2019	16	0	0	0	0	0	5	5	6
2014	12	0	0	0	0	0	3	5	4
2009	18	0	0	0	0	0	6	5	7
2004	13	0	0	0	0	1	4	4	4
Total from Listed Causes									
2019	1,005	8	9	13	23	50	149	296	457
2014	1,023	10	3	10	15	51	152	294	488
2009	1,026	4	6	11	30	59	141	284	491
2004	951	6	3	8	18	54	140	260	462

CASE 2

HILLSBORO HEALTH

Hillsboro Health is a 501(c)(3) corporation created in 2015 by the merger of Hillsboro County Home Health Agency (HCHHA) and Valley Hospice. HCHHA—originally named Middleboro Visiting Nurses Association—was founded in 1946 as a nonprofit home health agency to provide healthcare services to the county's population. Valley Hospice began serving residents in the county in 1980, providing palliative care and support for the terminally ill and their families. Volunteers provided most of the hospice services. Until the merger, Valley Hospice had been unable to qualify for Medicare certification. In 2013, it realized that it lacked the needed capital and expertise to become Medicare certified, so it sought a merger partner. Today, Hillsboro Health is an integrated healthcare organization providing home care, hospice, and community health services.

The formal merger agreement that created Hillsboro Health was agreed upon by both HCHHA and Valley Hospice boards and signed on January 2, 2015. The original affiliation/merger feasibility team was composed of four individuals—the two board presidents and the two executive directors of both organizations. Once approved, in accordance with the bylaws of the existing organizations and state regulations, the merger was effective 90 days later.

The merger agreement stipulated the mission and vision statements as well as the governance structure of Hillsboro Health. Under the merger, Hillsboro Health absorbed all assets and liabilities of Valley Hospice, with the stipulation that a board-restricted fund would be established with these assets to be used in the future to assist in fulfilling Hillsboro Health's hospice mission. In addition, the agreement also stipulated that Hillsboro Health would employ the executive director of Valley Hospice for 18 months.

MISSION AND VISION

The following mission and vision of Hillsboro Health were approved by the board of directors in March and January 2015, respectively:

Our Mission

We strive to provide comprehensive quality home health care and support services, for the purpose of restoring, advancing, and maximizing the level of independence to individuals and families in their place of residence. We believe that all clients will thrive in the comfort of their own home and attain the highest quality of life while respecting their need for dignity and compassionate care.

We provide continuity in care for the terminally ill and their families. We strive to maintain the comfort and dignity of the client through palliative care, with relief of physical symptoms and provision of emotional and spiritual support. We value the quality of life to the end of life while recognizing the ongoing needs of the client, family, and staff with emotional and bereavement support.

Our Vision

Hillsboro Health strives to set the standard of excellence in home care and hospice by demonstrating cutting-edge results in client outcomes; performance improvement; and client, family, physician, and employee satisfaction.

GOVERNANCE

Overall responsibility for Hillsboro Health rests with its board of directors. The 15-person corporate board meets quarterly to review the status of the agency. All directors serve for a five-year term and may be reelected by the board. The executive committee nominates individuals for membership on the board, and the new board then elects its officers. The election of directors is done by the full board at its June meeting. New directors and officers take their positions beginning July 1st. Last year, a consultant recommended that the board cease being self-perpetuating and establish mandatory term limits. The board is still considering this concept.

The executive committee—composed of the president, vice president, secretary, and treasurer—meets monthly and as needed with the chief executive officer (CEO) to resolve special issues and plan board meetings. Every April, the executive committee prepares a slate of nominees for new board members. The finance and audit committee meets monthly with the executive director to review the financial status of the agency. It also reviews the annual budget and recommends it to the full board for approval. The professional advisory committee meets monthly to review issues related to clinical care and quality standards.

At the time of the merger, the number of board members was expanded to accommodate former board members from Valley Hospice. Under the merger agreement, approved by both boards, Hillsboro Health has a 15-member corporate board and two six-member advisory boards. Initially, former board members of Valley Hospice were assigned three slots on the Hillsboro Health corporate board: Jack Donnelly (former board president), Reverend Philip Martin (former board vice president), and Ruth Berrie (former board member).

The current leadership of the Hillsboro Health corporate board is as follows:

- Janet Myer, the president. She lives in Middleboro and is a senior vice president at Middleboro Trust Company. This year marks her eighth consecutive year as board president, and she has one year remaining on her five-year term. Myer was instrumental in the reorganization of HCHHA several years ago and led the merger discussions and negotiations between HCHHA and Valley Hospice.

- David Ruseski, the vice president. He lives in Mifflenville and is the owner of Ruseski Auto Sales in Middleboro and Jasper. He has been a member of the board for 14 years and a long-term member of the finance and audit committee.

- Mary Steel, JD, the secretary. She lives in Middleboro and maintains a solo law practice in Mifflenville. She has been on the board for 12 years.

- Steve Meadows, the treasurer. He lives in Statesville and is the senior partner in the accounting firm of Meadows and Associates in Middleboro. He has served on the board for 14 years. As treasurer, he is a member of the finance and audit committee.

The 11 other members of the Hillsboro Health corporate board are as follows; the (number)* indicates the number of years served on the HCHHA or Valley Hospice board and the number of years remaining on current board term:

Hillsboro Health Board of Directors

Members	*Residence*
Ruth Berrie, RN (9, 3)*	
Retired	
Former director, Faith-Based Nursing Program, State University	
Former member, Valley Hospice board	Statesville
Nancy Blau (3, 2)	
Retired	
Former Hillsboro County commissioner	
Member, Middleboro School Board	Middleboro
William Bond (15, 5)	
Vice president, Finance, Master Tractor, Inc.	Mifflenville
Marquis Cushing, MD (12, 1)	
Retired	
Former internist	Jasper
Jack Donnelly (12, 5)	
Editor, *Middleboro Sentinel*	
Former president, Valley Hospice board	Mifflenville
Carl Fisher (9, 1)	
Retired Major General, US Army	
Member, board of the local chapter of AARP	
Farmer	Boalsburg
Melissa Giles, JD (2, 3)	
Legislative aide to US Representative James Giles	Jasper
Walker Hahn, CPA (7, 2)	
Principal, Financial Planning Services of Capital City	
Principal, Connors and Smith, Inc.	Jasper
Marsha Logic, JD (10, 4)	
Attorney, Jasper Legal Assistance Clinic	Jasper
Reverend Philip Martin (17, 4)	
Methodist Church of Middleboro	
Former vice president, Valley Hospice board	Middleboro
Alicia Tierry (0, 5)	
Art historian and curator, Middleboro Art Gallery and Association	Middleboro

Every month, the members of the board of directors are provided with operational and financial data on Hillsboro Health's "dashboard." As a condition of board service, each member must agree to protect people's confidentiality and guarantee no conflicts of interest. All board members are expected to support Hillsboro Health's fund-raising and community activities and to participate in board development activities. Other than Dr. Marquis Cushing, no other physician serves on Hillsboro Health's corporate board because physician interest in doing so has been minimal.

Community advisory boards were created at the time of the merger to ensure that the community had direct input into the programs of the Home Care Services Division and the Hospice and Palliative Care Division. Hillsboro Health managers in charge of these programs meet with the advisory boards and are responsible for maintaining effective and open communications with these members, giving them updates on program accomplishments and plans. Most members of the advisory boards are former board members of HCHHA or Valley Hospice. They meet semiannually and participate in the annual strategic planning work session of the corporate board. Members serve three-year terms and are then reappointed by the Hillsboro Health CEO with the approval of the corporate board. Vacancies are filled as needed and are up to the recommendation of the CEO.

Following are the current membership lists of the two advisory boards; the (number)* indicates the number of years remaining on current board term:

Home Care Services Community Advisory Board

Members	Residence
Janet Doe, RN (3)* Retired Former director of school nursing, Middleboro School Department	Middleboro
Martin Happy, MD (3) Principal, Happy Point Medical Consultants	Mifflenville
Candice McCory, RN (2) Director, Disease Prevention, Hillsboro County Health Department	Middleboro
Matty O'Brien, OTD (2) Professor emeritus of occupational therapy, State University	Middleboro
Michele Regan, RN (1) Director, Nursing and Patient Services, Jasper Gardens	Jasper
Helen Vosper, RN (1) Retired Former director, Nursing, MIDCARE and Webster Health System	Middleboro

Hospice and Palliative Care Community Advisory Board

Members	*Residence*
Cindy Donnelly (3)	
Former member, Valley Hospice board	
Former newspaper reporter, *Middleboro Sentinel*	Mifflenville
Alice Meadows (3)	
Vice president, Middleboro Golf Course	Middleboro
Lois Metz, LISW (2)	
Independent social work practitioner	Middleboro
Grace Niebauer (2)	
Homemaker	Harris City
Trustee, MIDCARE	
Victoria Seed (1)	
Vice president, Mid-State Oil Company	Jasper
Matilda Strawbridge, LCSW (1)	
Retired	
Former director, Social Services, Capital City General Hospital	Statesville

The board of directors is organized using standing committees:

Executive Committee	Elected by the Full Board
	President: Janet Myer
	Members: David Ruseski—Vice President
	Mary Steel—Secretary
	Steve Meadows—Treasurer
	Staff: Martha Washington
Finance and Audit Committee	Appointed by the Board President
	Chair: William Bond
	Members: Jack Donnelly, Walker Hahn, David Ruseski, Steve Meadows
	Staff: John Gochnaur
Professional Advisory Committee	Appointed by the Board President
	Chair: Marquis Cushing
	Members: Ruth Berrie, Marsha Logic
	Staff: Catherine Newfields

Fund-Raising Committee   Appointed by the Board President
                                            Chair: Carl Fisher
                                            Members: Nancy Blau, Walker Hahn
                                            Staff: Angela Lopez, Mary Care

Publicity and Public Relations Committee Appointed by the Board President
                                            Chair: Philip Martin
                                            Members: Melissa Giles, Alicia Tierry
                                            Staff: Martha Washington, Gomez Pile

For three years before the merger, HCHHA experienced a decline in operating margins. In 2013 and 2014, it sustained its first losses from operations. The finance and audit committee is especially concerned by such a downward trend in financial performance from operations as well as the impending significant changes in reimbursement mandated by Medicare and Medicaid. Whether HCHHA could financially afford a merger and the added expenses associated with becoming Medicare-certified as a hospice was the main issue discussed during the merger process. William Bond, chair of the finance and audit committee, indicated that "a good year for our home care programs is a margin of 1 to 3 percent. Medicare funding is a complex system, especially for a small agency." Janet Myer supported this point and indicated that the decision to merge with Valley Hospice was to, first and foremost, make a Medicare-certified hospice available in the county and to build a more robust infrastructure to navigate the current and anticipated environment in all aspects of home care. She said, "We merged at exactly the right time. The need was mutual. Valley Hospice did not have the resources and expertise to bring a Medicare-certified hospice to our area. We needed to further develop and broaden our services and our management team."

The fund-raising as well as publicity and public relations committees jointly sponsor community fund-raising activities. Annually, Hillsboro Health sponsors the Holiday Ball and the Memorial Day 5K family road race in Middleboro and the Labor Day 10K road race in Jasper. The committees also continue the traditions of Valley Hospice and sponsor monthly "leadership circle" community meetings and dinners to inform the public of the organization's accomplishments and ask for financial support.

MERGER AGREEMENT AND STRATEGIC PLAN

Although Hillsboro Health was created on January 1, 2015, it did not become official until the merger was signed on January 2. Aside from the points previously mentioned, the merger agreement stipulated that no Valley Hospice employee would be discharged within six months of the merger. Hillsboro Health agreed to honor all of Valley Hospice contractual obligations. Due diligence for the merger was provided by Capital City Consulting, which guided Hillsboro Health through the approval process and asset transfer. The consultants also provided a two-year strategic plan that covers all aspects of the agency.

Capital City Consulting recommended that HCHHA sell the Hartsdale House—the site of its offices—before the merger because this facility, while a community landmark, was not essential to its operations and represented a needless drain on its resources. The Hartsdale House is a spacious home on the border of Middleboro's central business district. It is noted for its antiques, classical style, and approximately 11 acres adjacent to the Middleboro Golf course. It is a community landmark and is featured in area travel brochures. The Hartsdale family donated this location to HCHHA in 1969 with a restricted endowment "to ensure its physical upkeep and maintenance in perpetuity."

Capital City Investment Partners and the Hillsboro Historic Land Trust jointly purchased the Hartsdale House on January 2, 2015, for $1.2 million. The contract requires that the new owners maintain the property in accordance with the conditions in the original gift and current stipulations of the Middleboro Historic District Commission. The house is slated to become a destination hotel and conference center. In January 2015, Hillsboro Health moved its main offices to leased space in Middleboro.

MANAGEMENT TEAM

CHIEF EXECUTIVE OFFICER

Martha Washington, RN, was hired in 2010. She has a four-year renewable contract, which the corporate board recently extended (after a formal review) for another four years and with an increase in salary. Prior to being CEO, she served as regional director for a large for-profit chain of home health agencies, managing the affairs of 13 separate agencies. In the past, she was the director of marketing for a large medical products firm headquartered in Capital City and was a visiting nurse for ten years with a large visiting nurse association (VNA) in a major midwestern city. Today, she is the vice president of the State Home Health Association board and maintains an active presence in the state legislature to lobby for home care issues. Her management style emphasizes the delegation of clearly expressed responsibilities.

Since her arrival, Washington has reorganized the organization in accordance with its mission. With board approval before her appointment, she opened an additional office in Jasper to support all programs in that area. She also expanded and added services. To date, her accomplishments include the development of the Private Duty Services program; the HCHHA merger with Valley Hospice; and the increased use of technology and information systems to support home care services, including the installation of an agencywide medical record system and medical information system. Her direct reports include the chief operating officer, chief financial officer, chief quality improvement officer, and project assistant.

CHIEF OPERATING OFFICER (COO)

Catherine Newfields, RN, was hired by HCHHA in 2011 to manage the Home Care Services Division. She was promoted to her current position at the time of the merger. Before that, she was an assistant professor of community health nursing at State University and worked for 17 years in all aspects of home care, including briefly as executive director of a small VNA. As COO, her direct reports include the program directors of Home Care Services, Private Duty Services, Community Health Services, and Hospice and Palliative Care as well as the directors of Administration, Information Systems Management, and Marketing.

CHIEF FINANCIAL OFFICER (CFO)

John Gochnaur, CPA, manages the fiscal resources of Hillsboro Health. He joined Hillsboro Health in 2016 and became the first employee it recruited using an executive search firm. Prior to that, he was chief financial officer of a VNA in a large midwestern city. He has more than 20 years of experience with home health and hospice and has been a speaker at regional meetings of home care financing. Since joining Hillsboro Health as CFO, he has been elected to the fiscal affairs committee of the State Home Health Association. A native of Middleboro, he has a daughter who teaches in the Middleboro School Department.

MEDICAL DIRECTOR

Since the merger, Dr. Jane Campbell has served as Hillsboro Health's medical director, working closely with the Home Care and Hospice divisions. She is trained in internal medicine and is board certified in geriatric medicine, with a subspecialty certification in hospice and palliative care. Although born and raised in Statesville, she completed her training at an East Coast medical school and her residencies in both the United States and England. Prior to this position, she was the deputy medical director of a large VNA in an adjacent state.

CHIEF QUALITY IMPROVEMENT OFFICER (CQIO)

As CQIO, Judith Herman, RN, is responsible for all aspects of quality improvement and utilization review at Hillsboro Health. She is a graduate of State University and holds a master in nursing quality improvement from a private university. She has approximately 15 years of experience in quality improvement in home health care and worked with the CEO in another organization before coming to HCHHA. Along with Selma Kessler, she cochairs Hillsboro Health's information systems development committee.

PROGRAM DIRECTOR OF HOME CARE SERVICES

Although Roberta (Bobbie) Allen, RN, worked for HCHHA for ten years, she was promoted into her position at the time of the merger two years ago. Previously, she worked in home care and with the VNAs in Capital City; Washington, DC; and the rural Midwest. She is active in the State Nurses Association and sponsors an intern from the nursing graduate program at State University.

PROGRAM DIRECTOR OF PRIVATE DUTY SERVICES

Michael Carlstead, LPN, was a home health aide and licensed practical nurse for more than 30 years, and 24 of those years were with HCHHA. At Hillsboro Health, he oversees the Private Duty Services Division and program development and growth. Aside from providing essential nursing services to the community, the division has consistently helped subsidize Hillsboro Health's other programs and services. He completed his nursing training 18 years ago but just recently earned a bachelor in business administration from a small college that offers distance education for active professionals. He plans to retire in six months.

PROGRAM DIRECTOR OF COMMUNITY HEALTH SERVICES

Angela Lopez, RN, serves in this capacity only part-time, having been appointed to the position right after the merger and the retirement of the former program director. She has worked for the agency (before and after the merger) for five years. Previously, she was an intern and program assistant for the Hillsboro County Health Department and for the state's Office of Health Promotion. She has a bachelor in community health nursing from State University and a master in public health from a major midwestern university.

PROGRAM DIRECTOR OF HOSPICE AND PALLIATIVE CARE

Prior to the merger, Middleboro native Mary Care, RN, CHPN, was the part-time executive director of Valley Hospice for three years. She brings to her full-time role at Hillsboro Health more than 24 years of experience working in hospice and palliative care programs, certifications in all aspects of hospice and palliative care nursing, and professional knowledge of community-based and inpatient hospice services. At Valley Hospice, she was the leading force behind the merger and the development of a Medicare-certified program. Under her leadership, Valley Hospice created an effective and extensive network of trained community volunteers who provided palliative and bereavement care as well as assisted with fund-raising.

DIRECTOR OF ADMINISTRATION

Steve Graham is responsible for all aspects of Administration, including inventory management, human resources management, telecommunication systems management, facilities management, and all vendor contracts. Prior to joining HCHHA 18 years ago, he was employed in a similar position with the local cable company.

DIRECTOR OF INFORMATION SYSTEMS MANAGEMENT

Selma Kessler, the chief information officer, was recruited through a regional executive search firm at the time of the merger. Her knowledge of and experience with healthcare hardware and software systems are vast, including overseeing the development and implementation of information systems at a VNA in the eastern part of the state. She holds a graduate degree in medical information systems and business processing from a private university on the West Coast. She and her husband are originally from Mifflenville.

DIRECTOR OF MARKETING

Gomez Pile was promoted into this position right after the merger. Before the merger, she was the part-time marketing and public relations assistant for Valley Hospice. Also, she was the regional marketing manager for a retail pharmaceutical chain in Capital City and a market representative for a national pharmaceutical corporation. She holds a master in marketing from State University.

ORGANIZATIONAL STRUCTURE

Hillsboro Health is organized into four divisions on the basis of mission, clientele, and reimbursement. Each division is a unique service line. Two—Home Care Services and Hospice and Palliative Care—rely on Medicare financing. Two others—Private Duty Services and Community Health Services—do not rely on Medicare funding. Each division has a program director who reports to the COO, and each division has a budget. Hillsboro Health adopted a flexible budgeting system when it was created two years ago.

The functional units of the organization are finance, quality improvement, information systems management, administration, and marketing. These units support the operations of the four divisions.

HOME CARE SERVICES DIVISION

This division provides nursing and other services—occupational therapy, physical therapy, and speech therapy—to clients in their homes. Medicare, Medicaid, self-pay, and private insurance fund the division. Years before the merger, HCHHA continually pursued contracts with local managed care organizations. As a result of these efforts, contracts are still in place with Central States Good Health Network and with a commercial health maintenance organization.

Medicare requires the beneficiary to be "confined to the home under the care of a physician. Services are based on an approved care plan established, certified, and periodically reviewed by a physician." Medicare pays Hillsboro Health a predetermined base payment using Home Health Resource Groups based on the Outcome and Assessment Information Set. The rate is established for each 60-day episode of needed care. In addition, Medicare covers the need for skilled nursing on "an intermittent basis" as well as the needs for physical therapy, speech-language pathology, and occupational therapy. As such, Medicare covers part-time or intermittent skilled nursing services, part-time or intermittent home health aide services, physical therapy, speech-language pathology, occupational therapy, medical social services, medical supplies, and durable medical equipment.

Registered nurses (RNs) assess and monitor all clients. They are responsible for treatment planning, administration of medications, and other nursing services. Home health aides work as team members in implementing treatment plans and assisting with self-care activities within the context of Medicare and Medicaid regulations. Therapists and other contract professionals—such as physical therapists, occupational therapists, speech therapists, social workers, and nutritionists—are available to consult and to implement treatment plans. Staff members have reported that, for a few years now, clients served by this program immediately following a hospital discharge have required more intensive services than in the past.

The division also provides pediatric care to children who are born prematurely, who are recovering from surgery, or who are experiencing a chronic disease. Special therapy is also available. Typically, these services are covered by health insurance plans, Medicare, and Medicaid.

When interviewed, Bobbie Allen, the program director, indicated that "staff turnover is a real, and sometimes very critical, issue. I believe our staff—especially our RNs—work harder and are paid less than those in a hospital." She said that matching staff talents with client needs creates staffing issues. Currently, all RNs are certified to administer IV therapies and some have special training and certification in palliative care and gerontology. Allen is concerned that hospitals in Capital City are referring their clients who live in Jasper to the Capital City VNA and Hospice and not to Hillsboro Health. She admitted to feeling annoyed when she hears a radio commercial extolling the services of the Capital City VNA and Hospice as she drives into Jasper. She shared that a frequent challenge for her division is getting the required physician recertification every 60 days for clients with Medicare.

The division is considering the following national data as a basis for planning:

National Utilization Statistics—Home Health Care
(Discharge means a case is closed by the home health agency [HHA].)

Clients Served by an HHA Within the Past Three Years	*Rate per 10,000 Population*
Under 65 years	16.4
65 years or older	277.0

Home Health Care Clients Discharged in the Past 12 Months	
Under 65 years	91.0
65 years or older	1,439.3

At Time of HHA Discharge, Client …	*Percentage*
Remained in community	71.5
Transferred to another setting	20.5
Died	2.3
Unknown	5.7

Hillsboro Health's data indicate that this division's experience closely parallels the national utilization patterns (see tables 2.1 and 2.2) and that few cases extend over a long time, making the division's mean service time significantly higher than the median values. Current efforts are underway to compare the division's service times with national statistics. A recent study done by a student at State University found that, on average, every Hillsboro Health Medicare home visit involved an average of 14.2 miles.

On the web at ache.org/books/ Middleboro2

When asked about her assessment of the agency, Allen questioned the impact of the four-division model, stating that "health promotion and education should not be isolated in a specific division—such as Community Health Services—but instead woven into all services provided by Hillsboro Health." She added, "sometimes our silos get in our way." She points out that the division needs the opportunity to expand its emergency preparedness and that Medicare's rule that requires a person to be "homebound" to be eligible continues to prevent the division from meeting the needs of a number of individuals. "Too often we have to explain to senior citizens that they do not qualify for Medicare Home Care because they are not homebound as defined by Medicare," she reported.

HCHHA equipped all clinical staff with a computer tablet for data entry and report generation. The tablets directly interface with the agency's master information system, which includes the client's medical record. The goal of this electronic point-of-care documentation system is to eventually eliminate all paper records, especially charts that need to be done in or during the home visit. Going beyond this practice, Hillsboro Health provided all clients served by the Home Care Services Division with a free tablet to enable them to maintain contact with staff, to facilitate client education, and to be the basis of expanded telemedicine applications.

Allen said, "My most significant management issue is cost control. Our financial margins are very small. We need to track and manage everything. Fortunately, I have access to a number of qualified colleagues who are responsible for quality reporting, billing, cost reporting, and information systems. Another difficulty we face is getting physicians to recertify a client's condition by face-to-face examination, and it can be a source of payment delay."

When asked about productivity, she volunteered that the "clinical staff is highly skilled and productive, but over the past two years, a number of our senior staff members have retired. When replaced, our productivity has increased." The division uses the following productivity guidelines: Nurses are expected to generate, on average, 30 points per week. For a routine visit, the time estimate is 1.25 hours. This breaks down to 45 minutes for the actual visit, 15 minutes for documentation, and 15 minutes for travel time. "We expect around 30 points per week," she said. "This leaves sufficient time for case conferences, meetings, and in-service education." Allen indicated that points need to be constantly monitored as clients are increasingly needing more time, especially for education.

Home Care Services Division Productivity Guidelines

Type of Visit	Time Estimate (Hours)	Points
Admission	2.50	2.0
Routine	1.25	1.0
Discharge	1.50	1.2

Recertification or Resumption	2.50	2.0
Nonbillable	1.25	1.0
Supervisory	0.625	0.5

PRIVATE DUTY SERVICES DIVISION

Begun in 2012 at HCHHA, the Private Duty Services program provides assistance with activities of daily living (ADLs) and other in-home services as needed. Medicare does not pay for these services; all funding comes from Medicaid, self-pay, or private insurance. The division and its programs were developed for both service and financial reasons. A formal marketing study completed in 2011 indicated a strong demand for these types of services in Middleboro and surrounding communities. To date, initial demand for these services has surpassed expectations. All services are purchased hourly, daily, or weekly. Medicaid sets its own hourly rates by service.

Program offerings include the following:

◆ Basic nursing care or assistance, such as medication administration and blood pressure screening, provided by licensed practical nurses and home health aides

◆ Physical, occupational, and speech therapy provided by professional therapists

◆ Social work services provided by licensed social workers

◆ 24/7 companion services provided by personal care attendants or others

◆ Light housekeeping, grocery shopping, meal preparation, laundry, and other in-home duties provided by homemaker/housekeeper aides

◆ Assistance with ADLs and respite care provided by personal care attendants

Clients can select from a menu of services—and prices—that meet their needs. No medical authorization is required.

When interviewed, Michael Carlstead, the program director, stated, "We never seem to have enough staff to meet our clients' needs. Not everyone is suited to do this type of work." He attributed the high staff turnover to low pay and modest benefits. Reflecting on his own experience, he said, "The paperwork really gets me down. In the past 20 years, the paperwork has just increased and never seems to end. But I love my loyal and great staff and I really enjoy working with them. I will miss them all when I retire."

Clients contract for a specific number of hours per week and are billed at the end of the week. Most clients pay with a credit card, but some pay with cash or check. Clients with an outstanding balance for more than two weeks are reviewed and potentially dropped from the program. For Medicaid to pay, the client must be Medicaid eligible and the service plan must be approved by Medicaid before services are provided.

Carlstead expressed concerns about the human resources dimension of the agency: "It is essential that we have current information on the professional status of all of our employees; sometimes we don't. Sometimes, we need more staff who have had the required background checks and who have undergone a formal review of their credentials. Credentialing and background checks are an issue that could get us into trouble. Another issue we face is the poor and potentially unhealthy condition of a client's home because of that person's inability to care for the home or because of too many family pets."

Although no significant competition for private duty services has developed in Middleboro, he is aware that in the past 18 months three national franchised agencies have opened in Jasper. "Competition in our southern market is getting to be fierce," he noted.

COMMUNITY HEALTH SERVICES DIVISION

The range of services offered by the Community Health Services Division depends on the funding it receives directly from state, county, town, and other grants. Following are the current programs it runs:

◆ *Maternal and child health program.* It provides educational, direct services, and health screening to expectant and new mothers with children under one year old as well as child home care visits to qualifying infants under one year old. Bilirubin photo light therapy is also available as needed. Funding for this program is provided by state Medicaid and an annual grant. All recipients of state public assistance are eligible to receive the service without charge, while others may pay with a modest contribution. Classes and clinics are held in Middleboro and Jasper if a grant is received from the state, county, or town. The Prenatal Program—which has been well received in the community— includes a home visit from a maternity nurse to evaluate the health of both mother and child and to provide counseling on breast-feeding, diet, and infant care.

◆ *High blood pressure screening program.* It provides not only screening but also referrals to physicians as appropriate. Screenings are done in public locations, such as shopping centers, churches, and schools. Funding for this program is obtained from United Way through an annual application. Recently, United

Way has requested a comprehensive assessment of the cost-effectiveness of the program as a condition of continued funding.

◆ *Community health activities program.* It provides physicals; immunizations; drug and alcohol testing; and, by appointment, smoking cessation and health education to high-risk individuals. CPR and first-aid classes are available per a grant from the county's chapter of the American Red Cross. All services take place at Hillsboro Health's offices in Middleboro and Jasper. Physicals and immunizations required for students of public elementary and secondary schools are free of charge to residents. Special classes are held in topics such as nutrition, foot care, and post-stroke care and recovery. Financial support for this program comes primarily from annual, voter-approved town appropriations.

◆ *Senior health clinics program.* It provides services such as foot care, blood pressure monitoring, earwax removal, injections, medication management support, immunizations, and preventive care. Funded by the State Office on Aging, this program is free to seniors older than aged 65; a modest fee is charged for seniors younger than aged 65. Clinics are held monthly in Jasper and Middleboro and approximately once every two months in other towns in Hillsboro County.

◆ *Head lice program.* It provides lice education, prevention, and treatment to schoolchildren and their family. The program relies on referrals from school nurses. Services are available in Hillsboro Health's offices and by appointment. The program is completely financed by an annual grant from the Retail Pharmacy Association of Hillsboro County.

Community Health Services Division is expected to cover all of its direct costs and an appropriate share of its indirect costs. Unique to the division is the need to write grant applications for private, state, and local funds and to attend town meetings to secure funding for its programs. When interviewed, Angela Lopez, program director, indicated that she is concerned that many community needs are left unfulfilled because of a lack of funds. She also noted that even if state and town funding were adequate today, Hillsboro Health may have a problem making ends meet in the future. United Way has already expressed concern that Hillsboro Health had been "so active and successful in its own fund-raising that future allocation decisions—or money coming from United Way—would be weighed carefully against the more substantial needs of other worthy organizations." A recent letter to the editor printed in the *Middleboro Sentinel* highlights Hillsboro Health's need to raise funds. The letter was written by an angry family member of a low-income program participant who had to pay for services; it noted, "The agency is supposed to be there for the community, and it turns a large profit every year! And we support them through United Way."

The division's relationship with the Hillsboro County Health Department is tenuous. "We probably need to meet more often," Lopez admitted. "They typically want us to take on contracts for less than our costs. We have issues with them."

According to Lopez, the services offered by Hillsboro Health differentiate it from similar agencies and make it especially attractive when—or if—an accountable care organization (ACO) is developed in Middleboro. "Although our services are modest, they are important, particularly at a time when the Hillsboro County Health Department and other voluntary health agencies in town struggle to deliver the types of services we provide," she added. "For example, in Jasper, we just put on a program to train babysitters in conjunction with the school system and the local chapter of the Red Cross. It was an overwhelming success."

Neither of the two hospitals in Middleboro financially contribute to the division's programming as part of their community benefit responsibility, and program coordination with the hospitals is also a problem. The agency's offices in Jasper receive modest municipal funding from the town, which cannot be said for the City of Middleboro. "Our smaller towns continue to do their best. But the city council in Middleboro continues to reduce its contribution and ask why the Hillsboro County Health Department cannot do what we do. We have serious and growing financial issues that will continue to limit our services," Lopez said.

HOSPICE AND PALLIATIVE CARE DIVISION

This division offers hospice and palliative services throughout Hillsboro County.

Hospice care is supported by a number of private health insurance plans as well as Medicare. To be eligible for Medicare funding, the individual must be certified as having a terminal illness with a medical prognosis of six months or less. Electing hospice care precludes the individual from receiving Medicare support for curing the terminal illness. Physician services, nursing care, medical equipment and supplies, drugs for pain and symptom management, hospice aide and homemaker services, physical therapy, occupational therapy, speech-language pathology services, social worker services, dietary counseling, spiritual counseling, grief and loss counseling, and short-term inpatient care for pain control and symptom management and for respite care are all covered by Medicare.

Medicare-supported hospice is available for two periods of 90 days and an unlimited number of subsequent 60-day periods. Medicare pays a daily rate for each day a client is enrolled in the hospice benefit period. Daily payments are made regardless of the amount of services furnished on a given day. The client pays for all eligible costs associated with the plan of care. Four payment levels are used: routine home care, continuous home care, inpatient respite care, and general inpatient care. Adjustments to these rates include a service-intensity add-on, to acknowledge the extra costs associated with the last seven days of life.

As a Medicare-certified hospice, the division is required to report to Medicare a number of quality measures related to opioid use in treatment, pain screening and assessments, and dyspnea screening and treatment as well as related quality indicators.

Medicare and Medicaid do not pay for palliative care. At the time of the merger, Hillsboro Health made the decision to provide palliative care regardless of the person's ability to pay as long as the need for such care is endorsed by the agency's hospice care team (including its physician, nurse, and social worker). Because a significant number of palliative care clients eventually become eligible for hospice, this decision was deemed appropriate.

Following are recent national statistics on hospice care in the United States:

National Hospice Statistics, 2018

Percentage of all deaths occurring under the care of a hospice	41.9%
Median length of hospice service	19.7 days
Mean length of hospice service	63.0 days
Proportion of clients under hospice for longer than 180 days	11.5%

Palliative care, in contrast to hospice care, is intended to make the client feel better. People who receive curative care (e.g., radiation therapy, chemotherapy, surgery) frequently need the benefits of palliative care to address the discomfort, symptoms, and stress of serious illness and curative treatments. People with cancer, congestive heart failure, chronic obstructive pulmonary disease, kidney failure, and AIDS frequently need palliative care. The palliative care team comprises nurses and social workers and, sometimes, registered dietitians, music therapists, and counselors. Volunteers are used as appropriate.

When interviewed, Mary Care, the program director, sounded pleased with the division's success: "Our Medicare-certified services have surpassed our original expectations. In less than three years, we have grown in scope and sophistication. Today, we offer a full range of services and are able to manage the complex financial systems and quality reporting. We were fortunate to hire Dr. Cecily Saunders as the hospice's medical director. Dr. Saunders has more than 20 years' experience in hospice and palliative care. Identifying and hiring the staff we needed to provide Medicare services was a challenge. The management team has been very supportive. In just two years, we have grown into our mission." When asked about the competition, she indicated that Jasper is a concern, saying, "There are three Medicare-certified hospices in Capital City, and all of them advertise that they serve all of Hillsboro County, especially Jasper residents."

At the time of the merger, using funds provided by the sale of Hartsdale House, Hillsboro Health decided not to begin a freestanding inpatient service. Instead, it signed five-year collaborative agreements with the two local hospitals to reserve and renovate two of their private rooms for Hillsboro Health's hospice clients. Under these agreements, when the rooms are used, Hillsboro Health pays the hospital for service and can augment the hospice client's care team as needed. In the past two years, 62 percent of Hillsboro Health's hospice clients died in their place of residence (including the nursing home), 28 percent died in a dedicated private room at the local hospital, and another 10 percent died as a hospital inpatient.

SUCCESSES AND CHALLENGES

The merger that formed Hillsboro Health required a significant upgrade to many management systems, but issues still remain. Martha Washington, the CEO, explained, "The coordination between our clinical personnel and business office still needs to be improved. For example, last year, in more than 20 cases, we failed to adhere to the 60-day physician review requirements. Also, too often, we begin providing home care services even before we have the signed physician's certificate. This jeopardizes and delays our qualification under Medicare."

The sale of the Hartsdale House provided the agency with significant capital to establish the Hospice and Palliative Care Division and expand the expertise of the management team. It has also allowed the provision of palliative care to clients who need it but may not have the ability to pay. "It is our belief that if we forge an effective relationship with our palliative care clients, they will select us if they are in need of hospice services down the road," she noted.

She added, "Our financial margins are small, and we are very dependent on community fund-raising, something that Valley Hospice excelled at and helped us build upon their bases. I am very grateful that almost all of the former volunteers with Valley Hospice are now working with our hospice program. They have embraced Hillsboro Health's expanded mission and vision and help us significantly access community philanthropy and provide superior service."

Although all employees are assigned to a specific division or functional area, the agency uses a flexible staffing model. A number of workers are cross-trained so that some can work effectively in more than one division. The management systems are sufficiently robust to appropriately charge the division that benefits from an employee's work. For example, if a home health aide assigned to the Hospice and Palliative Care Division works in the Private Duty Services Division, the latter is charged for the associated staff expenses. This staffing flexibility and a collaborative team of program directors have been essential in Hillsboro Health's growth in some areas and in its contracts with other organizations. Every two weeks, the senior management team meets formally to review operations and to problem-solve. For the full board meetings, only Washington, the CFO, the medical director, and the COO usually attend.

When asked about any fallout from the merger, she expressed her disappointment that Mary Bird, her former special projects assistant, elected to resign when she was not hired into a position with more responsibility. Aside from that, she recalled that the months before and after the merger were a whirlwind: "The plan provided by Capital City Consulting was insightful, and the senior consultant met with us as needed. Many today are surprised by our ability to successfully accomplish such a bold and provocative plan in a relatively short time."

The continued application of technology and telemedicine is essential to the agency's mission and vision. "Government funding will never pay us what it should, so we need to find ways to provide the best-quality service with what funding is available to us," she explained. "Our primary challenge in the future will be to hold on to our markets as more and more competition develops. How either or both of the community hospitals in our service area will position themselves in this changing market is an open question."

Hillsboro Health's current marketing program has not established a strong relationship with primary care physicians in Middleboro and beyond. Washington is aware of this shortcoming, noting, "In home health, marketing is more than advertising. We need to better secure our clients at the source—namely, their primary care physician. As the local hospitals have acquired more primary care practices, the physicians and nurse practitioners have looked first to the hospital for services; we are, at best, second."

She foresees steadily declining revenue and funding for the Community Health Services Division. She and the board believe the division gives them an advantage if Hillsboro Health were to join an ACO in the future. "The general public just did not seem to realize that the 'grey tsunami' is upon us. Patients are being discharged from hospitals quicker and sicker, and this situation—coupled with the Affordable Care Act—has created a complex situation for home health," she noted. "I am optimistic that hospitals, primary care providers, nursing homes, and home health agencies working together as an ACO will improve health and lower costs. Our goal is to be the home care provider of choice as an ACO is developed to serve this community."

On a recent Sunday morning public affairs show broadcast on Middleboro's TV Channel 32, Washington, as a guest panelist, was asked about how NGOs (nongovernment organizations) could make people's lives better. She framed her answer around Hillsboro Health's specific core competencies. "As healthcare providers, we need to reduce hospital admissions and readmissions and the need for emergent care. We also need to accurately diagnose patients' needs and treat and care for them with the highest level of professionalism," she began. "It is also essential that we accurately code cases for reimbursement and provide payers with all the needed documentation to ensure timely payment. We have to meet realistic productivity benchmarks and become even smarter in providing clinical care using comprehensive information about our patients." This TV appearance garnered her an invitation to be a keynote speaker at the upcoming State Conference of Home Health Leaders in Capital City.

Although some members of the corporate board still want Hillsboro Health to remain the sole provider of home health, private duty, and hospice and palliative care services in Middleboro, Washington has told the board the goal is unrealistic. Instead, she is focused on continuing the agency's highly positive reputation. "We are known for our prudent administration of funds, high quality of care, and can-do attitude. Healthcare professionals throughout the county view us as a highly professional place to work," she said. "Our Medicare-certified hospice has identified us as a key and essential player in the state's healthcare system and a champion for the needs of our citizens. That's what I hope we can retain—this positive public image. It has multiple advantages."

Tables 2.3 through 2.10 show the services provided and the resources invested by Hillsboro Health.

*On the web at
ache.org/books/
Middleboro2*

Table 2.1

Hillsboro Health Service Area Utilization by Town

On the web at ache.org/books/ Middleboro2

Division	Boalsburg	Carterville	Harris City	Jasper	Middleboro	Mifflenville	Minortown	Statesville	Total
Home Care									
Client Census	37	42	187	310	853	205	57	105	1,796
RN Visits	695	861	4,659	10,356	16,521	3,985	990	4,382	42,449
LPN Visits	14	16	71	118	324	78	22	40	682
HH Aide Visits	339	460	1,711	2,239	8,240	1,878	622	962	16,450
PT Visits	153	147	622	720	2,384	594	199	201	5,020
OT Visits	21	24	105	125	532	116	32	59	1,014
ST Visits	3	3	20	41	72	17	4	20	189
SW Visits	10	11	51	74	231	56	25	28	487
Private Duty									
Client Census	8	10	34	137	134	39	11	30	403
RN In-Home Hours	17	21	72	290	284	83	23	64	854
LPN In-Home Hours	111	389	1,323	5,731	5,015	1,518	400	1,196	15,683
PCA In-Home Hours	227	359	1,930	9,026	10,918	2,569	425	986	26,440
HH Aide In-Home Hours	65	80	93	11,450	13,583	2,752	301	117	28,441
Other In-Home Hours	4	7	39	322	232	68	15	11	698
Community Health									
Ante/Postpartum Visits	1	2	19	164	102	26	2	14	330
Child Health Visits	3	6	21	190	107	30	2	22	380
Prenatal Class Enrollee	6	10	19	28	19	17	16	4	119
High BP Screening	32	45	23	2,800	3,773	324	103	356	7,456
Hospice & Palliative Care									
Palliative Care Clients	1	2	5	14	40	9	2	10	83
Hospice Clients	2	3	16	50	128	23	7	27	256

Note: BP: blood pressure; HH: home health; LPN: licensed practical nurse; OT: occupational therapist; PCA: personal care attendant; PT: physical therapist; RN: registered nurse; ST: speech therapist; SW: social worker.

Table 2.2
Hillsboro
Health Services
Provided

*On the web at
ache.org/books/
Middleboro2*

Division	2019	2018	2017	2016
Home Care				
Unduplicated Client Census	1,796	1,582	1,578	1,498
RN Visits	42,449	42,404	39,477	38,334
LPN Visits	662	678	980	823
HH Aide Visits	16,450	13,540	12,445	10,343
PT Visits	5,020	4,697	4,630	4,240
OT Visits	1,014	993	897	899
ST Visits	189	165	174	178
SW Visits	487	472	434	445
Total Visits	**64,325**	**60,899**	**57,037**	**53,262**
Private Duty				
Unduplicated Client Census	403	312	260	225
RN In-Home Hours	854	1,044	1,534	1,267
LPN In-Home Hours	15,683	14,555	13,165	12,564
PCA In-Home Hours	26,440	22,657	19,345	16,745
HH Aide In-Home Hours	28,441	19,737	17,018	11,788
Other In-Home Hours	698	416	212	180
Total Hours	**72,116**	**58,409**	**51,274**	**42,544**
Community Health				
Ante/Postpartum Visits	330	412	500	499
Child Health Visits	380	412	456	450
Prenatal Class Enrollees	119	140	123	130
Children Seen—Middleboro	501	598	534	612
Children Seen—Jasper	301	222	305	317
High Blood Pressure Screening				
People Screened	7,456	6,867	7,234	7,124
MD Referrals	398	423	407	456
Senior Health Clinics				
Clients Seen—Middleboro	923	902	920	934
Clients Seen—Jasper	254	243	289	389

continued

Division	2019	2018	2017	2016
Hospice and Palliative Care				
Palliative Care Unduplicated Client Census	83	65	53	21
Number of Veterans Served	10	12	7	5
3-Year Average, % Palliative Care Patients Who Died, Died at Home	63.1%	67.0%	59.4%	51.0%
Hospice Care Unduplicated Client Census	256	231	204	161
Hospice Median Length of Service (Days)	19.1	19.4	22.3	28.2
Hospice Mean Length of Service (Days)	69	67.4	66.3	48.2
% Patients in Hospice Over 180 Days	11.3	11.1	12.3	8.3
Bereavement Service (Hours) Provided to Families and Friends	723	617	590	320
Total Volunteer Hours	**2,119**	**2,008**	**1,634**	**1,045**
Mean Hours per Volunteer	44	46	50	55
Home Nursing and Aide Visits	5,489	5,156	4,356	3,054
Home SW and Chaplain Visits	927	892	740	501
% Families Who Reported Their Bereavement Needs Were Met	88.0%	85.0%	91.0%	94.0%
% Discharged Hospice Patients with 3+ Types of Advanced Planning Instruments	68.9%	71.3%	80.2%	41.0%

Table 2.2
Hillsboro
Health Services
Provided
(continued)

*On the web at
ache.org/books/
Middleboro2*

Note: HH: home health; LPN: licensed practical nurse; MD: physician; OT: occupational therapist; PCA: personal care attendant; PT: physical therapist; RN: registered nurse; ST: speech therapist; SW: social worker.

Table 2.3
Hillsboro
Health Home
Care Utilization
by Principal
Diagnosis

Principal Diagnosis	Percentage of All Cases
Diseases of the Circulatory System	25.5
Heart Disease	12.6
Diseases of the Musculoskeletal System and Connective Tissue	12.6
Diabetes Mellitus	10.8
Diseases of the Respiratory System	8.6
Essential Hypertension	7.0
Injury and Poisoning	6.6
Diseases of the Skin and Subcutaneous Tissue	6.2
Neoplasm	3.5
Total	**93.40**

Table 2.4
Hillsboro
Health Hospice
Admission
by Principal
Diagnosis

Principal Diagnosis	Percentage of All Cases
Cancer	35.1
Heart Disease	30.0
Parkinson's Disease/ALS	9.7
Lung Disease	9.3
Debility Unspecified	4.0
Renal Failure	3.8
Alzheimer's Disease	3.1
Other	5.0
Total	**100.0**

Age (Years)	Percentage of All Admissions
Under 35	0.0
35–64	11.2
65–74	17.7
75–84	25.4
85 or older	43.7
Total	**100.0**

Table 2.5
Hillsboro Health Hospice Patient Age at Time of Admission

Level of Care	Percentage of All Admissions
Routine Care	95.2
General—Inpatient	1.8
Continuous Care	2.6
Respite Care	0.4
Total	**100.0**

Table 2.6
Hillsboro Health Hospice Services by Level of Care

Table 2.7
Hillsboro Health
Statement of
Revenues and
Expenses

*On the web at
ache.org/books/
Middleboro2*

	2019	2018	2017	2016
Revenues				
Home Care				
Medicare—Net	4,922,576	4,733,050	4,566,254	4,217,339
Medicaid—Net	130,330	129,667	126,448	120,445
Other—Net	84,670	89,337	92,550	85,383
Subtotal	**5,137,576**	**4,952,054**	**4,785,252**	**4,423,167**
Private Duty				
Revenue—Gross	4,544,223	4,532,778	4,406,354	4,014,629
Bad Debt	−44,675	−45,230	−44,120	−31,445
Contract Allowances	−8,440	−8,934	−8,738	−7,324
Subtotal	**4,491,108**	**4,478,614**	**4,353,496**	**3,975,860**
Community Health				
From State and Towns	208,750	240,000	240,000	270,000
United Way	20,000	20,000	60,000	60,000
Other	1,935	1,257	1,458	1,500
Subtotal	**230,685**	**261,257**	**301,458**	**331,500**
Hospice and Palliative Care				
Medicare	2,658,338	1,955,737	1,245,334	850,334
Other	345,223	280,330	205,229	120,450
Subtotal	**3,003,561**	**2,236,067**	**1,450,563**	**970,784**
Total Revenue	**12,862,930**	**11,927,992**	**10,890,769**	**9,701,311**
Expenses				
Salaries and Wages	7,872,680	7,284,476	6,369,780	5,568,340
Benefits	2,125,624	1,966,808	1,719,840	1,465,552
Supplies	603,556	600,334	590,202	502,338
Equipment—Medical	601,339	452,994	498,330	325,440
Equipment—Office	6,022	6,930	215,302	345,600
Rental—Middleboro	328,400	328,400	328,400	300,000
Rental—Jasper	145,600	145600	145,000	145,000
Computer Systems	180,000	180,000	180,000	150,000

continued

	2019	2018	2017	2016
Travel	175,330	182445	179202	180,339
Computer Services	129,445	112,405	110,393	113,245
Consulting	0	300	300	184,330
Insurance	56,729	56,240	59,450	120,404
Advertising and PR	54,894	55,402	45,020	35,200
Legal/Audit	55,088	55,700	59,400	85,300
Telecommunications	23,445	24,355	23,656	22,679
Printing and Postage	15,450	14,330	14,200	13,720
Board Expenses	15,000	14,780	14,983	14,902
Memberships	10,200	10,100	10,300	10,450
Depreciation Expense	138,240	136,283	132,550	143,560
Total Expenses	**12,537,042**	**11,627,882**	**10,696,308**	**9,726,399**
Gain or (Loss) from Operations	**325,888**	**300,110**	**194,461**	**−25,088**

Table 2.7
Hillsboro Health
Statement
of Revenues
and Expenses
(continued)

*On the web at
ache.org/books/
Middleboro2*

Notes: (1) Years ending December 31. (2) Numbers are in US dollars. (3) PR: public relations.

Table 2.8
Hillsboro Health
Balance Sheet

*On the web at
ache.org/books/
Middleboro2*

	2019	2018	2017	2016
Current Assets				
Cash and Cash Equivalents	492,393	439,229	393,330	309,223
Accounts Receivable (Net)	2,245,612	2,165,528	1,840,202	1,430,350
Prepaid Insurance	21,450	17,340	14,230	12,343
Inventory	125,339	173,400	180,340	129,470
Total Current Assets	**2,884,794**	**2,795,497**	**2,428,102**	**1,881,386**
Property/Equipment				
Gross, Property, and Equipment	3,264,667	3,139,299	2,990,383	2,858,330
(Less Accum. Depreciation)	853,062	714,822	578,539	445,989
Net Property and Equipment	2,411,605	2,424,477	2,411,844	2,412,341
Other Assets				
Investments (at Market)	8,661,228	8,262,746	7,786,581	7,410,474
Total Assets	**11,072,833**	**10,687,223**	**10,198,425**	**9,822,815**
Liabilities and Net Assets				
Current Liabilities				
Accounts Payable	718,225	723,445	615,330	634,559
Salaries Payable	154,284	198,303	193,448	154,229
Accrued Items	278,445	255,683	306,492	325,127
Current Portion of Long-Term Debt	91,600	91,600	91,600	91,600
Total Current Liabilities	**1,242,554**	**1,269,031**	**1,206,870**	**1,205,515**
Noncurrent Liabilities				
Loan Payable	525,234	600,234	675,234	750,234
Total Liabilities	**1,767,788**	**1,869,265**	**1,882,104**	**1,955,749**
Net Assets				
Donor Restricted Funds	930,112	923,459	945,282	985,223
Hospice Restricted Funds	1,134,226	1,066,172	980,879	912,217
Home Care Restricted Funds	4,745,998	4,659,506	4,521,449	4,295,376
Unrestricted Funds	2,494,709	2,168,821	1,868,711	1,674,250
Total Net Assets	**9,305,045**	**8,817,958**	**8,316,321**	**7,867,066**
Liabilities + Net Assets	**11,072,833**	**10,687,223**	**10,198,425**	**9,822,815**

Notes: (1) Years ending December 31. (2) Numbers are in US dollars.

Position	2019		2018		2017		2016	
	Salary	FTE	Salary	FTE	Salary	FTE	Salary	FTE
Administration								
Chief Executive Officer	160,500	1.0	154,080	1.0	150,998	1.0	141,938	1.0
Chief Operating Officer	135,200	1.0	129,792	1.0	127,196	1.0	119,564	0.5
Chief Financial Officer	145,300	1.0	139,488	1.0	136,698	1.0	128,496	0.6
Chief QI Officer	78,910	1.0	75,754	1.0	74,239	1.0	69,784	0.5
Director of ISM	71,300	1.0	68,448	1.0	67,079	0.7	63,054	0.0
Medical Director	180,000	1.0	172,800	1.0	169,344	0.8	159,183	0.8
Director of Administration	41,589	1.0	39,925	1.0	39,127	1.0	36,779	1.0
Director of Marketing	62,445	1.0	59,947	0.9	58,748	0.7	55,223	0.5
Other Finance Staff	32,400	4.2	31,104	4.0	30,482	3.5	28,653	3.0
QI Staff	32,000	4.0	30,720	4.0	30,106	3.0	28,299	2.0
ISM Staff	65,337	2.0	62,724	2.0	61,469	1.0	57,781	0.5
Other Administration Staff	22,600	6.0	21,696	6.0	21,262	4.5	19,986	4.5
Home Care								
Program Director	82,450	1.0	79,152	1.0	75,986	1.0	72,946	1.0
RN	60,347	38.6	55,519	35.2	51,078	35.0	46,991	33.0
LPN	41,204	0.6	40,380	0.6	39,572	0.5	38,781	0.5
HH Aide	25,188	18.3	24,684	19.2	24,191	20.0	23,707	20.2
Physical Therapist	70,990	5.0	68,860	4.0	66,794	4.0	64,791	3.0
Occupational Therapist	88,738	1.0	86,963	1.3	85,224	1.5	83,519	1.5
Speech Therapist	48,838	0.5	44,931	0.5	41,336	0.7	38,030	0.7
Social Worker	73,563	1.0	69,149	1.0	65,000	1.0	61,100	1.0
Administrative Staff	32,200	3.0	31,556	3.0	30,925	3.0	30,306	3.0

Table 2.9
Hillsboro Health Agency Staffing (Salary and FTE)

continued

Table 2.9
Hillsboro Health
Agency Staffing
(Salary and FTE)
(continued)

Position	2019 Salary	2019 FTE	2018 Salary	2018 FTE	2017 Salary	2017 FTE	2016 Salary	2016 FTE
Private Duty								
Program Director	62,400	1.0	59,280	1.0	56,340	1.0	53,523	1.0
RN	60,347	0.5	55,519	1.0	51,078	1.0	46,991	1.0
LPN	41,204	9.5	40,380	7.5	39,572	5.5	38,781	5.5
Occupational Therapist	88,738	0.5	86,963	1.0	85,224	1.0	83,519	1.0
PCA	20,197	24.8	18,985	27.5	17,846	28.2	16,775	30.4
Other	26,880	0.8	28,990	0.8	28,990	0.8	28,990	0.8
Administrative Staff	17,330	1.0	31,556	1.0	30,925	1.0	30,306	1.0
Community Health								
Program Director	62,440	1.0	61,816	1.0	61,197	1.0	60,585	0.9
RN	60,347	1.5	55,519	2.0	51,078	2.5	46,991	3.0
Administrative Staff	17,330	1.0	31,556	1.0	30,925	0.5	30,306	0.5
Hospice and Palliative Care								
Program Director	78,200	1.0	74,290	1.0	70,576	1.0	67,047	0.8
RN	60,347	14.5	55,519	13.5	51,078	9.5	46,991	9.0
HH Aide	25,188	2.5	24,684	2.0	24,191	2.0	23,707	2.0
PCA	20,197	10.4	18,985	10.0	17,846	8.0	16,775	6.0
Occupational Therapist	88,738	0.5	86,963	0.5	85,224	0.5	83,519	0.5
Social Worker	48,838	5.0	69,149	4.0	65,000	3.0	61,100	2.0
Other	48,440	2.0	40,440	2.0	40,440	2.0	40,440	1.0
Administrative Staff	32,490	2.5	31,556	2.5	30,925	2.5	30,306	2.0
Total		**173.2**		**169.0**		**156.9**		**147.2**

Notes: (1) Salaries are in US dollars. (2) Full-time equivalent (FTE) positions are paid for 2,080 hours per year. (3) All full-time employees work 1,896 hours per year and receive two weeks of paid vacation and 13 paid holidays. (4) All salaries are expressed as the average salary for that position. (5) Benefit costs are in addition to salary costs. (6) HH: home health; ISM: information systems management; LPN: licensed practical nurse; PCA: personal care attendant; QI: quality improvement; RN: registered nurse.

	Hillsboro Health Home Care	State Average	National Average
Managing Daily Activities			
How often patients improved at walking or moving around	53%	54%	58%
How often patients improved at getting in and out of bed	48%	58%	54%
How often patients improved at bathing	58%	68%	66%
Managing Pain and Treating Symptoms			
How often the home health team checked patients' pain	100%	96%	98%
How often the home health team treated patients' pain	100%	98%	98%
How often patients had less pain when moving around	70%	62%	67%
How often the home health team treated patient symptoms of heart failure (weakening of the heart)	100%	99%	98%
How often patients' breathing improved	54%	60%	63%
Treating Wounds and Preventing Pressure Sores (Bed Sores)			
How often patients' wounds improved or healed after an operation	82%	87%	89%
How often the home health team checked patients for the risk of developing pressure sores	100%	96%	99%
How often the home health team included treatments to prevent pressure sores in the plan of care	100%	88%	97%
How often the home health team took doctor-ordered action to prevent pressure sores	100%	93%	95%
Preventing Harm			
How often the home health team began patients' care in a timely manner	92%	92%	91%
How often the home health team taught patients (or family caregivers) about their medications	96%	94%	91%
How often patients improved at taking their medicines correctly by mouth	47%	46%	51%

Table 2.10
Hillsboro Health Home Care Services Quality Scorecard

continued

	Hillsboro Health Home Care	State Average	National Average
How often the home health team checked patients' risk of falling	98%	91%	98%
How often the home health team checked patients for depression	99%	97%	97%
How often the home health team determined whether patients received a flu shot for the current flu season	78%	78%	75%
How often the home health team determined whether patients received a pneumococcal vaccine	80%	79%	87%
For patients with diabetes, how often the home health team got doctor's orders, gave foot care, and taught patients about foot care	100%	92%	92%
Preventing Unplanned Hospital Care			
How often home health patients needed any urgent, unplanned care in the emergency dept. without being admitted into the hospital	17%	16%	17%
How often home health patients had to be admitted into the hospital	16%	15%	13%
How often home health patients, who had a recent hospital stay, had to be readmitted into the hospital	Worse than Expected		
How often home health patients, who had a recent hospital stay, received care in the emergency dept. without being readmitted into the hospital	Same as Expected		
Patient Survey Results			
How often the home health team gave care in a professional way	88%	89%	88%
How well the home health team communicated with patients	87%	88%	85%
Whether the home health team discussed medicines, pain, and home safety with patients	83%	85%	83%
How patients rated the overall care from the home health agency	82%	87%	84%
Likelihood patients would recommend the home health agency to friends and family	79%	80%	79%

CASE 3

PHYSICIAN CARE SERVICES, INC.

Physician Care Services (PCS), Inc. was founded as a tax-paying corporation on January 1, 2000. Currently, three physicians each own 20 percent and one physician owns 40 percent of the stock. PCS currently offers urgent care and occupational health services in two locations—at the Alpha Center located in Mifflenville (just outside the city limits of Middleboro) and at the Beta Center located in Jasper (close to the Jasper Industrial Park and suburban neighborhoods). The Alpha Center opened in January 2000. Initially, it treated only occupational health clients, but this policy changed in 2004 when services began to be offered to private-pay (retail) clients. The Beta Center opened in January 2006 and treats private-pay and occupational health clients.

At these centers, ambulatory medical care is provided on a walk-in basis, but no emergency services are available. If an individual who needs emergency care arrives, the center calls an ambulance to transport the person to the nearest hospital emergency department (ED). Over the past two years, approximately 2 percent of PCS arrivals were immediately dispatched to a hospital. PCS refers people covered by Medicaid to other service providers.

PCS specializes in offering services deemed "convenient" by the general public. It does not provide continuing medical care. Its physicians refer to other physicians in the area if their clients need continuing or specialized medical care. Although clients often return to the centers for services, PCS does not offer chronic illness management. Client satisfaction is PCS's highest operational goal.

CLIENT SERVICES

OCCUPATIONAL HEALTH CLIENTS

Occupational health clients are employees sent to a PCS center by their employer for treatment of a work-related injury (which is usually covered by workers' compensation insurance) and for pre-employment or annual physicals and health testing (which are paid directly by the employer). Because they have special work conditions—usually involving the use of hazardous chemicals or materials—some local organizations contract with PCS to conduct comprehensive physicals in accordance with the US Department of Transportation (DOT) requirements and other federal and state laws and regulations. The local industry considers PCS a cost-effective and convenient alternative to a hospital ED and thus uses PCS in lieu of employing an in-house physician. Corporate clients expect PCS to assist with all case management related to worker injury, and they hold PCS accountable for providing to their workers timely, appropriate, and cost-effective services.

Physicals for OSHA (Occupational Safety and Health Administration) compliance are currently priced between $300 and $500 per physical. Physicals for local police and fire include pulmonary function tests (PFTs), laboratory tests, and electrocardiograms (EKGs) and are currently priced between $250 and $350 per physical, depending on contractual volume. Pre-employment physicals include a urine dip test and are typically priced between $90 and $125 per physical. Charges for these services are billed directly to the employer.

National studies have found a relationship between the types of industries in a community and the types and amount of demand for ambulatory occupational healthcare, including workers' comp services. Five years ago, Carlstead Rayon—a textile corporation in Middleboro—stopped using PCS and signed a long-term occupational health contract with MIDCARE.

PRIVATE-PAY CLIENTS

PCS offers private-pay clients general medical care, except obstetrics and gynecology services. Private-pay clients are attracted to PCS because they do not need an appointment and they can pay with cash, check, or credit card at the time of service. PCS also works with these four health insurance plans in the area: Statewide Blue Shield, American Health Plan, Cumberland River Health Plan, and Central State Good Health Plan.

At the time of service, private-pay clients with these insurance plans are screened by staff to verify their coverage and determine whether they have satisfied any required deductibles. If deductibles have been met, the clients pay just the copay amount and the full bill is electronically sent to their insurance plan. If deductibles have not been met, the clients pay the charge for the service and the amount is entered into the insurance company's system as partial fulfillment of any outstanding deductible. A recent study suggested that these four insurance companies and Medicare cover approximately 85 percent of PCS's private-pay clients. If clients are not covered by one of these four insurers, they are given a bill to claim reimbursement directly from their own insurance plan. In addition, PCS bills Medicare. Clients covered by Medicaid are referred to a nearby hospital ED, and so are clients who have a history of bad debt at PCS or who are unable to pay at the time of service. PCS maintains an aggressive credit and bad-debt collection policy.

Eighty percent of private-pay clients live within a 30-minute travel distance from a PCS center. Approximately 65 percent have a primary care provider (PCP). At the time of service, private-pay clients are asked whether a record of their care at PCS should be sent to their PCP. If authorized by clients, the staff sends an electronic record to the PCP.

Tables 3.1 through 3.4 provide detailed data on client utilization.

On the web at ache.org/books/ Middleboro2

ORGANIZATIONAL STRUCTURE AND MANAGEMENT TEAM

The Alpha Center is in a small shopping center on the main road between Middleboro and Mifflenville. The Beta Center is on the first floor of a new office building adjacent to a large shopping mall in Jasper. Ample parking is available in both locations, and attractive, visible signage helps visitors find their way in each center. The centers are open 60 hours per week, from 8 a.m. to 7 p.m. on weekdays and from 9 a.m. to 1 p.m. on Saturdays. They are closed on Sundays and on some holidays, such as Memorial, Independence (July 4), Thanksgiving, Christmas, and New Year's days. Each center operates in 6,000 square feet of rental space and has four fully furnished patient examination rooms as well as a well-equipped imaging center. Currently, the centers have some excess space.

Three years ago, PCS made its imaging services available to all PCPs in the community. Using electronic ordering, a PCP can order an X-ray at PCS and choose whether to receive a radiologist's report within 12 hours or to directly receive the image electronically. PCS charges for the X-ray, and the patient is responsible for any additional charges such as the reading fee. This service has become an attractive and cost-effective alternative to hospital-based and affiliated radiographic services. Health insurance companies have continued to promote this option with PCPs.

For patient care, the minimum staffing at each center is one receptionist, one medical assistant, one physician or nurse practitioner, and one radiographic technician. Additional staff members (e.g., nurse practitioners, physician assistants) are scheduled on the basis of anticipated high-volume days. Typically, the nurse practitioners work on Saturdays and assist with physicals and other services as needed. Physician assistants are also used to assist on high-volume days.

The central administrative and billing office is an additional 2,500 square feet and is located adjacent to the Alpha Center. The central office staff includes the president, medical director, director of nursing and clinical care, business manager, and receptionist/billing personnel.

CHARGES

Each center uses the same schedule of prices. The basic visit charge (CPT 99202) is currently $125. Current detailed prices are as follows; at PCS, the current procedural terminology (CPT) codes are also known as evaluation and management or E and M codes:

CPT Code	Description	Price ($)
99201	Office visit, brief, new	96
99202	Office visit, limited, new	125
99203	Office visit, intermediate, new	150
99204	Office visit, comprehensive, new	176
99211	Office visit, minimal, established	65
99212	Office visit, brief, established	96
99213	Office visit, limited, established	160
99214	Office visit, intermediate, established	190
99215	Office visit, comprehensive, established	210

Additional charges are levied for ancillary testing and specialized physician services, such as suturing. A client returning for a medically ordered follow-up is charged $96.

Based on CPT comparison, PCS fee levels are competitive within the area. No similar medical service exists within a 45-minute radius of both centers. In the past, as part of an advertising campaign to attract private-pay clients, PCS offered discounted physicals—such as $48 camp physicals for children and $69 family checkups.

The following are PCS's 15 most common diagnoses:

ICD-10-CM Diagnostic Codes	Description
461	Sinusitis, acute
462	Pharyngitis, acute
466	Bronchitis, acute
465	Laryngopharyngitis, acute

599	Urinary tract infection
786	Respiratory, nonspecific
382	Otitis media
789	Abdominal pain, nonspecific
724	Spinal stenosis
780	Syncope and collapse
477	Allergic rhinitis
372	Conjunctivitis, acute
034	Streptococcal sore throat
490	Bronchitis, nonspecific
845	Ankle sprain

The following are PCS's most frequently performed procedures:

ICD-10-CM Procedure Codes	Description
12001	Simple wound repair, 2.5 cm
10060	Incision/drainage abscess, simple
29125	Short arm splint, static
12002	Simple wound repair body, 2.6–7.5 cm
29515	Short leg splint
10120	Foreign body removal

National studies suggest that urgent care visits are at least $30 less than the charge for a visit to a PCP in private practice. Other studies indicate that urgent care visits cost $250 to $600 less than the cost of ED visits for the same ICD-10-CM/CPT/E and M code.

Some occupational health clients are charged a negotiated volume-based price, especially for physicals. PCS's medical director negotiates fees for specific physicals and tests ordered by an employer. Typically, an employer approaches PCS in need of a specific type of physical (such as the annual physical required by the DOT for all operators of school buses) or lab test for its employees. PCS submits a bid to perform a certain number of physicals or tests for a flat rate.

Tables 3.5 through 3.8 show detailed financial information about PCS.

On the web at ache.org/books/ Middleboro2

INFORMATION SYSTEM

Urgent Care Plus is the corporation-wide electronic health record certified by the Centers for Medicare & Medicaid Services (CMS). It meets or exceeds all CMS Meaningful Use criteria. As an integrated business, financial, and medical information system, Urgent Care Plus is installed in the computer terminals in the reception areas and examination rooms at both Alpha and Beta centers as well as in the central office.

Clinically, it is used for storing and processing client records, which assist with treatment; physician order entry; prescription or pharmacy records (eRx); laboratory results; and radiographic services records, from either PCS or other providers. It is updated within four days of a client's visit to PCS, is available to the client electronically, and can communicate with the statewide immunization registry. Administratively, the system is used for bookkeeping and billing, appointment services, case management, staff scheduling, and data management. Financially, it captures, stores, and reports all CPT codes and links medical procedures with revenue and expense information. It has a direct online link with participating insurance companies and with Medicare.

Using Urgent Care Plus, all clients may register online before arriving at a center. Once they complete the registration, they are given a case number and one hour to arrive for their appointment. If clients do not register before coming to a center, they may do so using a computer terminal in the reception area. Displays in the waiting area indicate the case number currently being seen and the approximate wait time. In addition, Urgent Care Plus allows employees who have direct deposit with a local bank to receive their biweekly pay stubs (with accrued balance of vacation and sick time) and annual W-2s electronically. Billing clerks also use the system to prepare and electronically submit clinical documentation for reimbursement to participating health insurance companies and Medicare.

PCS leases its hardware and software, so vendors provide hardware maintenance, software updates, and technical assistance. Paper medical records that existed before 2008 are retained in active files for ten years and then transferred to closed files.

MARKETING AND ADVERTISING

PCS promotes its retail services through newspaper advertisements and community events. For example, PCS sponsors a youth baseball team in Middleboro and an annual 5K road race in Jasper. The registration fees from the road race are donated to a charity selected by PCS's board of directors. Social media and search engine optimization direct potential clients to the PCS website, which allows clients to register for services and schedule appointments. Each year in March, PCS distributes a coupon that can be applied to the cost of individual physicals or physicals for all children in any one family; coupons must be redeemed by the end of May or June. After receiving a service, every client is given a short satisfaction survey, the results of which are posted on the PCS website.

Occupational health services are promoted by direct contact. At least once monthly, PCS contacts every company that uses its services to determine client satisfaction. Annually, PCS provides each corporate client with a comprehensive list of all of the occupational health services PCS offers as a basis to meet with the company's leadership.

Table 3.9 shows comparative data of charges for the regional market.

BOARD OF DIRECTORS

The PCS board, composed of the four physician owners, meets quarterly to review operations. The annual board meeting occurs in December, at which time the officers are elected for the coming year. As majority stockholder, Dr. Stephen J. Tobias is chair of the board of PCS. The board secretary is Dr. Jay Smooth, and the other board members are Dr. Rita Hottle and Dr. Laura Cytesmath. The owners have the option of buying any available stock at the current book value. An outsider can purchase stock only if all the owners refuse to exercise this option and if all the owners approve the purchase. PCS has paid a stock dividend in each of the past five years.

PRESIDENT, CEO, AND MEDICAL DIRECTOR

In addition to being board chair, Dr. Tobias is the president/CEO and medical director of PCS. He graduated from Private University Medical School and completed postgraduate medical education in general internal medicine at Walter Reed National Military Medical Center. He also holds a master in public health from State University and is board certified in general internal medicine, emergency medicine, and occupational health. As medical director, he is responsible for PCS's medical quality assurance programs and the recruitment and retention of qualified physician employees. Among his duties are securing the professional services to read X-rays, scheduling the other physicians and nurse practitioners, and seeing clients in the Alpha Center. Compensation for the medical director position began at PCS in 2008, so he receives a separate salary as medical director and as president/CEO. As president, he is responsible for the management of all resources and for strategic planning.

Dr. Tobias founded PCS. Before doing so, he was a full-time ED physician at MIDCARE. Originally, he tried to establish joint-venture urgent care centers with MIDCARE, but when those plans did not work, he recruited his colleagues—now the other PCS stockholders—to start PCS. On top of his PCS positions, he has consulting medical staff privileges in the department of medicine at MIDCARE and occasionally provides services in the hospital's ED.

A recent state court decision, which is currently under appeal, declared that physicians who work in an urgent care corporation constitute "real and bona fide" competition to a hospital's ED. If this decision is upheld, Dr. Tobias and other PCS physicians who have an employment arrangement with MIDCARE may be violating the noncompete clause in their contracts with MIDCARE.

CLINICAL STAFF

The PCS clinical staff comprises eight physicians, three nurse practitioners, and two physician assistants. All physicians are required to hold medical staff privileges at an area hospital and to be board certified. All are credentialed annually.

Staff Name	Medical Specialty	Certification
Physicians		
Bennet Casey, MD	Family Practice	Board Certified
Mark Welby, MD	Family Practice	Board Certified
Stephen Tobias, MD	Emergency Medicine	Board Certified
Jay Smooth, MD	Emergency Medicine	Board Certified
Rita Hottle, MD	Emergency Medicine	Board Certified
Laura Cytesmath, MD	Emergency Medicine	Board Certified
Micah Foxx, DO	Occupational Health	Board Certified
Regina Majors, MD	Occupational Health	Board Certified
Nurse Practitioners		
Carl Withers, ARNP	Family and Adult Health	
Jane Jones, ARNP	Family and Adult Health	
Gerri Mattox, ARNP	Family and Adult Health	
Physician Assistants		
Rutherford Hayes, PA		
Margaret Fishborne, PA		

Before 2007, PCS physicians were retained as independent contractors and received no benefits outside of their hourly wage. In 2007, nurse practitioners were added to the staff and physicians, and all other employees—who worked more than 1,200 hours—began to receive comprehensive benefits. Today, full benefits coverage (with deductibles and copays) is provided to a clinical staff member who works 1,400 or more hours. Anyone who works a minimum of 20 percent to 70 percent of the time receives a prorated coverage with the option to purchase additional coverage. Benefits include the following:

◆ Malpractice insurance, including tail coverage

◆ Stipend for continuing medical education

◆ Health insurance

◆ Dental insurance

◆ Life insurance

◆ Short-term disability

◆ Long-term disability

Physicians are paid $100 per hour, while nurse practitioners receive $50 per hour. These payment levels are within the appropriate market range. Like Dr. Tobias, Drs. Smooth, Hottle, and Cytesmath work as ED physicians at MIDCARE. Dr. Casey serves as an occupational health consultant to companies in the region and as an expert witness in occupational health cases in the state. Dr. Welby works at Convenient Medical Care, Inc. in Capital City. Dr. Foxx, who recently relocated to Jasper with her family, is available to work no more than six shifts per month, a condition she has established until her children reach school age. Dr. Majors also works as an ED physician in Capital City. Physician assistants at PCS are paid $40 per hour and assist on shifts that are anticipated to be high volume.

Once a month, Dr. Tobias creates a schedule for all clinical staff with the understanding that, if a physician is unable to work, he or she is responsible for securing a replacement from the qualified medical staff. Physicians and nurse practitioners work an entire shift (e.g., 11.5 hours on a weekday). Fridays and Saturdays are typically assigned to the nurse practitioners, while physician assistants are on call for busy days to assist physicians.

In 2014, PCS changed its protocol involving radiographic images. Currently, the physician on duty can waive having the X-ray read by a radiologist and instead include the physician's notes on the X-ray in the client's chart. If the X-ray is referred to a radiologist for reading, a report is received in 12 hours or sooner. Nurse practitioners are required to refer all X-rays they order for professional interpretation. As Dr. Tobias reported at that time, this has become the common standard in urgent care.

The clinical staff meets quarterly to review areas of concern. Dr. Tobias does random reviews of medical records to ensure compliance with standards of clinical practice. He is also responsible for all clinical staff credentialing issues.

Medical assistants at each center are trained to take limited X-rays, draw specimens for laboratory testing, do EKGs, and conduct simple vision and audiometric examinations. Each center is equipped to do the following:

◆ On-site X-ray

◆ PFT

◆ EKG

◆ Vision and audiometric testing

◆ Some laboratory testing (e.g., streptococcal screen, urine dip)

◆ Drug and breath alcohol testing

A regional laboratory processes more advanced laboratory work.

Two medical assistants are assigned to each weekday shift. One is assigned for seven hours per day (i.e., 35 hours per week), and the other is assigned for four hours per weekday and Saturdays (i.e., 25 hours per week). Their responsibilities include examination room preparation, assisting the physician or nurse practitioner, patient testing, case management, scheduling visits or follow-up care, and addressing patient questions. Each center maintains a pool of qualified medical assistants who are trained, evaluated, and scheduled by the director of nursing and clinical care.

CENTRAL OFFICE STAFF

Dr. Tobias is responsible for the overall management of PCS. Joan Washington, LPN, is the director of nursing and clinical care. She trains, supervises, and schedules the medical assistants as well as orders medical supplies, meets with occupational health employers as needed, and performs general administrative duties as assigned by Dr. Tobias. If needed, she substitutes as a medical assistant.

Hannah Coin is the business manager and has three full-time staff members. She schedules the receptionists who double as billing clerks at each center, and she manages all insurance billing and the general ledger, including accounts payable and accounts receivable. If needed, she or a member of her staff substitutes for a receptionist. Central office maintains a list of available (and trained) fill-in receptionists to cover absences and other needs.

RECEPTION STAFF

One full-time (35 hours per week) front-desk receptionist works in each center. Aside from answering phones, greeting visitors, and helping clients with registration, the receptionist is also responsible for setting appointments, billing, creating and maintaining records for occupational health clients, and managing cash receipts. One or more additional receptionists are hired for the remaining 25 hours per week.

THREATS AND OPPORTUNITIES

LEGAL ACTIONS

In 2015, Dr. Tobias discharged Nancy Stone, RN, from her position as director of nursing and clinical care. It was a hard decision, according to Dr. Tobias, as Stone was well liked by the employees. The problem was she could not get along with some of the physicians and had difficulty coping with multiple job responsibilities. By the end of her tenure, she was refusing to provide patient care at the Beta Center. She is suing Dr. Tobias and PCS for "wrongful discharge."

At the initial hearing for the case, Stone complained that she had "too many duties to do well and that PCS was more interested in getting clients in and out than providing quality medical care." She added that "meeting her job expectations was hard when the job lacked any formal job description." When interviewed, Dr. Tobias could not share much because of the ongoing legal action. He did admit that he felt compelled to act even though Stone is the sister of the vice president for human resources at Carlstead Rayon.

EXPANSION

PCS has plans to achieve even greater corporate profitability. It has earned its place in the regional medical care system and its future appears very solid. At the end of 2007, one of its original owners exercised his option to be bought out by another stockholder. Dr. Tobias bought that partner's shares, increasing his ownership in the corporation. Today, PCS is in the position to open a third—and even a fourth—center. It may purchase buildings to house its Alpha and Beta centers and add some services to better serve all of its clients. As Dr. Tobias explained, "We are a debt-free corporation that is beginning to earn serious profits. We have distinguished ourselves by the high quality of care we provide. Our clients are delighted with our deep commitment to patient care, convenience, and affordability. We have every reason to believe we will continue to prosper and expand."

The original real estate leases on the Alpha and Beta centers expired at the end of 2019. Dr. Tobias indicated that he timed the expiration of these leases to coincide with the year that PCS would be ready to make a major strategic move. Each current lease has a renewal clause for up to 36 months, with an escalation clause so that rents do not increase any more than 15 percent per year. He estimated that appropriate facilities could be acquired for $170 per square foot (including land, site improvements, and facilities) and that it would take approximately nine months from the time the contract is executed to the time the centers are fully operational.

FUTURE CHALLENGES

Dr. Tobias named waiting time as an issue that always warrants ongoing study. He also reported that the nonowner physicians frequently mention the need for a bonus plan to reward performance on "very busy days." At the most recent annual meeting of the board, he committed to hiring a consultant to address this issue.

Although he was very pleased that PCS clients generally report "complete satisfaction" with the quality of care provided at the centers—for which he repeatedly credited the competent clinical and administrative staff—he was concerned about the growth of the occupational health business. "Our early success with occupational health may be slowing," he said. "If we lose a significant amount of manufacturing in the region, we potentially lose our occupational health clients. Our future in occupational health will follow the local economy."

Unemployment in the region has already affected the demand for occupational health. Fewer people are being hired, and the unemployed lack health insurance. Fees paid by the workers' comp program have been fixed for 24 months. Dr. Tobias had expressed a great deal of optimism that the Affordable Care Act would significantly expand PCS's pool of private-pay clients.

Two years ago, PCS instituted an "appointment plan" for its occupational health clients. Under this plan, which has been succesful, before clients come for a service, they—or someone from their company—can call a center to determine the approximate wait time, make a decision if they want service, and register for service at an approximate time that day. This allows clients to reserve a specific place in the queue even before they arrive. On a normal day, every client who arrives at a center is given an approximate wait time by the receptionist and told that waiting is not required to preserve their scheduled appointment. While "first in, first out" is generally used, urgent care cases—especially injuries—are bumped ahead of nonemergency patients. Signage in the waiting area explains that some occupational health clients are served by appointment and those appointments override arrival order.

To attract more occupational health clients, PCS promotes its services in the regional market. It puts up billboards on main roads, advertises in local and state newspapers, maintains a reader-friendly website, and posts announcements on social media. In addition, the director of nursing and clinical care visits current and prospective occupational health clients and typically answers approximately 15 to 25 telephone inquiries per month regarding quotes for specific services, such as employee physicals.

PHYSICIAN CONCERNS

PCS physicians expressed concern about how Dr. Tobias schedules them. According to these physicians, they are never sure exactly how many shifts per month they will work and at which center. All prefer to work at only one center and indicated that this type of stability leads to a better medical care team.

Records suggest that certain physicians have productivity profiles that are significantly different from the productivity profiles of other physicians. On "busy days," revenue per visit drops, a trend that suggests that physicians do less ancillary testing when they are busy. The target for physicians and nurse practitioners is to see three to four clients per hour. Three physicians have also requested extra compensation for "very busy days," arguing that they receive the same hourly pay as physicians who work on slow days. Dr. Tobias does not think this claim is warranted.

Two (nonowner) physicians indicated that, because they are paid by the hour, they should be paid for treating clients who arrive right before closing time. Until this change, all staff members were paid only for the hours in their shift (e.g., 11.5 hours), which was sometimes fewer than the actual number of hours worked. Employees are expected to treat all clients who arrive during work hours, even if this extends their work time beyond closing time. All physicians reported that they feel their pay level is reasonable given their responsibilities.

Six occupational health nurses at the local corporations indicated that they were satisfied with PCS's clinical staff. Several nurses said they appreciated PCS—specifically, the medical assistants—for keeping them informed about certain clients and for being creative in explaining restrictions and suggesting "light duty," which is medically appropriate work an injured worker could perform for the employer until the worker is ready to resume regular duties.

New Services

Recently, Dr. Tobias returned from a professional meeting with statewide data that he deemed could assist PCS in better estimating its market in the future. These numbers are unrelated to workers' comp and occupational health visits:

Average Number of Ambulatory Care Visits per Year, by Age and Sex

Age (Years)	Male	Female
0–14	3.37	3.09
15–44	1.99	3.92
		(includes OB/GYN)
45–64	2.98	4.34
65+	4.51	5.19

At this meeting, he learned that other urgent care businesses use the following parameters—taken from a national study—in their fiscal and market planning:

◆ For every 15 percent increase in basic visit fee, there is a 25 percent reduction in utilization by private-pay clients without health insurance.

◆ Clients covered by insurance, including Medicare and commercial plans, are generally not price sensitive as long as the annual increase in basic visit fee does not exceed 20 percent.

◆ Annual increases in ancillary charges up to 15 percent do not affect the number of new visits by private-pay clients. Ancillary charge increases above 15 percent, however, may reduce return visits by as much as 45 percent, regardless of clients' payment source.

A discussion of these statistics and new ideas and opportunities is on Dr. Tobias's agenda for the next board meeting. His ideas for new services are as follows.

Prescription Drugs for Private-Pay Clients

This service is already available to clients covered by workers' comp insurance. State law permits physicians (and nurse practitioners) to dispense prescription drugs as long as they maintain adequate records. National firms that specialize in drug repackaging enable PCS to buy prepackaged prescription drugs to sell to clients. PCS has already established its formulary for workers' comp clients, and it has determined that by maintaining 12 specific drugs—in pill form—it can meet approximately 60 percent of the private-pay clients' demand for prescription drugs. The charge for workers' comp clients is directly billed to the employer as part of the overall cost of service.

Dr. Tobias indicated that PCS should extend this service to all of its clients. By only providing high-volume drugs, PCS can guarantee high inventory turnover. An appropriately sized initial inventory for private-pay clients can be capitalized for a center at a total cost of $1,000. All suppliers promise a next-day replenishment of inventory items. The shelf life of all drugs is more than one year. Even with a markup of 800 percent, PCS prescription prices are competitively priced in the region. The question is whether this service should be expanded to private-pay clients. By reviewing the medical records of current private-pay clients (nonphysicals), PCS has determined the following:

Average Number of Prescriptions Received

Age of Client (Years)	per Visit
0–14	1.20
15–44	0.80
45–64	1.10
65+	1.90

The average (supplier) cost per PCS prescription is estimated to be $5.00.

To offer this service, PCS has to purchase software—which costs $12,500 per year—to verify insurance coverage and copays and to process insurance payments. The initial thinking is to begin the service in six months, but questions remain about whether prescriptions may be refilled without a medical visit and how clients without a prescription plan card may be billed. An urgent care center in Capital City recently ended its pharmaceutical sales to private-pay clients because of a high number of refused claims by drug plans.

Drug Testing for All Employees and Job Applicants

The director of human resources at a local company—a PCS occupational health client— has informed PCS that the company's new labor contract includes this clause: "All workers and job applicants are subject to mandatory random drug testing, and anyone who fails or refuses the test will be immediately discharged or will not be hired." Thus, the company is sending workers and job applicants to PCS for drug testing.

Under the new state law and workers' comp regulations, drug testing is required for all workers who are injured at work. Also, employers can institute random drug testing. Some occupational health clients have even requested that PCS choose workers for testing using a random selection process. A process using employee Social Security numbers has been discussed. Other occupational health clients have suggested that PCS begin this service.

Currently, a test that screens for the presence of all common illegal drugs is available from a reference laboratory for a processing cost of $8 per test. The list price for this test is $42 and $63 if a certified medical review officer (MRO) reads it; Dr. Tobias is a certified MRO. The test requires about ten minutes of a medical assistant's time, specifically to maintain compliance with the chain-of-custody protocol during specimen collection.

Employee Physicals by Appointment

Increasingly, employers are issuing formal requests for proposals (RFP) for occupational health physicals that require appointments. For example, a current RFP from an employer in Jasper calls for 350 annual physicals that must be done between 3:15 p.m. and 4:30 p.m. on Mondays through Fridays. The physical must include the following:

	PCS List Price ($)
Medical history and examination	0
EKG	100
Chest X-ray	150

Urine (dip) test	20
Complete blood count with differential	60
Vision (Snellen) screen	30
Audiometric test	80

Each physical takes approximately 80 minutes to complete. The estimated vendor cost for the physical (e.g., X-ray reading fees, laboratory charges) is $125.00. PCS's bid for this contract will be evaluated by the employer on the basis of the total price and ability to meet its time parameters.

Currently, this employer uses MIDCARE's ED for all occupational health needs. Dr. Tobias thinks the board must develop policies regarding these types of RFPs.

Ambulatory Physical Therapy (PT)

National studies estimate that approximately 30 percent of occupational health clients and 5 percent of private-pay clients are referred to physical therapy (PT) for treatment. PCS may have the opportunity to move into this ambulatory PT market.

Providers typically receive from workers' comp $195 for an initial PT evaluation and, on average, $125 per PT visit. On average, each workers' comp case generates 5.75 visits—one initial visit and 4.75 additional visits. Most commercial and managed care plans pay $60 per visit and $100 for an initial evaluation.

Dr. Tobias recommends that PCS, depending on estimated demand, offer PT service for one or both centers (e.g., 7 a.m. to 2 p.m. on Monday, Wednesday, and Friday; 11 a.m. to 7 p.m. on Tuesday and Thursday). Staffing could include one full-time PT ($80 per hour or $75,000 plus benefits per year) and one part-time PT assistant (PTA) at approximately $25 per hour. PTs can simultaneously manage between two and five clients—as well as supervise a PTA who provides the direct therapy—given specific treatment plans. Dr. Tobias also indicates that PCS may be able to contract for the needed PT and PTA from local nursing homes. The PT must do the initial patient evaluation and establish the treatment plan but need not be on-site to supervise the PTA.

Equipment for each center can be purchased and installed for approximately $30,000 (five-year depreciation, no salvage value). Operational costs, such as laundry and medical supplies, are estimated to add approximately $15 per visit. The one-time information system upgrade for ambulatory physical therapy costs $6,500. Other costs need to be estimated. A consultant has recommended that PCS service only workers' comp clients initially, but Dr. Tobias insists that full coverage be considered.

MANAGEMENT POLICY ON WAITING

Waiting is defined by clients as the time spent in a reception area, not the time spent in an examination room waiting to see the clinical staff. National studies indicate that approximately 70 percent of urgent care clients wait 20 minutes.

Dr. Tobias plans to tell the board members that PCS must begin to address this problem, but first they have to better understand the current waiting times and issues. A consultant has told PCS that its service times for private-pay clients are approximately 20 percent of gross billed charges. For example, a visit that costs (gross billed charges) $100 takes approximately 20 minutes—20 percent of 100—of service time. For all workers' comp cases and employer-paid physicals, service time is approximately 25 percent of gross billed charges.

As demand increases during the day, the clinical care team sequentially sees patients in multiple examination rooms. Typically, a visit begins with a brief encounter with the medical assistant, who records vital signs, takes a medical history, and records the reason for the visit. Then, the physician or nurse practitioner enters the room (with the chart) and performs an additional examination. Specific medical tests may be ordered. The medical assistant administers these tests (e.g., X-ray) or collects blood or urine for laboratory processing. The physician or nurse practitioner ends the visit by providing a specific diagnosis and treatment plan, additional medical orders, or a referral.

OTHER CONCERNS

At a recent board meeting, one member asked whether PCS will ever be for sale and, if so, how it can be best positioned for sale. He believes the corporation cannot be a long-term successful player in the increasingly competitive medical marketplace. "I am very concerned that the big box stores will add walk-in services to go along with their pharmacies," he said. "I just do not see how we can compete. Our market area is just too volatile!" Dr. Tobias has always indicated that he would be willing to sell PCS for "the right price." He has also stated that when the economy and manufacturing in the region pick up, PCS's occupational health business should rebound along with its overall profits.

Three-year renewable leases are used to secure needed medical equipment (e.g., X-rays, computers) and most furniture. In 2017, PCS's accountant recommended that it borrow funds to purchase needed equipment and stop using leases. To do this, each center would require between $200,000 and $250,000 worth of new equipment. Currently, PCS maintains a line of credit with a commercial bank in Capital City. Its cost of capital is 2.5 percent above the *Wall Street Journal* prime rate. Based on its annual credit review, PCS has been informed that its cost of capital could increase by 1.5

percentage points over the next 18 months. The bank stated that there is a serious flaw in the management and organization of PCS, saying, "PCS has become too dependent on Dr. Tobias in his many roles. His duties need to be divided between two or more qualified professionals." If PCS does not address this situation, its creditworthiness will be significantly downgraded. Over the past seven years, this situation has been noted in the bank's annual audit/management letter.

Officials in Jasper have requested a meeting with PCS to discuss emergency planning and expanded services. Their specific questions include whether the Beta Center would expand its hours on Saturday (until 9 p.m.) and offer services on Sunday afternoon (until 4 p.m.). The officials cited the majority of urgent care centers across the nation that offer services on Saturdays (8 a.m. to 9 p.m.) and Sundays (9 a.m. to 7 p.m.). A formal response to this inquiry is due within the next two weeks.

	Total Visits	Alpha Center PP Visits	Alpha Center OH Visits	Beta Center PP Visits	Beta Center OH Visits	Alpha Ctr Gross Charges ($)	Beta Ctr Gross Charges ($)	Total Gross Charges ($)
2019								
January	1,209	702	85	192	230	120,490	101,630	222,120
February	1,030	502	70	207	251	88,190	110,555	198,745
March	1,039	549	65	204	221	93,905	100,385	194,290
April	1,100	581	90	187	242	104,045	104,830	208,875
May	1,030	580	45	167	238	94,000	100,730	194,730
June	1,067	593	50	195	229	96,985	101,725	198,710
July	1,195	660	52	219	264	107,140	116,460	223,600
August	1,276	703	60	217	296	115,135	126,580	241,715
September	1,031	506	65	209	251	87,670	110,835	198,505
October	948	503	33	205	207	80,195	95,975	176,170
November	905	529	25	168	183	82,205	82,995	165,200
December	816	525	47	119	125	86,465	57,285	143,750
Total	**12,646**	**6,933**	**687**	**2,289**	**2,737**	**1,156,425**	**1,209,985**	**2,366,410**
2018								
January	1,006	512	80	202	212	84,720	88,698	173,418
February	993	498	66	214	215	80,100	91,041	171,141
March	1,048	540	73	217	218	87,135	92,313	179,448
April	1,102	586	76	203	237	93,930	96,442	190,372
May	1,041	578	55	163	245	88,755	94,122	182,877
June	1,011	578	65	133	235	90,705	87,502	178,207
July	995	555	68	117	255	88,185	91,698	179,883
August	1,266	691	51	269	255	103,230	109,786	213,016
September	1,092	596	60	202	234	92,160	95,408	187,568
October	1,029	547	76	199	207	88,665	86,816	175,481
November	955	523	54	178	200	81,135	82,182	163,317
December	969	504	40	190	235	75,840	94,285	170,125
Total	**12,507**	**6,708**	**764**	**2,287**	**2,748**	**1,054,560**	**1,110,293**	**2,164,853**

Table 3.1
PCS Utilization Report

On the web at ache.org/books/ Middleboro2

continued

Table 3.1
PCS Utilization
Report
(continued)

*On the web at
ache.org/books/
Middleboro2*

	Total Visits	Alpha Center PP Visits	Alpha Center OH Visits	Beta Center PP Visits	Beta Center OH Visits	Alpha Ctr Gross Charges ($)	Beta Ctr Gross Charges ($)	Total Gross Charges ($)
2017								
January	976	503	70	213	190	77,684	79,612	157,296
February	1,038	565	69	200	204	85,430	81,920	167,350
March	1,077	610	66	205	196	90,620	80,300	170,920
April	1,173	606	66	294	207	90,108	94,416	184,524
May	1,036	526	65	200	245	79,678	93,400	173,078
June	1,036	543	45	203	245	78,054	93,772	171,826
July	1,224	651	81	227	265	98,718	102,348	201,066
August	1,161	593	71	229	268	89,394	103,436	192,830
September	1,099	520	85	289	205	82,710	93,236	175,946
October	1,015	549	48	201	217	79,392	85,684	165,076
November	958	525	61	194	178	78,790	73,896	152,686
December	949	501	68	193	187	77,048	76,292	153,340
Total	**12,742**	**6,692**	**795**	**2,648**	**2,607**	**1,007,626**	**1,058,312**	**2,065,938**
2016								
January	866	413	60	200	193	59,534	72,780	132,314
February	887	475	53	145	214	65,590	72,025	137,615
March	978	497	87	189	205	74,306	74,657	148,963
April	954	476	59	205	214	66,788	78,805	145,593
May	1,015	545	73	165	232	77,450	78,965	156,415
June	1,026	563	72	160	231	79,394	78,140	157,534
July	948	521	75	107	245	74,978	75,791	150,769
August	1,064	514	83	207	260	75,592	90,991	166,583
September	950	423	64	188	275	61,434	92,744	154,178
October	970	509	78	156	227	74,102	76,648	150,750
November	950	503	85	145	217	74,654	72,805	147,459
December	910	494	73	156	187	71,432	66,248	137,680
Total	**11,518**	**5,933**	**862**	**2,023**	**2,700**	**855,254**	**930,599**	**1,785,853**

Note: OH: occupational health; PP: private-pay.

	Monday	Tuesday	Wednesday	Thursday	Friday	Saturday	Total
Alpha Center							
August			22	16	20	18	76
	48	34	32	28	27	16	185
	53	37	29	24	25	22	190
	47	33	33	22	21	20	176
	40	27	24	25	20		136
September						17	17
	H	35	23	14	29	16	117
	40	27	28	16	29	12	152
	38	28	20	18	25	10	139
	39	25	29	19	21	13	146
October	37	24	19	15	15	7	117
	30	26	16	14	11	13	110
	29	27	14	12	10	13	105
	35	25	21	14	18	12	125
	32	27	20				79
November				16	22	12	50
	29	22	30	16	19	10	126
	34	28	16	17	22	9	126
	30	31	33	H	24	11	129
	28	37	23	15	20		123
Beta Center							
August			15	17	19	9	60
	28	26	14	16	21	12	117
	28	30	18	10	19	9	114
	29	25	15	14	21	13	117
	28	24	18	15	20		105
						10	10
September	H	33	18	17	13	6	87
	42	17	15	16	18	9	117
	33	26	22	12	18	10	121
	29	27	26	13	19	11	125
	24	20	14	10	15	7	90
October	20	18	12	11	11	13	85
	19	17	15	11	10	13	85
	25	15	17	13	14	12	96
	22	17	17				56
				14	12	7	33
November	19	13	18	13	9	6	78
	14	16	14	15	12	8	79
	20	17	20	H	14	12	83
	21	17	15	12	13		78

Table 3.2
PCS Monthly
Detailed
Utilization

Note: H: holiday.

Table 3.3
PCS Alpha
Center Client
Records,
August 6–9

*On the web at
ache.org/books/
Middleboro2*

Day	Num	Art	Age	Town	Sex	First	Ins	Phy	Charge ($)
1	1	815	23	1	2	1	1	2	140
1	2	817	64	2	2	2	1	2	140
1	3	819	34	1	2	3	1	2	145
1	4	820	45	1	2	2	3	2	96
1	5	822	17	6	2	1	1	2	130
1	6	822	56	4	1	3	2	2	96
1	7	830	19	6	1	3	2	2	96
1	8	833	7	4	1	3	1	2	130
1	9	855	56	1	2	1	1	2	130
1	10	905	32	2	2	1	1	2	138
1	11	910	34	4	1	2	1	2	140
1	12	915	23	1	2	1	2	2	140
1	13	925	21	7	2	2	2	2	135
1	14	1000	54	6	1	3	1	2	96
1	15	1012	51	1	1	1	2	2	140
1	16	1025	56	1	2	2	1	2	135
1	17	1105	49	4	1	2	1	2	135
1	18	1108	23	4	1	1	2	2	130
1	19	1203	45	2	1	2	2	2	140
1	20	1209	71	1	1	2	3	1	130
1	21	1215	71	1	1	2	3	2	140
1	22	1230	23	4	1	3	2	2	96
1	23	1245	28	1	1	3	2	2	96
1	24	1250	45	2	2	1	1	2	145
1	25	1255	47	1	2	2	9	1	180
1	26	1320	45	1	2	3	1	2	96
1	27	1345	22	2	1	1	2	2	130
1	28	1355	19	1	2	1	2	2	140
1	29	1420	34	1	2	2	2	2	130
1	30	1430	25	1	1	2	2	2	135
1	31	1435	68	1	1	2	3	2	140

continued

Day	Num	Art	Age	Town	Sex	First	Ins	Phy	Charge ($)
1	32	1435	43	1	1	2	1	2	130
1	33	1512	3	2	1	1	1	2	130
1	34	1517	50	7	1	2	1	2	140
1	35	1537	63	2	1	2	1	2	140
1	36	1539	21	2	2	2	1	2	145
1	37	1545	56	1	1	2	2	1	150
1	38	1550	66	1	2	2	3	2	155
1	39	1555	19	1	1	1	1	2	140
1	40	1600	50	2	1	1	2	2	145
1	41	1600	43	2	1	2	2	2	130
1	42	1610	68	1	1	2	3	2	150
1	43	1625	50	2	1	2	2	2	140
1	44	1630	23	1	1	2	1	2	160
1	45	1645	18	1	1	3	1	2	96
1	46	1705	27	2	1	2	2	2	144
1	47	1740	45	2	2	2	2	2	130
1	48	1750	61	2	1	1	2	2	140
2	1	800	57	4	2	1	1	2	140
2	2	805	42	1	2	2	1	2	130
2	3	810	40	1	1	1	1	2	145
2	4	815	34	2	1	3	2	2	96
2	5	815	45	4	1	2	9	1	150
2	6	824	23	1	2	1	1	2	130
2	7	833	35	8	1	1	8	2	170
2	8	845	23	1	2	2	2	2	130
2	9	905	55	1	2	2	2	2	150
2	10	910	19	1	1	3	1	2	96
2	11	925	21	4	2	2	1	2	140
2	12	1010	33	2	1	1	2	2	145
2	13	1030	33	1	2	2	2	2	135
2	14	1055	33	2	1	1	2	1	150

Table 3.3
PCS Alpha Center Client Records, August 6–9 *(continued)*

On the web at ache.org/books/ Middleboro2

continued

Table 3.3
PCS Alpha
Center Client
Records,
August 6–9
(continued)

On the web at
ache.org/books/
Middleboro2

Day	Num	Art	Age	Town	Sex	First	Ins	Phy	Charge ($)
2	15	1120	68	2	1	3	3	2	96
2	16	1205	61	1	2	3	2	2	96
2	17	1215	35	1	1	1	2	2	130
2	18	1215	4	1	1	1	1	2	160
2	19	1309	29	7	1	1	1	1	130
2	20	1310	25	6	2	1	1	2	139
2	21	1320	23	2	2	1	1	2	140
2	22	1400	55	8	1	1	2	2	145
2	23	1420	21	7	2	1	1	1	143
2	24	1421	21	1	2	1	2	2	140
2	25	1425	23	2	2	1	1	2	150
2	26	1507	50	2	2	2	2	2	130
2	27	1515	67	2	1	1	3	2	150
2	28	1555	4	1	1	3	2	2	96
2	29	1610	30	1	2	1	2	1	150
2	30	1620	24	2	1	1	1	2	150
2	31	1630	28	2	1	3	3	1	96
2	32	1650	37	1	1	2	2	2	140
2	33	1705	25	2	2	2	1	2	150
2	34	1720	22	1	2	1	1	2	150
3	1	800	56	1	2	1	8	2	215
3	2	810	77	1	1	2	9	1	170
3	3	830	54	1	1	1	1	2	150
3	4	845	32	1	1	3	3	2	96
3	5	905	24	2	1	1	1	2	135
3	6	930	45	1	1	2	8	2	170
3	7	1000	2	4	1	1	1	2	180
3	8	1015	34	1	1	1	1	2	150
3	9	1025	66	1	2	2	3	2	150
3	10	1100	44	1	1	3	2	1	96
3	11	1145	37	1	1	1	1	2	140

continued

Day	Num	Art	Age	Town	Sex	First	Ins	Phy	Charge ($)
3	12	1200	50	2	2	1	2	2	145
3	13	1205	56	2	2	2	1	2	150
3	14	1220	32	4	1	2	1	2	145
3	15	1245	29	7	1	2	1	2	148
3	16	1310	26	4	1	1	2	1	150
3	17	1330	23	1	2	1	1	2	140
3	18	1345	21	6	2	2	1	2	140
3	19	1400	25	1	1	1	1	2	96
3	20	1420	28	1	2	1	2	2	140
3	21	1450	69	1	2	2	3	2	150
3	22	1510	52	2	1	1	1	2	140
3	23	1530	50	2	2	2	2	2	156
3	24	1545	24	1	2	2	2	2	130
3	25	1555	21	7	2	3	1	2	135
3	26	1620	22	7	1	2	2	2	140
3	27	1630	23	4	1	3	2	2	96
3	28	1645	17	7	2	2	2	1	130
3	29	1650	14	2	1	1	1	2	130
3	30	1650	25	2	1	1	2	2	140
3	31	1700	31	2	2	3	1	2	96
3	32	1720	45	1	2	2	1	2	96
4	1	800	55	1	1	2	1	2	130
4	2	815	61	2	1	1	1	2	150
4	3	815	17	1	2	1	8	2	130
4	4	830	4	2	1	1	2	2	175
4	5	900	25	4	2	1	9	1	200
4	6	920	7	1	1	3	2	2	96
4	7	945	36	8	2	1	9	1	291
4	8	1000	44	2	2	1	9	1	225
4	9	1020	24	1	2	1	2	2	143
4	10	1045	18	2	1	1	1	2	140

Table 3.3
PCS Alpha Center Client Records, August 6–9 (*continued*)

On the web at ache.org/books/ Middleboro2

continued

Table 3.3
PCS Alpha
Center Client
Records,
August 6–9
(continued)

*On the web at
ache.org/books/
Middleboro2*

Day	Num	Art	Age	Town	Sex	First	Ins	Phy	Charge ($)
4	11	1130	28	2	1	2	1	2	142
4	12	1200	34	1	2	1	1	2	146
4	13	1215	32	1	2	1	2	2	160
4	14	1215	9	2	2	1	1	2	140
4	15	1235	44	1	2	1	8	2	196
4	16	1245	47	1	2	1	2	2	150
4	17	1250	34	4	1	1	8	2	190
4	18	1310	29	6	2	2	2	2	160
4	19	1340	28	1	2	3	2	2	96
4	20	1420	44	1	2	1	2	2	150
4	21	1530	12	1	1	2	1	2	160
4	22	1545	50	2	2	2	1	2	140
4	23	1545	26	1	2	3	2	1	96
4	24	1600	39	2	2	2	2	1	170
4	25	1600	69	2	2	3	3	2	96
4	26	1630	30	1	2	2	1	2	145
4	27	1700	38	1	1	2	3	2	96
4	28	1720	13	1	1	2	1	2	150
5	1	815	22	1	2	1	9	1	190
5	2	825	23	2	2	1	1	2	135
5	3	915	19	9	2	1	2	2	150
5	4	940	36	7	1	2	2	2	125
5	5	1000	45	2	1	1	9	1	180
5	6	1000	23	2	1	2	9	1	180
5	7	1045	60	1	1	3	3	2	96
5	8	1130	59	1	2	2	8	2	200
5	9	1215	52	4	1	1	2	2	150
5	10	1230	35	4	2	3	2	2	96
5	11	1240	21	7	2	1	1	2	130
5	12	1250	66	2	2	2	3	2	96
5	13	1310	45	2	2	1	8	2	150

continued

Day	Num	Art	Age	Town	Sex	First	Ins	Phy	Charge ($)
5	14	1320	23	1	1	1	1	2	140
5	15	1350	21	1	2	1	3	2	96
5	16	1440	37	1	1	2	9	1	145
5	17	1510	40	6	2	3	2	1	96
5	18	1540	50	9	1	2	2	2	140
5	19	1620	66	8	2	2	3	2	130
5	20	1650	45	2	2	1	2	2	140
5	21	1715	54	2	2	2	1	2	145
5	22	1730	74	1	1	3	3	2	130
5	23	1730	3	1	2	2	2	2	135
5	24	1800	19	2	1	1	1	1	130
5	25	1820	47	2	2	1	2	1	140
5	26	1830	57	2	2	2	1	2	130
5	27	1845	35	2	1	3	2	1	130
6	1	800	12	2	1	1	1	2	140
6	2	800	27	1	2	2	2	2	132
6	3	810	44	2	1	1	2	1	140
6	4	820	55	2	2	3	1	2	96
6	5	910	23	3	1	1	1	2	125
6	6	930	19	2	2	2	2	1	140
6	7	1015	7	7	2	2	2	2	150
6	8	1045	70	9	1	1	3	2	140
6	9	1050	24	8	1	1	1	1	130
6	10	1100	17	9	2	3	2	2	96
6	11	1120	19	2	2	3	1	2	96
6	12	1130	24	1	1	1	2	2	125

Table 3.3
PCS Alpha Center Client Records, August 6–9 *(continued)*

On the web at ache.org/books/ Middleboro2

continued

Table 3.3
PCS Alpha
Center Client
Records,
August 6–9
(continued)

On the web at
ache.org/books/
Middleboro2

Day	Num	Art	Age	Town	Sex	First	Ins	Phy	Charge ($)
6	13	1145	16	2	2	2	2	2	130
6	14	1215	44	8	1	1	2	2	140
6	15	1230	48	2	2	3	2	2	96
6	16	1245	8	1	1	2	1	2	96
Total	**185**								**25,328**

Notes:
Day:

1	Monday	3	Wednesday	5	Friday
2	Tuesday	4	Thursday	6	Saturday

Num: Arrival order (i.e., 1 is first person to arrive)

Art: Arrival time, using 24-hour clock or "military time"

Age: Client age, in years

Town:

1	Middleboro	3	Jasper	5	Statesville	7	Boalsburg	9	Other
2	Mifflenville	4	Harris City	6	Carterville	8	Minortown		

Sex:

1   male

2   female

First: Is this your first ever visit to a PCS center?

1   Yes

2   No, and it is not a medically ordered return visit

3   No, it is a medically ordered return visit

Ins: Insurance coverage/payment

1	Commercial insurance	3	Medicare	9	Employer pays
2	Cash, check, or credit card	8	Workers' comp		

Phy: Physical?

1   Yes

2   No

Charge: Gross billed charges in US dollars

Day	Num	Art	Age	Town	Sex	First	Ins	Phy	Charge ($)
1	1	800	44	3	2	2	8	2	385
1	2	810	32	3	1	1	1	2	160
1	3	810	45	3	2	1	8	2	270
1	4	845	66	3	1	3	3	2	96
1	5	845	21	5	1	1	8	2	180
1	6	845	7	9	2	3	1	2	180
1	7	900	34	3	2	1	2	2	180
1	8	915	51	3	2	1	8	2	350
1	9	915	59	3	2	1	1	2	180
1	10	930	40	3	1	1	8	2	390
1	11	1005	23	5	1	2	9	1	375
1	12	1015	32	3	2	1	8	2	280
1	13	1035	40	5	2	2	1	2	190
1	14	1045	75	5	2	2	1	2	220
1	15	1015	22	3	1	1	9	1	350
1	16	1105	30	3	2	1	1	2	160
1	17	1115	36	3	2	1	1	2	165
1	18	1130	50	3	1	1	2	2	145
1	19	1145	67	9	2	1	3	2	150
1	20	1145	23	3	1	3	2	2	96
1	21	1200	54	3	2	2	1	2	150
1	22	1200	19	3	1	1	2	2	220
1	23	1215	56	3	2	2	1	1	150
1	24	1220	23	3	1	1	1	2	160
1	25	1330	34	3	1	1	8	2	310
1	26	1430	25	9	1	1	1	2	150
1	27	1800	49	3	2	2	9	1	300
1	28	1810	69	3	2	1	3	2	170
2	1	800	70	9	2	2	3	2	135
2	2	845	44	3	1	3	9	1	300
2	3	915	25	3	1	1	9	1	300
2	4	930	32	3	2	1	1	2	160
2	5	930	37	9	2	2	8	2	275
2	6	1015	40	3	1	1	8	2	325

Table 3.4
PCS Beta Center
Client Records,
August 6–9

*On the web at
ache.org/books/
Middleboro2*

continued

Table 3.4
PCS Beta Center
Client Records,
August 6–9
(continued)

*On the web at
ache.org/books/
Middleboro2*

Day	Num	Art	Age	Town	Sex	First	Ins	Phy	Charge ($)
2	7	130	23	3	1	1	1	2	190
2	8	1045	19	3	2	1	9	1	300
2	9	1050	25	4	1	1	9	1	275
2	10	1115	45	3	2	2	2	2	190
2	11	1130	50	3	1	1	2	2	160
2	12	1145	27	9	1	1	9	1	270
2	13	1215	29	3	2	2	1	2	190
2	14	1230	30	9	2	2	9	1	300
2	15	1310	45	3	1	1	8	2	325
2	16	1325	29	3	2	2	1	2	150
2	17	1420	40	9	1	1	1	2	160
2	18	1500	55	3	1	1	8	2	200
2	19	1520	45	3	2	2	1	2	150
2	20	1550	56	3	1	1	1	2	140
2	21	1610	8	9	1	1	1	2	96
2	22	1640	56	3	1	2	2	2	165
2	23	1720	23	9	1	1	1	2	165
2	24	1730	50	3	1	2	9	1	320
2	25	1800	56	3	2	1	9	1	260
2	26	1830	44	5	2	2	2	2	250
3	1	1250	47	3	1	1	9	1	300
3	2	1305	56	3	2	2	9	1	310
3	3	1310	23	9	2	1	1	2	155
3	4	1345	58	5	2	2	9	1	275
3	5	1400	44	5	1	1	1	2	160
3	6	1430	12	3	1	1	1	2	175
3	7	1500	40	3	2	1	8	2	375
3	8	1520	39	5	1	2	8	2	250
3	9	1545	50	5	1	1	9	1	375
3	10	1610	46	5	2	1	9	1	375
3	11	1630	45	3	2	1	8	2	325
3	12	1645	23	3	1	2	9	2	375
3	13	1705	48	3	1	2	8	2	325
3	14	1730	32	3	1	2	1	2	160

continued

Day	Num	Art	Age	Town	Sex	First	Ins	Phy	Charge ($)
4	1	800	23	3	1	1	9	1	350
4	2	845	19	3	1	1	8	2	300
4	3	920	44	3	2	2	8	2	290
4	4	1030	32	3	1	2	2	1	350
4	5	1110	50	5	1	2	2	2	350
4	6	1150	43	3	2	2	9	1	375
4	7	1250	50	5	1	1	8	2	400
4	8	1300	9	3	2	3	2	2	96
4	9	1345	45	3	2	1	1	2	190
4	10	1500	56	3	1	1	9	1	300
4	11	1515	75	3	1	2	3	2	150
4	12	1600	46	3	1	2	8	2	300
4	13	1640	48	3	1	1	9	1	300
4	14	1700	40	3	1	1	9	1	300
4	15	1720	23	9	1	1	8	2	425
4	16	1810	30	9	1	1	2	2	150
5	1	810	50	3	1	1	1	2	160
5	2	845	27	5	1	1	8	2	280
5	3	900	22	9	1	1	2	2	120
5	4	1015	18	3	1	1	9	1	300
5	5	1030	23	3	2	2	1	2	140
5	6	1045	64	9	2	1	8	2	260
5	7	1130	45	9	1	2	9	1	300
5	8	1130	23	3	2	2	1	2	160
5	9	1145	12	3	2	2	8	2	260
5	10	1215	35	5	2	2	9	1	300
5	11	1230	23	5	1	2	9	1	300
5	12	1330	29	3	2	1	1	2	160
5	13	1345	40	3	2	1	9	1	300
5	14	1400	35	3	2	1	2	2	180
5	15	1420	46	3	2	2	2	2	170
5	16	1430	24	9	1	1	1	2	170
5	17	1520	59	9	1	1	9	1	300

Table 3.4
PCS Beta Center Client Records, August 6–9 *(continued)*

On the web at ache.org/books/ Middleboro2

continued

Table 3.4
PCS Beta Center
Client Records,
August 6–9
(continued)

*On the web at
ache.org/books/
Middleboro2*

Day	Num	Art	Age	Town	Sex	First	Ins	Phy	Charge ($)
5	18	1530	60	3	1	1	8	2	325
5	19	1540	45	2	1	1	8	2	240
5	20	1700	33	3	2	3	8	2	96
5	21	1710	21	5	1	1	1	1	160
6	1	900	19	5	2	3	1	2	200
6	2	900	34	3	1	2	8	2	240
6	3	915	45	3	1	2	2	2	170
6	4	940	34	3	2	1	9	1	300
6	5	950	12	9	3	1	1	2	160
6	6	1000	34	3	2	1	1	2	180
6	7	1030	55	3	2	2	1	2	170
6	8	1045	45	3	2	2	8	2	220
6	9	1100	60	3	1	2	9	1	350
6	10	1130	55	3	2	1	8	2	270
6	11	1200	14	9	2	1	1	2	140
6	12	1200	23	3	2	1	9	1	350
Total	**117**								**27,855**

Notes:

Day:
| 1 | Monday | 3 | Wednesday | 5 | Friday |
| 2 | Tuesday | 4 | Thursday | 6 | Saturday |

Num: Arrival order (i.e., 1 is first person to arrive)

Art: Arrival time, using 24-hour clock or "military time"

Age: Client age, in years

Town:
| 1 | Middleboro | 3 | Jasper | 5 | Statesville | 7 | Boalsburg | 9 | Other |
| 2 | Mifflenville | 4 | Harris City | 6 | Carterville | 8 | Minortown | | |

Sex:
1 male
2 female

First: Is this your first ever visit to a PCS center?
1 Yes
2 No, and it is not a medically ordered return visit
3 No, it is a medically ordered return visit

Ins: Insurance coverage/payment
| 1 | Commercial insurance | 3 | Medicare | 9 | Employer pays |
| 2 | Cash, check, or credit card | 8 | Workers' comp | | |

Phy: Physical?
1 Yes
2 No

Charge: Gross billed charges in US dollars

Record	Date	MD/ARNP	Day	Ctr	Revenue ($)	Visits
	August			**Alpha**		
1	1	3	3	1	3,784	22
2	2	4	4	1	2,560	16
3	3	4	5	1	3,520	20
4	4	7	6	1	2,340	18
5	6	1	1	1	6,355	48
6	7	1	2	1	4,588	34
7	8	3	3	1	4,445	32
8	9	4	4	1	4,263	28
9	10	7	5	1	3,705	27
10	11	7	6	1	1,972	16
11	13	1	1	1	7,420	53
12	14	1	2	1	5,291	37
13	15	3	3	1	5,278	29
14	16	4	4	1	3,744	24
15	17	4	5	1	4,125	25
16	18	7	6	1	3,080	22
17	20	1	1	1	6,768	47
18	21	1	2	1	4,587	33
19	22	3	3	1	6,105	33
20	23	4	4	1	3,850	22
21	24	3	5	1	3,360	21
22	25	7	6	1	3,120	20
23	27	1	1	1	5,680	40
24	28	1	2	1	3,942	27
25	29	3	3	1	4,032	24
26	30	4	4	1	4,000	25
27	31	8	5	1	3,221	20
	September			**Alpha**		
28	1	7	6	1	2,601	17
29	H	1	1	1	0	0
30	4	1	2	1	5,005	35
31	5	3	3	1	4,186	23

Table 3.5
PCS Revenue
Generation
by Physician,
Center, and Day
of Week

*On the web at
ache.org/books/
Middleboro2*

continued

Table 3.5
PCS Revenue
Generation
by Physician,
Center, and
Day of Week
(*continued*)

*On the web at
ache.org/books/
Middleboro2*

Record	Date	MD/ARNP	Day	Ctr	Revenue ($)	Visits
32	6	4	4	1	2,002	14
33	7	4	5	1	4,495	29
34	8	11	6	1	2,240	16
35	10	1	1	1	5,640	40
36	11	1	2	1	3,780	27
37	12	3	3	1	4,788	28
38	13	4	4	1	2,464	16
39	14	3	5	1	4,234	29
40	15	7	6	1	1,692	12
41	17	1	1	1	5,396	38
42	18	1	2	1	4,004	28
43	19	3	3	1	3,600	20
44	20	4	4	1	3,312	18
45	21	4	5	1	3,900	25
46	22	7	6	1	1,390	10
47	24	1	1	1	5,850	39
48	25	1	2	1	3,550	25
49	26	3	3	1	4,930	29
50	27	4	4	1	3,040	19
51	28	3	5	1	3,465	21
52	29	7	6	1	2,106	13
	October			**Alpha**		
53	1	1	1	1	5,180	37
54	2	1	2	1	3,432	24
55	3	3	3	1	3,040	19
56	4	3	4	1	2,310	15
57	5	4	5	1	2,100	15
58	6	7	6	1	931	7
59	8	1	1	1	4,260	30
60	9	1	2	1	3,640	26
61	10	3	3	1	2,744	16
62	11	4	4	1	2,128	14
63	12	3	5	1	4,010	11
64	13	7	6	1	1,690	13

continued

Record	Date	MD/ARNP	Day	Ctr	Revenue ($)	Visits
65	15	1	1	1	4,118	29
66	16	1	2	1	3,510	27
67	17	3	3	1	2,338	14
68	18	4	4	1	1,788	12
69	19	3	5	1	1,500	10
70	20	7	6	1	1,690	13
71	22	1	1	1	5,040	35
72	23	1	2	1	3,500	25
73	24	3	3	1	3,255	21
74	25	4	4	1	2,156	14
75	26	7	5	1	2,520	18
76	27	11	6	1	1,440	12
77	29	1	1	1	4,576	32
78	30	1	2	1	3,888	27
79	31	3	3	1	3,411	20
	August			**Beta**		
80	1	6	3	2	3,975	15
81	2	6	4	2	4,760	17
82	3	5	5	2	5,415	19
83	4	8	6	2	1,350	9
84	6	3	1	2	6,440	28
85	7	3	2	2	6,110	26
86	8	6	3	2	3,780	14
87	9	6	4	2	4,160	16
88	10	5	5	2	5,145	21
89	11	11	6	2	1,740	12
90	13	3	1	2	6,244	28
91	14	3	2	2	7,320	30
92	15	6	3	2	4,590	18
93	16	6	4	2	2,650	10
94	17	5	5	2	5,244	19
95	18	8	6	2	1,404	9
96	20	3	1	2	7,048	29

Table 3.5
PCS Revenue Generation by Physician, Center, and Day of Week (*continued*)

On the web at ache.org/books/ Middleboro2

continued

Table 3.5
PCS Revenue
Generation
by Physician,
Center, and
Day of Week
(continued)

*On the web at
ache.org/books/
Middleboro2*

Record	Date	MD/ARNP	Day	Ctr	Revenue ($)	Visits
97	21	3	2	2	6,000	25
98	22	6	3	2	3,975	15
99	23	6	4	2	3,584	14
100	24	5	5	2	6,216	21
101	25	8	6	2	1,950	13
102	27	3	1	2	7,000	28
103	28	3	2	2	6,360	24
104	29	6	3	2	5,040	18
105	30	6	4	2	3,960	15
106	31	9	5	2	5,120	20
	September			**Beta**		
107	1	8	6	2	1,470	10
108	3	H	1	2	0	H
109	4	3	2	2	6,930	33
110	5	6	3	2	4,446	18
111	6	6	4	2	5,100	17
112	7	9	5	2	3,926	13
113	8	8	6	2	888	6
114	10	3	1	2	9,030	42
115	11	3	2	2	4,420	17
116	12	6	3	2	4,260	15
117	13	6	4	2	4,880	16
118	14	6	5	2	4,806	18
119	15	8	6	2	1,305	9
120	17	3	1	2	7,029	33
121	18	3	2	2	6,240	26
122	19	6	3	2	5,874	22
123	20	6	4	2	3,336	12
124	21	3	5	2	5,670	18
125	22	8	6	2	1,400	10
126	24	3	1	2	6,409	29
127	25	3	2	2	6,615	27
128	26	6	3	2	6,656	26

continued

Record	Date	MD/ARNP	Day	Ctr	Revenue ($)	Visits
129	27	6	4	2	3,380	13
130	28	6	5	2	5,225	19
	October			Beta		
132	1	3	1	2	4,872	24
133	2	3	2	2	4,300	20
134	3	6	3	2	3,920	14
135	4	6	4	2	2,900	10
136	5	5	5	2	2,025	15
137	6	8	6	2	2,275	7
138	8	3	1	2	4,400	20
139	9	3	2	2	3,906	18
140	10	6	3	2	3,600	12
141	11	6	4	2	2,937	11
142	12	8	5	2	3,267	11
143	13	5	6	2	1,885	13
144	15	3	1	2	3,857	19
145	16	3	2	2	4,352	17
146	17	6	3	2	3,840	15
147	18	6	4	2	3,080	11
148	19	8	5	2	3,240	10
149	20	10	6	2	1,735	13
150	22	3	1	2	5,250	25
151	23	3	2	2	3,300	15
152	24	6	3	2	4,641	17
153	25	6	4	2	3,640	13
154	26	8	5	2	4,214	14

Table 3.5
PCS Revenue Generation by Physician, Center, and Day of Week *(continued)*

On the web at ache.org/books/ Middleboro2

continued

Table 3.5
PCS Revenue
Generation
by Physician,
Center, and
Day of Week
(continued)

*On the web at
ache.org/books/
Middleboro2*

Record	Date	MD/ARNP	Day	Ctr	Revenue ($)	Visits
155	27	5	6	2	1,740	12
156	29	3	1	2	4,554	22
157	30	3	2	2	3,723	17
158	31	6	3	2	4,522	17

Notes:

Code	MD/ARNP	Day	Center
1	B. Casey, MD	Monday	Alpha
2	M. Welby, MD	Tuesday	Beta
3	S. Tobias, MD	Wednesday	
4	J. Smooth, MD	Thursday	
5	R. Hottle, MD	Friday	
6	L. Cytesmath, MD	Saturday	
7	C. Withers, ARNP		
8	J. Jones, ARNP		
9	M. Foxx, DO		
10	R. Majors, MD		
11	G. Mattox, ARNP		

Revenue: Total gross billed charges
Visits: Number of paying patients
H: Holiday

	2019	2018	2017	2016
Revenue				
Client Services—Gross	2,366,410	2,164,853	2,103,574	2,065,938
Contractual Allowances	72,565	73,233	53,657	50,565
Patient Revenue—Net	2,293,845	2,091,620	2,049,917	2,015,373
Other Revenue—Imaging	246,454	202,445	195,887	180,366
Total Revenue	**2,540,299**	**2,294,065**	**2,245,804**	**2,195,739**
Expenses				
Salaries and Wages	1,292,372	1,134,229	995,224	953,779
Staff Benefits	339,904	306,242	268,710	257,520
Administrative Expenses	18,330	17,339	10,494	10,056
Advertising	34,000	34,000	37,182	30,004
Collection Fees	1,267	845	342	659
Computer Support	42,668	40,282	34,256	33,289
Consultants	1,529	1,270	948	805
Equipment Leases	10,400	10,400	10,400	10,400
Insurance	28,100	24,100	24,100	18,560
Laboratory	64,882	66,676	70,232	79,393
Laundry and Housekeeping	12,830	12,256	8,156	3,474
Legal/Audit	8,100	8,450	8,450	7,850
Medical Supplies	61,450	58,220	57,354	58,556
Office Supplies	18,437	29,348	28,420	28,556
Printing and Postage	4,222	4,038	4,002	3,300
Professional Fees	23,955	23,425	23,302	23,884
Rent	78,500	78,750	58,900	58,900
Repairs and Maintenance	3,167	2,966	1,529	2,349
Telephone	2,766	2,454	3,262	2,550
Utilities	18,925	16,800	13,560	13,720
Interest	350	1,654	1,378	2,055
Depreciation	22,556	20,560	20,585	18,363
Bad Debt Expenses	2,437	2,556	2,768	2,989
Total Expenses	**2,091,147**	**1,896,860**	**1,683,554**	**1,621,011**
Income (Loss) Before Taxes	**449,152**	**397,205**	**562,250**	**574,728**
Federal Tax	175,169	154,910	219,277	224,144
State Tax	40,424	35,748	50,602	51,725
Income (Loss) After Taxes	**233,559**	**206,547**	**292,370**	**298,858**

Table 3.6
PCS Statement
of Operations

*On the web at
ache.org/books/
Middleboro2*

Notes: (1) Fiscal years 2016–2019. (2) Numbers are in US dollars.

Table 3.7
PCS Balance
Sheet

*On the web at
ache.org/books/
Middleboro2*

	2019	2018	2017	2016
Assets				
Current Assets				
Cash, Operating	52,383	58,445	73,494	68,334
Accounts Receivable—Net	139,385	134,450	138,450	140,230
Inventory	3,339	4,125	5,233	28,734
Prepaid Expenses	3,078	4,565	4,021	5,688
Total Current Assets	**198,185**	**201,585**	**221,198**	**242,986**
Investments	762,353	741,220	682,334	673,030
Property, Plant, and Equipment (PPE)				
Equipment and Leasehold Improvements—Gross	360,445	359,516	356,284	322,464
Less Accumulated Depreciation	283,712	261,156	240,596	220,011
Leasehold Improvements—Net	552,363	552,363	552,363	552,363
Net PPE	629,096	650,723	668,051	654,816
Total Assets	**1,589,634**	**1,593,528**	**1,571,583**	**1,570,832**
Liabilities and Net Assets				
Current Liabilities				
Accounts Payable	49,668	56,929	67,393	83,272
Accrued Expenses	29,000	27,387	30,100	45,662
Accrued Payroll Taxes	23,446	29,395	27,445	28,449
Total Current Liabilities	**102,114**	**113,711**	**124,938**	**157,383**
Long-Term Liabilities				
Notes Payable	19,449	24,600	25,020	24,030
Total Liabilities	**121,563**	**138,311**	**149,958**	**181,413**
Net Assets				
Common Stock				
Authorized and Issued	720,000	720,000	720,000	720,000
Retained Earnings	748,071	735,217	701,625	669,419
Total Net Assets	**1,468,071**	**1,455,217**	**1,421,625**	**1,389,419**
Net Assets + Liabilities	**1,589,634**	**1,593,528**	**1,571,583**	**1,570,832**

Notes: (1) For fiscal year ending December 31. (2) Numbers are in US dollars.

	Salary ($)	Benefits ($)	Total ($)
President: Tobias	20,000	1,000	21,000
Medical Director: Tobias	20,000	1,000	21,000
Subtotal	**40,000**	**2,000**	**42,000**
Clinical Staff			
Alpha Center			
Casey, Tobias (FB)	143,520	50,476	193,996
Smooth (PB)	47,840	10,525	58,365
Withers, Jones (MB)	43,240	3,892	47,132
Subtotal	**234,600**	**64,892**	**299,492**
Beta Center			
Welby, Cytesmath (FB)	143,520	50,232	193,752
Hottle (PB)	47,840	10,525	58,365
Foxx, Majors (MB)	43,240	3,027	46,267
Subtotal	**234,600**	**63,784**	**298,384**
Nurse Practitioner—Alpha Center	10,530	2,106	12,636
Nurse Practitioner—Beta Center	10,530	2,106	12,636
Subtotal	**490,260**	**132,888**	**623,148**
Professional Staff			
Medical Assistants	92,280	29,530	121,810
Receptionists/Billing Clerks	86,128	27,561	113,689
Radiographic Technician	48,204	15,425	63,629
Other	2,400	528	2,928
Subtotal	**229,012**	**73,044**	**302,056**
Administrative Staff			
Director of Nursing and Clinical Care	64,000	20,480	84,480
Business Manager	62,500	20,000	82,500
Business Office Staff (4 FTEs)	120,000	24,000	144,000
Other	52,000	2,600	54,600
Subtotal	**298,500**	**67,080**	**365,580**
Total	**1,292,372**	**339,904**	**1,632,276**

Table 3.8
PCS Compensation for Twelve Months

Notes: (1) Numbers are in US dollars. (2) FB: full benefits; FTEs: full-time equivalents; MB: minimum benefits, based on hours worked; PB: partial benefits.

Table 3.9
PCS Market
Analysis of
Basic Visit
Charges

	2019	2018	2017	2016
MIDCARE ED	240	240	200	200
Webster Health System ED (Quick Med)*	140	140	140	125
Convenient Medical Care*	135	135	135	120
Capital City General ED	180	180	170	150
Medical Associates*	125	125	125	115
PCS*	125	125	125	115

Notes: (1) Charges in US dollars. (2) * Comparisons based on CPT 99202. (3) ED: emergency department.

MIDDLEBORO COMMUNITY MENTAL HEALTH CENTER

Middleboro Community Mental Health Center (MCMHC) was founded in 1964 as a 501(c)(3) nonprofit organization and funded in part by the Community Mental Health Act of 1963. Today, it provides a comprehensive menu of mental health services and programs—including emergency and education—for adults and children and their families. It also runs a central office called Gardner Place as well as a four-bed group home called Justin Place in northwest Middleboro.

As a state-designated facility, MCMHC is required to offer an array of services, including 24-hour emergency services, assessment and evaluation, intake and referral, therapy, case management, community-based rehabilitation, outpatient psychiatric care, and disaster mental health support. The state designates catchment areas for community mental health centers, and the area for MCMHC—and for another center located between Jasper and Capital City—is Hillsboro County. Services provided outside the catchment area, other than emergency services, may reduce the resources used to treat residents within the catchment area. Every five years, the state conducts an assessment for redesignation, and MCMHC is due for its review in two years.

MCMHC maintains contracts with several private insurance carriers. It also receives reimbursement for serving Hillsboro County residents who are covered by Medicaid. To be eligible for the Medicaid program, a person must be determined to have conditions and circumstances that contribute to a mental health diagnosis.

HISTORY

Using federal funds, MCMHC began operations in 1964 in a small rental office in Middleboro. Its aim was to provide mental health services primarily to children and families who were unable to obtain such care elsewhere. Previously, mental health services in and around the city were delivered in a noncoordinated manner by area hospitals and by Swift River Psychological Services, which MCMHC acquired in 1967.

MCMHC purchased a building on the north side of Middleboro in 1971. It owes the expansion of its programs and services to changes in mental health legislation through the 1970s, which culminated in the passage of the Mental Health Systems Act (Public Law 96–398) in 1980. This act strengthened the linkages among mental health programs and services; awarded grants for serving specific populations, including the severely mentally ill and severely emotionally disturbed; and expanded mental health education. Just one year later—in 1981—under the Reagan administration, the act was repealed and replaced by a block grant program. These block grants sharply decreased federal funding for mental health services.

Amendments to the Medicare program in 1987 increased outpatient mental health benefits for the first time in more than two decades, enabling MCMHC to introduce programs for severely mentally ill adults. Service delivery remained at a steady level for many years, until President Clinton signed the Children's Health Act (Public Law 106–310) into law in 2000. This act established standards for the care and treatment of children and youth in community-based facilities. As a follow-up to this act, President George H. W. Bush called for the expansion of community health centers, including mental health services, in 2002.

Since 2002, MCMHC has continued to develop its programs and services, albeit modestly. In 2005, it moved its offices into Gardner Place, located in the central business district of Middleboro. In 2007, it purchased Justin Place, located on the northwest side of the city.

Inpatient behavioral healthcare across the state is extremely limited. Only one such facility exists in the state—the 154-bed State Behavioral Health Hospital situated nearly 150 miles northeast of Middleboro.

MISSION

The mission of MCMHC is as follows:

Our mission is to provide an array of appropriate mental and behavioral programs and services to residents of Hillsboro County. Our programs and services promote the well-being and quality of life of our community by preventing and managing the challenges to mental and behavioral health.

GOVERNANCE

MCMHC is licensed as a nonprofit community mental health center. Under its corporate umbrella are all of its programs and services as well as its two properties—Gardner Place and Justin Place.

The organization is governed by a board of directors that comprises 17 members. Members are elected to four-year terms and may serve a maximum of three consecutive terms. The board as a whole meets monthly, and its subcommittees meet on a separate schedule. The executive committee meets with the executive director every two weeks, while the other committees meet at least quarterly. Current members of the MCMHC board are as follows; the (number)* indicates the number of years remaining on current board term:

MCMHC Board of Directors

Members	Residence
John Regis, JD (1)*, *Chair*	
Attorney	Middleboro
Josephine Crawford, PhD (2), *Vice Chair*	
Clinical psychologist	Statesville
Blanche Stacy, LCSW (3), *Secretary*	
Retired social worker	Middleboro
George Blanchford, CPA (2), *Treasurer*	
President, Blanchford Public Accountants	Jasper
Althea Actor, MD (1)	
Psychiatrist	Middleboro
Geraldine Connelly (3)	
Management consultant	Jasper
William Dawson (1)	
President, Hyland Motors	Middleboro

Johanna Gilliam (4)
   Dental assistant   Mifflenville

Sadie Grant, CISSP (2)
   Manager, Information Technology, River Industries   Middleboro

Bennett Hauser (2)
   Human resources manager, Jersey Products   Jasper

Jackson Hebert (1)
   Senior account executive, TV Channel 32   Boalsburg

Stephanie Jervis-Washburn
   Executive director, MCMHC   Middleboro

Stephen Rodgers, JD (4)
   Attorney   Middleboro

Penelope Sanchez-Rosario, NCC AP (3)
   Substance abuse counselor   Statesville

Virginia Shaw, PsyD (3)
   Pediatric clinical psychologist   Jasper

Joan Stemsrud, RN (4)
   Retired nurse   Carterville

Martha Washington, RN (2)
   CEO, Hillsboro Health   Middleboro

Bertram Yang (2)
   Vice principal, Middleboro High School   Middleboro

Assignments to the board's standing committees are as follows:

- Executive (Regis, Crawford, Stacy, Blanchford)

- Finance (Connelly, Hebert, Blanchford, Regis)

- Nominating (Shaw, Grant, Hauser, Gilliam)

- Quality and Compliance (Yang, Regis, Actor, Washington, Stemsrud)

- Planning (Actor, Dawson, Sanchez-Rosario, Shaw, Rodgers)

- Development (Regis, Crawford, Stacy, Blanchford, Dawson, Connelly)

According to the term-limit clause of the organization, the following members are now serving their final term: Regis, Actor, Dawson, and Hebert. In addition, Blanchford has indicated he will not serve beyond his current term when it ends in two years. All other members are eligible to serve at least one more term and have not voiced a plan to step down. MCMHC is considering increasing the size of the board and adding another term to the current limit of three. Dr. Crawford, vice chair of the board, explained the reasoning behind this idea: "It really takes two or three terms to understand the organization, and then it's time to leave. It's important that we retain continuity on the board. Also, it would be nice to have more board members from smaller towns outside of Middleboro. Some of the most serious mental health issues can be found in rural areas, so it's important for us to address those needs. After all, we are here for the entire county, not just Middleboro."

Development or fund-raising is an area of increasing concern for MCMHC. Historically, it has been able to manage healthy total margins mostly because of substantial contributions from two Middleboro families. One of those families informed the board three years ago that it has shifted its charitable priorities and the coming year will mark the end of its generous donations. MCMHC's governance has yet to develop a strategy to make up for this financial loss.

MANAGEMENT TEAM AND ORGANIZATIONAL STRUCTURE

Stephanie Jervis-Washburn has been the executive director of MCMHC since 2015. She holds a master in marriage and family therapy (MFT) from an East Coast university and obtained her master in healthcare administration from State University. Prior to joining MCMHC, she worked for ten years as a marriage and family therapist in a small private group in Capital City. Active in professional organizations, she serves on the education subcommittee and the executive committee of the American Association for Marriage and Family Therapy as well as the executive committee of the Governor's Blue Ribbon Commission for Child Mental Health. She has extensive lobbying experience and is well-regarded in her profession.

Since arriving at MCMHC, Jervis-Washburn has focused on reorganizing the management structure and offering new service and educational programs for the community. Her background in MFT has, not surprisingly, led to the development of robust MFT programs, which are considered models in the state. She is frequently asked to consult with other organizations that are pursuing similar initiatives. Although the MFT programs have been popular and successful, they have caused concern among some board members and senior staff, who think her laser focus on MFT could diminish the quality of other MCMHC programs and services.

Another area of attention for Jervis-Washburn has been strengthening the administrative foundation of the organization, including finance and information technology. As she noted, "An organization such as ours must be incredibly sensitive to changes in reimbursement. We have survived because of our ability to respond to—I dare say, predict—the changes coming down the road in, for example, Medicaid reimbursement, which accounts for a large portion of our revenue. Programs like Medicaid are becoming more difficult to predict, given the current political environment locally and nationally. We need to be alert to opportunities that may expand our payer mix to nongovernmental sources, although many private and commercial payers do not compensate well—if at all—for community-based services such as ours. It's an ongoing struggle."

To this end, and with the board's instruction, Jervis-Washburn has been working to secure external or nonstate funding, such as federal and private grants. Small grants, usually obtained from the state, have always represented a portion of MCMHC's financial base. Typically, such grants are allocated for a particular program or service and are generally noncompetitive, given that they are awarded to all designated community mental health centers. Last year, she submitted the organization's first grant application to the Substance Abuse and Mental Health Services Administration (SAMHSA), aiming to design and implement a countywide program to address the growing adolescent opioid epidemic. Unfortunately, the proposal was declined. Jervis-Washburn is undeterred, however, and intends to submit the proposal to other funders and to be more proactive with grant writing in general.

Rodgers, a member of the board, urged her to explore the possibility of MCMHC taking on some aspects of the Drug Court for Hillsboro County. While not necessarily a financially attractive venture, the organization's involvement in the court can have a positive impact on the county and will be consistent with MCMHC's mission.

Giving priority to information technology has paid off, as the organization's transition to the *Diagnostic and Statistical Manual of Mental Disorders*, 5th edition (DSM–5), has gone relatively smoothly. "Like most centers, we are still struggling a bit with the fine points of DSM–5, but overall we are doing relatively well," Jervis-Washburn said. "Changes in the area of autism spectrum disorders are still somewhat controversial for some of our clinicians, but this is not a problem unique to our organization. The autism spectrum is the one area we need to address more thoroughly."

In part because of its advanced information systems and its positive reputation for service provision, MCMHC has been approached by a Capital City–based organization to cocreate a tri-county accountable care organization. "This is an opportunity we are definitely evaluating, although we may not be ready to assume the financial risk for our patient population," she admitted.

Within the past several years, Jervis-Washburn has substantially changed the organizational structure of MCMHC. She now has only one direct report—the senior director Shanique Harrison, PhD. In addition, she meets regularly with Dr. Ivan Stanzl, the medical director, regarding clinical issues.

SENIOR DIRECTOR

Dr. Harrison was named senior director in 2015 when the previous clinical head retired after nearly 20 years in office. As a clinical psychologist with special training in dialectical behavior therapy for adolescents, she was a team leader in MCMHC's Adult Services Program, but before this she worked at a small mental health facility in Capital City for five years and was a faculty member in the psychology department at State University for seven years. She is active in the mental health community and has recently become a member of a regional committee—sponsored by the National Alliance on Mental Illness—that addresses the stigma of mental illness.

Dr. Harrison's appointment to senior director was somewhat divisive because several staff members who had worked for the organization longer than she had were passed over for the position. Although she is aware of the controversy, she has made deliberate efforts to be collaborative in her decision making. With direction from Jervis-Washburn and support from the board, she has made the following changes in her short tenure:

♦ Split MCMHC into two divisions—Administrative Services and Clinical Services—that are each headed up by a director

♦ Combined all children and family programs into a single unit that is headed by a manager who reports to the director of Clinical Services (in the past, each of these programs had a direct reporting relationship to the clinical head)

DIRECTOR OF ADMINISTRATIVE SERVICES

Clement Gray, a longtime employee of MCMHC, is the director of the division. He received a bachelor of science in business administration from State University and is an active member of the Healthcare Financial Management Association.

The division of Administrative Services comprises Human Resources, Information Technology, Planning and Marketing, Properties, and Finance. Information Technology, Properties, and Finance are headed by a manager with specialized training and background in his area of responsibility. Human Resources is headed by an acting manager, and Gray has been acting as manager of Planning and Marketing. Given his experience and expertise, he is often called in to assist in Finance, a responsibility he enjoys but one that takes him away from his extensive assigned duties. As a result, he is "somewhat overwhelmed" and has frequently expressed to Dr. Harrison his difficulties.

The tacit discord between the two divisions is also a cause for frustration. "Everybody works really hard around here, but the clinical people believe they work just a little bit harder and what they do is more important than what we administration people do. Without us, there would be no resources and no information to get the clinical job done," he explained. "Many of our clinicians believe that their way of caring for a client is the only way to go. At times, they minimize the views of other staffers—who are as highly qualified but may not have gone through the same academic or theory-based training as the clinicians. People get pretty passionate about this."

Gray reported that maintaining a sustainable reimbursement structure is among the concerns that "keep him up at night," although he does meet with Dr. Harrison and the director of Clinical Services to commiserate and strategize. Another challenge is managing the human resources and professional needs of the large—and still growing—workforce that includes individuals with a wide variety of educational backgrounds and disciplines.

He thinks the organization does not pay enough attention to planning and marketing efforts, saying, "We get so focused on the clinical needs of our clients that we don't leave time as an organization to look ahead. Right now, that's working OK—mostly because we have dedicated people and because our IT system works so well. But I'm not sure how long that will last."

Property Manager

Three years ago, MCMHC hired Charles McKenny to handle all facility-related issues at both Gardner Place and Justin Place. A longtime, residential property manager, he maintains a small staff of one building engineer and three housekeepers; turnover has been high among the housekeepers. The board and Jervis-Washburn have instructed McKenny, who reports directly to Gray, to look for multiunit housing properties for possible purchase and conversion into condominiums for clients in the final phase of treatment. He believes many such properties are available in Middleboro and the northern communities of Hillsboro County but are limited in the southern area.

At Gardner Place, space is at a premium and the staff has been very adept at using the space creatively to adapt to the growing needs of the organization, but McKenny noted, "The building is out of space. It's not possible to double up any of the current offices or areas because of the confidential nature of what goes on in here, and it's not possible to add space. So we continue to apply Band-Aids to the place and make do with what we got."

Director of Clinical Services

Simone Beauchamp, RN, has been an MCMHC employee for 14 years. Before she was promoted to director six months ago, she was the associate manager of Emergency Services. Known for her high-energy, roll-up-your-sleeves attitude, she is passionate about making a difference in the lives of those with mental health needs. Dr. Harrison just asked her to conduct a thorough analysis of the programs under Clinical Services.

Although Beauchamp has six months to complete the assignment, she has already started and noticed some issues, such as duplication of services delivered by Adult Services and Child and Family Services. She wonders whether restructuring the programs by the type of service delivered—as opposed to by the client's age and family status—may eliminate or minimize the duplication. She also sees a need to work more closely with the director of Administrative Services to understand the financial implications of programs and services on MCMHC operations.

Clinical Services comprises five programs: Adult Services, Child and Family Services, Emergency Services, Quality and Compliance Services, and Education Services. Each program is headed by an associate manager who has skills, training, and experience appropriate for the role's tasks and responsibilities.

Adult Services

The adult program is designed for clients aged 18 years or older and provides a wide range of treatments and approaches as well as coordination of clinical and psychiatric rehabilitation. Services are offered at a variety of locations, depending on the needs of the client. Most clients are seen in Gardner Place, but care may also be delivered in the client's home or another healthcare facility. Among the most common services clients receive are counseling and therapy (individual or group), dialectical behavioral therapy, functional support (which assists with identifying and managing the use of community-based resources apart from MCMHC), illness management and recovery, psychiatric nursing, family support, mental health education, and vocational assistance. In addition, supported living services are provided in Justin Place.

Four standing interdisciplinary teams develop and deliver treatment plans to program clients. Every team includes one team leader-clinician and at least one other clinician. To maintain the greatest degree of flexibility, the teams do not specialize in a specific treatment modality, and the general approach followed for assessment is essentially the same for each team. On occasion, however, teams do "take on the clinical philosophy" of their respective team leader, which has created conflict among team members and complicated client transitions. Additional team members may be drawn from a rotating team, which is composed of clinicians with specific skills and experience that may augment those of the interdisciplinary teams.

Child and Family Services

This program is geared toward children aged 18 years and younger as well as their families. Like Adult Services, it has three standing interdisciplinary teams comprising a team leader-clinician and at least one other clinician; it also draws additional team members from a rotating team.

Services are provided in several settings, including Gardner Place, private homes, schools, and community-based facilities. In the past five years, the program has grown in schools because of the dramatic increase in substance abuse—opioid use in particular— among teenagers. MCMHC board and management have had frequent and ongoing conversations with state legislators to push for increased drug prevention and education as well as funding for such programming. At a recent board meeting, board members asked Jervis-Washburn to move youth substance abuse to the top of the organization's priorities.

Complicating this issue is that the federal government affords privacy protection to adolescents who seek treatment. Because providers may be prohibited from informing parents or guardians that their children are in treatment, they cannot bill for services rendered because parents or guardians may receive an Explanation of Benefits from their insurers if providers submit a claim.

Mental health services for children and their families are extremely limited in Hillsboro County. Communities ask their schools for an array of mental health counseling and education, and, in turn, schools seek help from MCMHC and the few providers in the county. Coordination of services between MCMHC and the schools has become increasingly problematic, however—although not necessarily because of the ongoing opioid crisis. Accommodating the goals and resource capabilities of both the schools and the organization remains a very serious challenge for MCMHC and its leadership.

Emergency Services

This program maintains a four-person team responsible for providing services to individuals or organizations facing a crisis. Phone and face-to-face assessment as well as referral and intervention are available on a 24/7 basis. About 50 percent of all assessments lead to referrals, which are frequently directed to the hospital emergency department (ED), and about 10 percent of those referred to the ED are admitted into the hospital. About two-thirds of the hospital admissions are voluntary. In addition, the team provides counseling and other appropriate services to individuals who have experienced or are experiencing traumatic events.

Quality and Compliance Services

The team for this program is charged with ensuring that MCMHC is structured and operates in a way that is consistent with federal and state guidelines. Generally speaking, compliance principles and standards exist for many areas, such as

◆ employee qualification, responsibilities, and credentialing;

◆ continuing professional education;

◆   professional sanctions;

◆   confidentiality, safety, and maintenance of documentation, records, and other information;

◆   clinical reviews;

◆   billing and financial reporting;

◆   conflict of interest;

◆   disclosure and reporting of employee misconduct; and

◆   employee and client rights.

Mental health is a heavily monitored and regulated sector of the healthcare industry, and the guidelines change frequently. As a response, MCMHC has increased the program's full-time staff from one to two individuals.

Developing behavioral health quality measures is a relatively new phenomenon influenced by the Affordable Care Act (ACA) of 2010. The ACA led to the publication of the National Quality Strategy (NQS), which "serves as a catalyst and compass for a nationwide focus on quality improvement efforts and approach to measuring quality." Part of the NQS pertains to behavioral health issues.

MCMHC believes strongly in creating and tracking appropriate measures of quality of care and has been working with SAMHSA's National Behavioral Health Quality Framework. This guideline focuses on the development of federal- and state-specific behavioral health barometers. Table 4.1 shows Hillsboro County's barometer as compared with that of the United States. Measuring and monitoring quality data enable MCMHC to develop a well-informed strategic plan.

Education Services

A staff of two health educators make up this program. These staff members develop and present behavioral health education customized for a client group or organization. For example, last year at the request of Carlstead Rayon, Education Services designed and then conducted for Carlstead Rayon's employees a four-hour educational session on the topic of stress management, substance abuse prevention strategies, and mindfulness. The training was well-received by both management and employees of the company. However, corporate clients such as Carlstead Rayon are hard to secure and engage.

Jervis-Washburn still believes the program as a whole is valuable and a market for it exists. More important, she believes educating the community is part of MCMHC's responsibility. She is particularly interested in expanding school-based education services— on the topics of alcohol and substance abuse, sexuality, and peer pressure—because schools do not have the expertise and dedicated staff to conduct such programs for students. Funding for this plan is nonexistent, however. During a discussion at a board meeting, a board member asked, "While we're on this issue, I've been wondering why we have a separate Education Services unit. Can't it be merged or spread across the other programs? We already have educators in the other programs. Anyway, isn't it the job of health teachers to educate their students about drugs and sex and other things?"

On the web at ache.org/books/ Middleboro2

STAFFING

Table 4.2 displays MCMHC's staffing budget by program and position. In many cases, staff has the flexibility to work as needed in more than one division. The budget reflects the manner in which staff members are allocated among programs for accounting purposes.

MCMHC has a disadvantage in recruiting and retaining clinical staff for a number of reasons:

1. Compensation levels are somewhat lower than market level for many positions, although few employment opportunities are available in Hillsboro County for mental health clinicians.

2. Many positions can be filled adequately by an individual with a baccalaureate degree, but other positions—such as therapists—require graduate and even postgraduate degrees. Given the compensation shortfalls, attracting educationally qualified individuals is challenging. In addition, some positions require even a master's-level clinician to obtain two years of staff experience prior to working independently. It has not been unusual for master's-level clinicians to work for MCMHC for two to three years to gain experience and then move out of the area to an organization that offers higher compensation.

3. Many healthcare organizations compete to hire individuals who are qualified to prescribe medications (e.g., nurse practitioners), but MCMHC has often not been successful at recruiting and retaining such staff because it offers low compensation.

The board has assigned Jervis-Washburn, Dr. Harrison, and Gray to develop a long-term strategy to address these ongoing problems.

Four psychiatrists work at least part-time for MCMHC, but only two of them—Dr. Stanzl (the medical director) and Dr. Actor (a board member)—have affiliations at MIDCARE. The other two psychiatrists have admitting privileges at Capital City General Hospital.

Last year, MCMHC implemented a tracking system that requires all staff members to log their time by activity, on 15-minute intervals. Although not a significant change for some clinicians, the logging requirement was initially resisted by many other staff. Jervis-Washburn had to spend a substantial amount of time explaining the importance of the procedure for cost-finding, which is a long-term goal of the organization, in anticipation of bundled-pricing initiatives. Still, the feeling among many employees—including clinicians—was that the change represented management's lack of trust in their professionalism. The tracking system also highlighted the US Department of Labor's requirement for organizations to pay for overtime work.

According to Jervis-Washburn, the relationship between MCMHC and private-practice mental health providers in the county is excellent: "They know we provide very good client services and are not reluctant to refer to us. We have worked very well to coordinate our care with theirs. At times, though, it appears they prefer to send to us the uninsured or Medicaid clients and keep the private-pay clients for themselves. We have been working with them to reach a more equitable arrangement, but frankly I'm not optimistic." These are the four private mental health practices in the county:

1. *Sockalexis Center.* Located in Jasper, this group is staffed by four PhD psychologists, three master's-level social workers, and three substance abuse counselors. It has the contract to provide services to Jasper schools and is developing a substance abuse program as well as an employee assistance program for some employers in Jasper. It also has contacted Physician Care Services, Inc. to explore a partnership to provide occupational health services.

2. *Royman Oaks, LLC.* Located in Statesville, the practice is staffed by two master's-level clinical social workers and four occupational therapists. It focuses on employment counseling and job-placement assistance.

3. *Grosvenor Arms.* Located in Jasper, this seven-bed adult group home is staffed by three residential counselors, one part-time clinical psychologist, one master's-level clinical social worker, and an MFT.

4. *Greenwood Group.* Located east of Jasper, the group is staffed by a psychiatrist with admitting privileges at MIDCARE, a psychiatrist with admitting privileges at Capital City General Hospital, two PhD clinical psychologists, one master's-level clinical social worker, one MFT, four substance abuse counselors, and several health-and-wellness personnel. The practice has been successful in penetrating the commercially insured substance abuse market and has a reputation for providing high-quality care in its "upscale" office.

FINANCE

Medicaid is the major payer at MCMHC. As shown in table 4.3, Medicaid accounts for approximately 75 percent of net client service revenue. This percentage has increased slightly over the past three years. Commercial insurance, such as Blue Cross/Blue Shield, is the second largest source of client service revenue, but this percentage has decreased slightly over the same time period. Table 4.4 displays the organization's published charges for the most common services. At MCMHC, charges for services are set on a sliding schedule, according to income. The minimum fee is charged for clients who are at or under the federal poverty level.

Internal Revenue Service Form 990 requires that salaries be released for the key employees of the organization. These are the key employees at MCMHC:

Name	Position	Current Salary ($)
Birgitta Stanislavska, MD	Psychiatrist	174,000
Gerald Considine, MD	Psychiatrist	160,000
Stephanie Jervis-Washburn	Executive Director	124,286
Ivan Stanzl, MD	Medical Director	122,250
Shanique Harrison, PhD	Senior Director	90,000
Jorge Ramirez, PhD	Clinical Psychologist	88,000
Elizabeth Gretsch, PhD	Clinical Psychologist	85,000
Simone Beauchamp, RN	Director, Clinical Services	82,500
Sophie Juarez, PMHNP-BC	Nurse Practitioner	82,000
Clement Gray	Director, Administrative Services	80,000
Grace Walker, ACNP-BC	Nurse Practitioner	80,000
Scott Burford	Director, Information Technology	70,000

On the web at ache.org/books/ Middleboro2

Tables 4.5 and 4.6 are MCMHC's balance sheet and statement of revenues and expenses, respectively.

MARKETING

Table 4.7 displays the client volume by service for the past four years; the data reflect unduplicated client counts. Table 4.8 shows the results of a special study of the most frequently ordered services by program; psychotherapy takes that designation across all programs. As shown in table 4.9, the largest share of the organization's clients in all service areas comes from Middleboro; this is not surprising, given that MCMHC began and is still headquartered in the city. Jervis-Washburn has given Gray the task of drafting a strategic and marketing plan to enhance the organization's profile outside of Middleboro.

To date, the organization has never had a marketing program. It believed for a long time that its excellent reputation and long-standing history in the area would be enough to attract a solid client base. In addition, the board tended to favor good services over market share and profitability. Within the past five years, however, competitors have entered the area, bringing along with them aggressive marketing campaigns that target local employers and what Gray has called "the high-paying client who needs substance abuse help."

In addition to increasing penetration in existing markets, the board and management team are making plans to identify needs or demands that could catalyze new programs and services that will showcase the staff's strengths and expertise. As Jervis-Washburn put it, "We have done well through the years doing what we do, but potential programs, services, and clients are waiting for us to discover them. It is incumbent on us to find them and move forward on a select few."

Table 4.1
MCMHC
Behavioral
Health
Barometer

Factor		Hillsboro County (%)	United States* (%)
Marijuana Use for Past Month, Aged 12–17 Years		6.4	7.4
Nonmedical Use of Pain Reliever for Past Year, Aged 12–17 Years	Female	9.4	5.4
	Male	7.3	4.0
Illicit Drug Use for Past Month, Aged 12–17 Years			
Cocaine		1.0	0.2
Heroin		2.3	0.1
Psychotherapeutics		6.1	2.6
Major Depressive Episode for Past Year, Aged 12–17 Years	**Total**	**13**	**11.4**
	Female	19.8	17.3
	Male	6.9	5.7
Treatment for Major Depressive Episode for Past Year, Aged 12–17 Years		37.5	41.2
Serious Thoughts of Suicide for Past Year, Aged 18+ Years		4.3	3.9
Serious Mental Illness (SMI) for Past Year, Aged 18+ Years		5.3	4.1
Mental Health Treatment/Counseling for Past Year, Among Aged 18+ Years with SMI		57.9	68.5
Alcohol Dependence or Abuse for Past Year, Aged 12+ Years		6.5	6.4
Illicit Drug Dependence or Abuse for Past Year, Aged 12+ Years		3.4	2.7
Heavy Alcohol Use for Past Month, Aged 21+ Years		6.7	6.6
Substance Abuse Treatment (Alcohol) for Past Year, Aged 12+ Years		7.2	7.6
Substance Abuse Treatment (Illicit Drugs) for Past Year, Aged 12+ Years		13.3	14.6

Source: Substance Abuse and Mental Health Services Administration (SAMHSA). 2015. *Behavioral Health Barometer: United States, 2015.* HHS Publication No. SMA–16–Baro–2015. Rockville, MD: SAMHSA.

Administrative Services		
Position	**FTE**	**Payroll ($)**
Executive Director	1.00	124,286
Medical Director	0.75	122,250
Senior Director	1.00	90,000
Director, Clinical Services	1.00	82,500
Executive Assistant	1.00	48,500
Director, Admin. Services	1.00	80,000
Sr. Administrative Assistant	1.00	38,000
HR Assistant	1.00	43,500
IT Manager	1.00	70,000
IT Asst. Manager	1.00	50,000
Records Assistant	1.00	28,000
Finance Manager	1.00	60,000
A/R Assistant	1.00	45,000
Accountant	1.00	45,000
A/R Staff Reps.	2.00	58,000
Insurance Rep.	1.00	29,500
Facility Manager	1.00	48,000
Maintenance Staff	2.00	54,000
Housekeeping Staff	4.00	92,000
Facility Psychologist	0.40	40,000
Residential Counselors	3.00	93,000
Facility Assistant	0.50	18,500
Facility Therapist	0.50	18,500
Housing Coordinator	1.00	41,000
Total	**29.15**	**1,419,536**

Adult Services		
Position	**FTE**	**Payroll ($)**
Team Leaders	4.00	194,500
Records Assistant	1.00	29,000
Psychiatrist	0.80	174,000
Health/Wellness Mentors	5.00	178,000
Intake/Admission Staff	3.00	93,500
Receptionists	2.00	46,000
Psychiatric Nurse	0.40	37,500
Outreach Therapists	23.00	850,000
Other Therapists	12.00	435,000
Program Assistants	4.00	130,000
Administrative Assistants	2.00	47,000
Transcriptionists	2.00	52,000
Sr. Social Worker	1.00	49,000
QI Associate	0.80	37,000
Nurse Practitioner	1.00	82,000
Psychologist	1.00	85,000
Total	**63.00**	**2,519,500**

Quality and Compliance Services		
Position	**FTE**	**Payroll ($)**
QI Coordinator	1.00	43,000
QI Assistant	1.00	38,000
Total	**2.00**	**81,000**

Education Services		
Position	**FTE**	**Payroll ($)**
Administrative Assistant	1.00	27,500
Health Educators	2.00	86,000
Total	**3.00**	**93,500**

Table 4.2
MCMHC Staffing Budget

On the web at ache.org/books/ Middleboro2

continued

Table 4.2
MCMHC
Staffing Budget
(continued)

*On the web at
ache.org/books/
Middleboro2*

Child and Family Services		
Position	**FTE**	**Payroll ($)**
Team Leaders	3.00	145,000
Outreach Therapists	14.00	515,000
Psychiatrist	0.80	160,000
Spectrum Specialists	4.00	130,000
Intake/Admission Staff	2.00	59,500
Administrative Assistants	1.20	32,000
Program Assistants	2.50	75,000
Transcriptionists	1.50	39,000
Psychologist	0.50	58,000
Records Assistants	1.00	28,900
Receptionists	2.00	46,000
School Therapists	2.00	96,000
Other Therapists	10.00	367,000
QI Associate	0.80	37,000
Total	**45.30**	**1,788,400**

Summary		
	FTE	**Payroll ($)**
Administrative	29.15	1,419,536
Child and Family	45.30	1,788,400
Adult	63.00	2,519,500
Emergency	14.80	701,500
Education	3.00	93,500
Quality/Compliance	2.00	81,000
Total	**157.25**	**6,603,436**

Emergency Services		
Position	**FTE**	**Payroll ($)**
Intake/Admission Staff	3.00	90,000
Emerg. Technicians	5.00	254,000
Psychiatrist	0.10	18,000
Records Assistant	0.50	15,000
Psychologist	1.00	88,000
Administrative Assistant	1.00	25,000
Transcriptionist	1.00	25,000
Therapists	3.00	97,000
Nurse Practitioner	1.00	80,000
QI Associate	0.20	9,500
Total	**15.80**	**$701,500**

Notes: (1) For fiscal year ending December 31. (2) Numbers are in US dollars. (3) This table includes salary only. An additional 19% should be added to account for fringe benefits. (4) A/R: accounts receivable; FTE: full-time equivalent; HR: human resources; IT: information technology; QI: quality improvement.

Payer	Programs			
	Adult Services (%)	Child and Family Services (%)	Emergency Services (%)	Total (%)
Self-Pay	5.7	3.5	3.1	3.7
Commercial Insurance	16.9	9.6	15.3	14.5
Medicaid	59.8	86.9	77.2	74.8
Medicare	7.5	0	2.9	7

Table 4.3
MCMHC Payer Mix and Percentage of Client Service Revenue by Program

Note: For fiscal year ending December 31.

Service	CPT Code	Rate ($)	Minimum Fee ($)
Intake/Diagnostic Evaluation	90781	185	10
Individual Psychotherapy	90834	125	8
Group Therapy	90853	50	3
Marriage/Family Therapy	90846	145	10
Emergency Treatment/Visit	Variable	400	20
Psychological Testing	Variable	110	8
PhD Psychologist Consultation	Hourly	250	15
Master's-Level Consultation	Hourly	150	12
Other Therapy	Variable	75	7
Educational Program	Variable	400	N/A
Nursing Services	Variable	150	12
Psychiatric Services			
Injection Administration	96372	25	5
New Patient—Level 1	99201	65	10
New Patient—Level 2	99202	80	12
New Patient—Level 3	99203	107	13
New Patient—Level 4	99204	205	14
New Patient—Level 5	99205	297	15
Established Patient—Level 1	99211	48	6
Established Patient—Level 2	99212	65	9
Established Patient—Level 3	99213	95	10
Establshed Patient—Level 4	99214	155	11
Established Patient—Level 5	99215	225	12

Table 4.4
MCMHC Published Charges for Most Common Services

Notes: (1) Fees—in US dollars in this table—are for clients at the federal poverty level. A full fee is charged for clients at 200% of the federal poverty level and above. (2) Income verification is required before treatment (other than emergency). (3) CPT: current procedural terminology.

Table 4.5
MCMHC
Balance Sheet

*On the web at
ache.org/books/
Middleboro2*

	2019	2018	2017	2016
Assets				
Current Assets				
Cash	697,614	396,970	568,825	591,529
A/R Client Services	1,483,295	1,538,511	1,634,938	1,493,082
Less Allowances	(693,829)	(736,584)	(763,088)	(774,209)
Net A/R Client Services	789,466	801,927	871,850	718,873
Other A/R	35,829	36,893	50,909	39,204
Inventory	14,500	15,903	13,084	15,689
Prepaid Accounts	73,829	79,888	43,892	56,356
Total Current Assets	**1,611,238**	**1,331,581**	**1,548,560**	**1,421,651**
Other Assets, Limited Use				
Restricted Building Fund	5,764,003	5,182,698	3,998,920	2,757,183
Halloway Fund	400,000	400,000	400,000	400,000
Total Other Assets	**6,164,003**	**5,582,698**	**4,398,920**	**3,157,183**
Property, Plant, and Equipment				
Furniture and Equipment	1,542,050	1,587,354	1,387,444	1,328,637
Computer Leasehold	450,000	450,000	450,000	400,000
Total	**1,992,050**	**2,037,354**	**1,837,444**	**1,728,637**
Less Accum. Depreciation	(893,849)	(829,849)	(746,849)	(641,849)
Total	**1,098,201**	**1,207,505**	**1,090,595**	**1,086,788**
Total Assets	**8,873,442**	**8,121,784**	**7,038,075**	**5,665,622**
Liabilities				
Current Liabilities				
Accounts Payable	180,483	150,258	146,903	69,384
Notes Payable	125,000	154,900	108,690	98,045
Accrued Benefits and Taxes	274,594	218,504	194,856	235,043
Contracts and Grant Payable	34,590	46,390	47,930	53,892

continued

	2019	2018	2017	2016
Other Accrued Expenses	353,920	294,830	248,594	210,392
Total Current Liabilities	**968,587**	**864,882**	**746,973**	**666,756**
Long-Term Debt	250,000	275,004	302,982	352,483
Total Liabilities	**1,218,587**	**1,139,886**	**1,049,955**	**1,019,239**
Net Assets				
Fund Balance—Unrestricted	1,390,852	1,289,200	1,289,200	1,289,200
Restricted Fund—Halloway	400,000	400,000	400,000	400,000
Restricted Building Fund	5,864,003	5,292,698	4,298,920	2,957,183
Total Net Assets	**7,654,855**	**6,981,898**	**5,988,120**	**4,646,383**
Net Assets + Total Liabilities	**8,873,442**	**8,121,784**	**7,038,075**	**5,665,622**

Table 4.5
MCMHC
Balance Sheet
(continued)

*On the web at
ache.org/books/
Middleboro2*

Notes: (1) For fiscal years ending December 31. (2) Numbers are in US dollars. (3) A/R: accounts receivable.

Table 4.6
MCMHC
Statement of
Revenues and
Expenses

*On the web at
ache.org/books/
Middleboro2*

	2019	2018	2017	2016
Revenues				
Fees Billed	15,689,421	15,356,832	14,938,729	14,589,374
Less Adjustments	(5,177,509)	(5,221,323)	(4,929,781)	(4,960,387)
Net Fees Billed	10,511,912	10,135,509	10,008,948	9,628,987
Grant 1	50,000	75,000	115,000	109,000
Grant 2	45,000	45,000	50,000	50,000
State PH	36,000	45,000	59,000	75,000
Town/County	118,000	146,000	150,000	150,000
United Way	2,500	5,000	0	0
MIDCARE	45,000	50,304	41,000	45,980
WHS	11,000	8,500	2,500	5,600
Donations and Other	318,674	479,372	678,743	709,583
Total	**11,138,086**	**10,989,685**	**11,105,191**	**10,774,150**
Expenses				
Salaries/Wages	6,509,875	6,365,098	6,142,320	5,927,339
Benefits and Payroll Taxes	1,236,876	1,209,369	1,167,041	1,126,194
Rental	10,000	12,500	15,000	12,000
Insurance	140,000	142,000	150,000	145,000
Depreciation	64,000	83,000	105,000	105,000
Other	2,504,378	2,183,940	2,184,093	2,089,035
Total	**10,465,129**	**9,995,907**	**9,763,454**	**9,404,568**
Excess (Deficit) of Revenue over Expenses (Total)	**672,957**	**993,778**	**1,341,737**	**1,369,582**
Excess (Deficit) of Revenue over Expenses (Operating)	**46,783**	**197,672**	**290,695**	**224,722**

Notes: (1) Years ending December 31. (2) Numbers are in US dollars. (3) State PH: State Department of Public Health; WHS: Webster Health System.

Program	2019	2018	2017	2016
Adult Services	3,954	3,886	3,769	3,734
Child and Family Services	1,458	1,539	1,490	1,501
Crisis Calls	2,459	2,306	1,847	1,739

Table 4.7
MCMHC Clients Served by Program

Note: For fiscal year ending December 31.

Program	Percentage of Total Billed Hours
Adult Services	
Psychotherapy (Individual)	41.5
Family Support Services	26.5
Group Therapy	5.3
Psychiatric Evaluation/Management	7.8
Intake/Evaluation—Psychotherapy	9.9
Psychoeducation	1.8
Child and Family Services	
Psychotherapy (Individual)	55.5
Family Support Services	7.1
Intake/Evaluation—Psychotherapy	10.3
Family Therapy	18.1
Psychiatric Evaluation/Management	3.5
Psychological Testing	2.5
Emergency Services	
Crisis Psychotherapy	77.9
Emergency Services (Nonspecified)	7.1

Table 4.8
MCMHC Special Study of Most Common Services by Program

Table 4.9
MCMHC
Percentage of
Program Clients
by Residence

Town/City	Children and Family Services (%)	Adult Services (%)	Emergency Services (%)	Total (%)
Middleboro	42	41	64	46
Jasper	18	26	15	21
Harris City	17	9	5	8
Statesville	9	8	5	8
Mifflenville	9	8	4	6
Carterville	4	4	3	4
Minortown	1	2	1	1
Boalsburg	2	1	1	1
Others in Hillsboro County	3	2	0	2
Out of Hillsboro County	5	3	2	3
Total	**100**	**100**	**100**	**100**

Note: For fiscal year ending December 31.

WEBSTER HEALTH SYSTEM

Webster Health System (WHS)—formerly called Webster Hospital—constitutes a hospital and a for-profit organization that are jointly owned by the system and members of the medical staff. The hospital is accredited by the American Osteopathic Association and is an affiliate member of Capital City–based Osteopathic Hospitals of America, Inc. In its recent report to the American Hospital Association, the hospital indicated it employs 704 personnel; is licensed to operate 105 inpatient beds; and has met all the conditions necessary for Medicaid, Medicare, and Blue Cross insurance coverage. Currently, it staffs 85 inpatient beds and has a case-mix index of 1.2155. Table 5.1 lists the hospital's services.

HISTORY

PHYSICAL STRUCTURE

The original 1930s hospital was a three-floor brick structure built to accommodate 70 inpatient beds. Surrounding the facility were houses purchased by the hospital. Over the years, the building has undergone expansions and renovations. For example, in 1989, the space was reconfigured to increase the number of inpatient beds to 105, an addition that was later cut back to its current size of 85. The most recent modernization program was completed seven years ago. It installed modern features that make the hospital more attractive and rearranged spaces to make operations and care delivery more efficient. It also expanded the maternity unit so that, when possible, all maternity services—including labor and delivery—are contained in the mother's private room. The homes next to the facility have been converted into offices for the 12 members of the medical staff. All of the other land on the hospital campus remains undeveloped. The hospital and adjacent offices, each of which complies with current building standards and codes, sit on a 16-acre campus located in southeastern Middleboro next to the interstate highway.

WEBSTER HOSPITAL

Founded in 1930 by Dr. Edward W. Webster as a short-term, general acute care nonprofit, the hospital has had close ties with Osteopathic Medical Center (OMC) in Capital City even before Osteopathic Hospitals of America (OHA) was established. Dr. Webster was a senior osteopathic physician at OMC, and in 1929, upon arriving in Middleboro, he began a community campaign to found a hospital that would serve as an alternative to Middleboro Community Hospital. He was the first superintendent of Webster Hospital and was successful in establishing osteopathic medicine in Hillsboro County. The Webster family still financially supports WHS. In the past 20 years, his sons and grandsons have continued to increase its endowment.

Since 1930, the hospital's relationship with MIDCARE—then called Middleboro Community Hospital—has been strained. Here are some examples:

◆ In 1996, Webster Hospital and Middleboro Community Hospital dissolved their more than 30-year joint venture corporation for shared laundry services. Middleboro Community Hospital elected a provision in the original 1965 agreement to buy Webster Hospital's share of the joint venture, even though Webster Hospital wished to retain the partnership. At the time of the forced sale, Middleboro Community Hospital indicated that its need for laundry services could only be met if it fully owned the laundry corporation. Middleboro Community Hospital did offer to provide laundry services to Webster Hospital on an annual contract, but Webster Hospital determined that establishing its own laundry service would be more efficient.

◆ In 1998, Webster Hospital terminated a joint education agreement with Middleboro Community Hospital. Under this agreement, staff members of both hospitals received continuing education at both institutions.

◆ In 1999, a formal joint committee of the boards of each hospital explored the possibility of a merger of the two organizations. Although supported by both CEOs, the merger was deemed not feasible by the committee. Since that time, the two entities have had minimal contact and have been increasingly competitive with each other.

◆ In 2000, when Webster Hospital signed the affiliation agreement with OHA and became WHS, the president and board chair of Middleboro Community Hospital published an open letter in the *Middleboro Sentinel*. The letter indicated these leaders' disappointment that a community hospital in Middleboro was now going to be "directed by a medical center based outside of the community" in Capital City. The letter went on to say, "We wish it had been obvious to us that Webster Hospital needed help to continue its operations. We would have assisted with providing quality care at a reasonable price for our community, as we do now."

Today, the sole remaining agreement between the two hospitals is compelled by regulation. Under this agreement, WHS patients and others under the care of an osteopathic doctor may come to MIDCARE for ambulatory cancer treatment. This provision was required by the state when it issued to MIDCARE the certificate of need for this service.

OHA AFFILIATION

Established in 1990 and headquartered in Capital City, OHA was developed to provide corporate direction and control for osteopathic hospitals in the tri-state region. It is a nonprofit corporation with a regional network currently composed of 18 affiliated organizations. These affiliates are nonprofit, community osteopathic hospitals that provide tertiary care. Each hospital elects to affiliate with the system and retains its independent corporate status. OHA has a board of directors chaired by Harry Swift. Annually, the board votes to retain an affiliate member. The board also has the ability to sever an affiliation contract with just a three-month notice.

As an affiliate member of OHA, WHS is subject to OHA's affiliate program. Under this program, a hospital agrees to do the following when it signs a formal affiliation contract (renewed annually):

◆ Retain the hospital's affiliate membership for at least three years, and elect one person to the OHA board of directors.

◆ Provide consulting and/or active privileges to all qualified physicians whom OHA recommends.

◆ Record all patient care information using the OHA medical records system, and share an abstract of this information with OHA.

◆ Purchase all supply items (medical and nonmedical) and durable medical equipment through OHA.

◆ Share with OHA a draft of the hospital's revenue and expense budget for the next fiscal year, and bring to the hospital's board OHA's comments on this budget.

◆ Allow OHA the first option for purchase if the hospital decides to change its ownership status.

◆ Pay OHA an annual affiliation fee of 0.5 percent of the hospital's gross charges or $1 million, whichever is less.

In return for this affiliation, a hospital receives the following services and benefits at no additional cost:

◆ Board education

◆ Development of the hospital's strategic plan and quality assurance system

◆ Access to capital for projects approved by OHA at the prime rate + 0.2 percent

◆ Continuing medical education

◆ Consulting services related to electronic health records, financial management, human resources administration, health benefit surveys, and new service development

◆ Tele-Med Services, a high-speed voice and video communications link between the attending physicians at an affiliated hospital and physicians at OMC

◆ Regional and community-specific advertising

Under the affiliation agreement, a hospital may lease from OHA a CEO at cost; use OHA-marked services, such as Quick Med; and book OMC Air Evac transportation at cost. Currently, 62 percent of all osteopathic hospitals in the tri-state area are affiliated with OHA.

OHA is organized into three separately operated corporations: OMC, OHA Hospital Services, and OHA Ventures.

OMC

Located in Capital City, OMC is a nonprofit, 210-bed medical center that provides a full range of acute and tertiary care services. It is a Level I trauma center as well as a designated teaching hospital that offers approved residencies in most medical specialties. Medical interns and residents visit WHS regularly as part of their community medicine training. Five years ago, in collaboration with State University, OMC launched degree programs for physician assistants and advanced nurse practitioners, with numerous specialties for the latter. Dr. Samuel Gilbert, an osteopath, is the president of OMC.

OHA Hospital Services, Inc.

This nonprofit corporation, based in Capital City, provides services to OMC and all OHA-affiliated hospitals. Currently, it offers the following services:

- ◆ Retirement planning

- ◆ Hospital risk-management programs

- ◆ Health services consulting

- ◆ Outplacement and recruiting

- ◆ Capital financing

- ◆ Meaningful use advisory

- ◆ EHR and medical record systems development and support

- ◆ Data warehousing

- ◆ Pharmacy contract management

OHA Hospital Services is headed by Garrett Fulerman.

OHA Ventures, Inc.

This Capital City for-profit is headed by Rose Flagstaff and currently specializes in managing medical groups. It also owns and operates medical office buildings. Three years ago, OHA Ventures introduced a joint purchase and management program that enables an OHA-affiliated hospital to copurchase and comanage individual medical practices with OHA Ventures. To date, no physician practice affiliated with WHS has elected to use OHA Ventures as a practice manager.

In the same period as the launch of the joint program, OHA Ventures independently began purchasing orthopedic, family practice, and cardiology practices of physicians affiliated with OHA-affiliated hospitals. As a result, all of these physicians become employees of OHA Ventures and are granted consulting status at OMC. Because OHA-affiliated hospitals are, generally, not interested in purchasing and managing medical practices, OHA Ventures had to justify this program to the OHA board. Flagstaff reasoned that the purchase would relieve physicians from the burden of practice management, allowing them to practice medicine instead, and would prevent osteopathic practices from being bought by allopathic hospital systems.

To date, OHA Ventures has purchased 24 medical practices and has three outstanding offers. In Hillsboro County, OHA Ventures owns three practices in Jasper: an OB/GYN practice (sold by Drs. Morton and Salt), a family practice (sold by Drs. Dadoveci, Child, Megg, Kidd, and Lady), and a pediatric practice (sold by four physicians not affiliated with WHS).

One hospital in another region of the state withdrew its OHA affiliation when OHA Ventures outbid it for an orthopedic practice. Three affiliates sued OHA Ventures for breach of contract, claiming these purchases violate the affiliate contractual relationship. The case was dismissed, with the court ruling that the "affiliate contract does not prohibit OHA or its subsidiaries from purchasing medical practices, especially given that the owners of the medical practices can entertain multiple offers, including offers from the affiliate member."

GOVERNANCE

WHS's board of trustees is composed of eight individuals. The 100 incorporators elect trustees on the basis of nominations by the board's nominating committee. Trustees are elected for four-year terms, with the stipulation that they may serve no longer than two consecutive terms. Current board trustees of WHS are as follows; the (number)* indicates the number of years remaining on current board term, and the (number)† indicates the trustee's second term:

WHS Board of Trustees

Members	*Residence*
Daniel Will (2)*†, *Chair*	
Attorney, Will & Associates	Middleboro
Harlan Crowe (3), *Vice Chair*	
President, Farmers and Merchants Bank	Mifflenville
Yolanda Nice (4), *Secretary*	
Director of Human Resources, U.S. Parts	Jasper

    Belinda Bond (1)[+], *Treasurer*
       Retired stockbroker   Boalsburg

    Eric Martin (4), *At-Large*
       President and CEO, Carlstead Rayon   Middleboro

    Tracy Meyer (2), *At-Large*
       Vice president of Finance, River Industries   Middleboro

    Samuel Mudd, DO (3), *At-Large*
       Retired physician   Middleboro

    Mike Webster (1), *At-Large*
       Proprietor, Webster Family Farm   Statesville

The standing committees of the board are as follows:

- Executive (Will, Crowe, Nice, Bond)

- Finance (Crowe, Bond, Martin)

- Joint Conference (Will, Dr. Taff, Swisher)

- Long-Range Planning (All Trustees)

- Medical Manpower/Credentials (Dr. Mudd, Meyer, Webster)

- Nominating (Nice, Crowe, Martin)

- Quality Assurance (Meyer, Will, Dr. Mudd)

    The board meets monthly, the executive committee meets twice a month, and other committees meet as needed (usually monthly). Every December, the board—along with the hospital auxiliary—sponsors a hospital fund-raising event called Holiday Ball at the Middleboro Golf Club.

MANAGEMENT TEAM AND ORGANIZATIONAL STRUCTURE

PRESIDENT AND CEO

Steve Swisher, CPA, was promoted to president and CEO nine months ago. Prior to this appointment, he was vice president of Administrative Services and chief financial officer (CFO) at WHS for 14 years. He holds a bachelor in accounting and a master of business administration from a midwestern university and is a member of the Healthcare Financial Management Association. Before coming to WHS, he was a senior fiscal analyst at Blue Cross and Blue Shield in Capital City.

The position of president and CEO became vacant when the well-loved and respected Edith Masterman retired from the job four years ago. WHS used a national executive search firm to identify qualified candidates. The first search yielded no candidates acceptable to the board, but the second search resulted in the hiring of Stella MacArthur. Twelve months later, however, she reached a mutual agreement with the board and resigned from the post. The board offered no reason for her immediate departure. During another lengthy search, Swisher was appointed acting president.

When interviewed, Swisher noted the board's concerns regarding changing market dynamics, especially in Jasper; the need to recruit new physicians for WHS's primary markets; the potential addition of specialized services; the system's financial challenges; and the development of a regional accountable care organization. He offered a "that's confidential" in response to reports that WHS's affiliation with OHA has become difficult, but he said this to clear up other rumors: "Our strength is our people, who are highly skilled and dedicated to our mission. We focus on keeping them happy, so I'm not aware of any behind-the-scenes union activity among our clerical and administrative staff. In regards to the turmoil associated with my office, there's none—no turmoil. We stumbled a few times during the recruitment process, but I think that may be due to our inexperience. Edith was so good at this job for so long that we relied too much on her instead of developing our own competencies and ensuring our policies match our changing needs. For example, we don't have an experienced governing board. That's because our bylaws dictate we remove the experienced trustees after serving only two terms on the board, so we lose the organizational knowledge and insights they gained during their tenure. That holds us back, and we have to address that and other issues if we want to create a strong vision and strategies for the future."

VICE PRESIDENT OF ADMINISTRATIVE SERVICES AND CFO

June Taylor, CPA, replaced Swisher in this position. She was promoted from the position of deputy chief fiscal officer, where she had been for ten years. She holds a bachelor in accounting and a master of business administration from State University and is a member of the Healthcare Financial Management Association.

As Swisher's direct report, she has extensive responsibilities, including overseeing these departments: Admitting, Business Office, Central Supply, Housekeeping, Laundry, Maintenance, Medical Records, Personnel, Purchasing, Security, and Telecommunications. In addition, Taylor is in charge of a laundry service contract between WHS and Hillsboro County Health Department. Several years ago, when WHS began searching for clients to use its excess laundry capacity (caused by the decrease in inpatient days), Taylor developed a contractual program that has WHS providing laundry services to Manorhaven, the long-term care facility owned and operated by Hillsboro County Health Department. She indicated that this contract, aside from being good business, keeps the hospital's laundry service an efficient operation with its current level of staffing.

Another one of her many duties is as chief personnel officer, which has become "an almost full-time job." She said, "Our HR staff have had a hard time filling openings because there seems to be a lack of qualified, acceptable professionals in our area. We're working hard to attract them."

Although Taylor remains optimistic about the future, she has worries. "The hospital's inpatient capacity has gotten about as small as it should," she said. "Too much smaller, and it will become less efficient." As a result, she advocates a competitive strategy to capture ambulatory and inpatient market share historically served by MIDCARE. "The good news is the hospital has a win–win relationship with the staff, including the medical staff. They know our needs, we know theirs, and we are committed to joint success," she added.

Five years ago, WHS installed an electronic health record system, with full support from OHA. All medical practices owned by WHS—through Webster Physicians—are connected to the system, while other affiliated practices can access the system by purchasing or leasing the software from WHS or OHA and then logging in through an online portal. Technical oversight of the system is provided by a private contractor and OHA Hospital Services. Taylor does not think the hospital needs a chief information systems officer at this time: "Our current arrangement with OHA for consulting services seems to be working well. We have their expertise, and the contractor is very responsive to our needs."

Vice President of Professional Services

Ellen Wilgus has been employed by WHS for 15 years and was director of Physical Therapy right before her appointment as vice president. She holds a bachelor in physical therapy from State University. She has served as president of the state chapter of the American Physical Therapy Association and remains active in professional organizations related to physical therapy and rehabilitation.

Wilgus reports to the president and has responsibility for the following departments: Anesthesiology, Dietary, Laboratory, Pharmacy, Physical Therapy, Radiology, Respiratory Therapy, and Social Services. The ever-increasing complexity of hospital management and the greater competition from MIDCARE are among her top concerns; she thinks WHS faces an uncertain future, even with its affiliation with OHA. "The hospital's decision to retain extra staff—and retrain them when needed—as it changes its primary orientation away from inpatient services made all the difference in the world," she explained. "Staff became creative problem solvers because they knew they were not going to lose their jobs." She also indicated feeling supported by her hardworking department heads and especially proud that the most recent accreditation review found no significant deficiencies in any of the departments she oversees.

Years ago, Wilgus headed the management task force that implemented the maternity unit redesign and expansion. For her exemplary performance on the task force, she earned an official commendation from the medical staff as well as a special recognition from the board and the former president. Currently, she leads the continuous quality improvement team's effort to shorten the length of inpatient hospital stays per diagnosis-related group.

VICE PRESIDENT OF CLINICAL SERVICES

Gretta Schmidt, RN, was hired to replace a retiring vice president. Prior to coming to WHS, she held numerous nursing positions at MIDCARE, including associate director of nursing, making her the first senior management member to have worked for a direct competitor; her selection was a unanimous decision approved by leadership. She graduated from MIDCARE School of Nursing, has a bachelor and master in nursing from State University, and is active in the state nursing association.

Like the other vice presidents, Schmidt reports to the president and is in charge of multiple departments, including Clinical Education, Pediatrics, Intensive Care, Medical Surgical Unit I, Medical Surgical Unit II, Medical Surgical Unit III, Emergency and Outpatient Departments, and Staff Development. WHS maintains a high nurse–patient ratio and is making progress in achieving an all-RN (registered nurse) nursing staff, something she is concentrating on.

When interviewed, Schmidt was careful with her remarks about MIDCARE, stating, "I'm unsure about the real issues between MIDCARE and this hospital. I sure am very impressed, though, by the high clinical competence of the nursing staff here. Nurse turnover is not as big an issue here as it is at MIDCARE." She is equally complimentary of the professional relationship between physicians and nurses. "Although there is no formal joint practice program, most aspects of joint practice characterize the nurse–physician relationship," she said.

VICE PRESIDENT OF MARKETING

David Story, who is from a prominent family in Middleboro, has been the marketing head at WHS for 12 years and, before that, was deputy director of marketing for a durable medical equipment firm in Capital City. He holds a liberal arts degree and a master of health administration from an eastern university and is a member of the American College of Healthcare Executives (ACHE).

His tenure at WHS has been productive from the beginning, and these successes have not been limited to marketing. He secured the certificate of need for the hospital's first CT (computed tomography) scanner. He recruited a number of physicians, many of whom are still on the medical staff. He, along with Swisher, negotiated a long-term financial loan with OMC to finance a project. Currently, he is working with Schmidt and the medical staff to examine the feasibility of establishing a women's health center at WHS. He also serves as the director of Webster Affiliate, Inc., the physician–hospital organization (PHO) he created to facilitate joint ventures—including joint medical practices—between the hospital and members of the medical staff.

MANAGEMENT INTERN

This advisory staff position is currently held by Justin Perkins, who recently earned a master of business and hospital administration from an eastern university and is completing a 24-month postgraduate fellowship program recognized by ACHE. Under the terms of this fellowship, the hospital has made no long-term employment commitment to him. A son of an osteopathic physician, Perkins was a unit manager at a large medical center before entering graduate school. Currently, he provides staff support to the president as well as to several board and hospital committees and has been managing WHS's Employee of the Month/Year program. He is a member of ACHE.

INTERNAL REVENUE SERVICE FORM 990 DISCLOSURE

According to WHS's recent IRS Form 990, the following are the ten highest-paid hospital employees:

Staff Name	Position	Current Salary ($)
Steve Swisher	President/CEO	328,500
June Taylor	CFO	303,000
Gretta Schmidt, RN	VP, Clinical Services	208,000
Jay Jill, RN	Associate VP, Clinical Services	162,040
Carla Fox	Associate VP, Administration	110,340
Ellen Wilgus	VP, Professional Services	105,370
Heidi Watkins	Associate VP, Finance	105,230
David Story	VP, Marketing	104,220
David Crow	Laboratory Director	94,500
Marvin Gardens	Pharmacy Director	93,440

Total compensation includes benefits, which are 40 percent above salary. The hospital does not directly employ any physicians in these specialties: emergency, radiology, pathology, and anesthesiology. These services are provided by contracted professional associations.

*On the web at
ache.org/books/
Middleboro2*

MEDICAL STAFF AND MEDICAL RESOURCES

Currently, the WHS medical staff has 110 physicians. All physicians are graduates of osteopathic schools of medicine and have completed internships and residencies in their respective areas of expertise. All active and consulting physicians must be board certified, unless this requirement is formally waived by the executive committee of the medical staff. See Table 5.2 for a full list of WHS's medical staff.

All consulting physicians are required to maintain active status on the medical staff of OMC in Capital City or another accredited hospital. At WHS, the majority of the active medical staff provides primary care. Patients who need higher-level procedures, tests, and medical interventions are referred or transferred to OMC or are served by consulting members of the OMC medical staff (who travel to WHS when needed). WHS maintains a helicopter landing pad on its roof to allow the rapid transfer of emergency patients to OMC using the OMC Air Evac transportation service. OMC Air Evac is also used to fly consulting physicians from OMC to WHS in an emergency. Air travel time from WHS to OMC—and vice versa—is approximately 26 minutes. When weather conditions do not permit air transfer, patients are moved in an ambulance to OMC or MIDCARE.

Following is a breakdown of the medical staff composition:

Services/Department	Active Physicians	Consulting Physicians	Total
Anesthesiology	4	0	4
Emergency	8	4	12
Medicine	37	14	51
Radiology & Pathology	6	6	12
Surgery	16	15	31
Total	**71**	**39**	**110**

CLINICAL SERVICES CONTRACTS

WHS has a contractual relationship with the following Capital City–based provider groups or professional associations (PAs) for the following services. These groups also support OMC and most OHA-affiliated hospitals:

◆ *Anesthesiology.* DO Anesthesiology Associates PA assigns to WHS four anesthesiologists and four nurse anesthetists as well as other staff as needed.

◆ *Emergency medicine.* DO Emergency and Occupational Health Associates PA assigns to WHS emergency physicians on a permanent basis along with other physicians as needed. WHS augments the emergency medicine staff with physician assistants.

- *Pathology.* DO Pathology Services PA assigns to WHS physicians who perform pathology services. As needed, additional pathologists are brought in or the procedure is done at OMC.

- *Radiology.* DO Radiology Services PA assigns to WHS radiologists and provides other clinical services. This group's main office and primary service locations are electronically linked so that its radiologists—wherever they may be working—can access patient data, read and interpret scans and images, and dictate reports.

DEPARTMENT OF MEDICINE

This department comprises physicians in private practice whose specialties include general and family practice, internal medicine, pediatrics, cardiology, and ENT (ear, nose, throat). Dr. Paul Tafy is the elected chair of the Department of Medicine.

DEPARTMENT OF SURGERY

This department comprises physicians in private practice whose specialties include general surgery, OB/GYN (obstetrics and gynecology), and orthopedic surgery. Dr. Doris Felix is the elected chair of the Department of Surgery.

SUBSIDIARY ORGANIZATIONS

Webster Affiliate, Inc.

This tax-paying PHO engages in projects of mutual interest to both WHS and members of its medical staff who are in private practice. WHS owns 70 percent of the Webster Affiliate stock and thus appoints two of the PHO's three board members. Currently, Webster Affiliate owns a number of medical offices and leases the facilities to the physicians for a fee.

Webster Physicians, Inc.

Owned solely by WHS, Webster Physicians is a tax-paying corporation that owns or operates medical practices for physicians affiliated with WHS. In addition, it provides contractual management services—such as information technology, maintenance, and billing—to other medical practices.

MEDICAL STAFF ORGANIZATION

Dr. George Taff (Department of Medicine) has been president of the medical staff for the past three years. The president is elected every two years and provided with a small stipend by WHS. Dr. Meagan Lincoln (Department of Pathology) is the vice president, and Dr. Charles Stein (Department of Surgery) is the secretary. The standing committees of the medical staff are utilization review and quality assurance, medical records, credentials, tissue, pharmacy and therapeutics, and executive.

Composed of the chairs of each standing committee and each department, the medical staff's executive committee meets monthly or as needed. The other committees also meet monthly. The entire medical staff meets quarterly. At its annual meeting, the medical staff votes on recredentialing.

In an interview with select members of the medical staff, Dr. Taff called the relationship among members of the medical staff "very professional" and noted that some of the older physicians seem uncomfortable with the speed but not the substance of many of the changes the medical staff and the hospital have rolled out over the years. Asked about the relationship between WHS and the physicians, he stated, "Collaboratively, the hospital has assisted us with expanding our reach to young, well-trained primary care doctors and with building appropriate referral bridges to OMC. Physicians feel included in the processes and decisions in this hospital, including its strategic planning. Many have been here for decades."

Dr. Taff shared that being president feels like a full-time job and that without the stipend he would be unable to meet many of its expectations. Still, he is on board to help WHS achieve its priorities. "The hospital has to continue to build up its primary care network, even if this means building offices and hiring more doctors. That should be a priority," he said. "The immediate priority of the PHO should be medical practice management. The previous priority of installing an information system that supports both the clinical and administrative sides is now a reality. I'm very impressed with how the hospital implemented the EHR and ensured its meaningful use. We are a model within the OHA system. Medically, the hospital needs to establish a much stronger presence outside of Middleboro, although that may be hard to do in Jasper given its upcoming highway, which will take people straight to the hospitals in Capital City."

Other physicians agreed with Dr. Taff. For example, Dr. Lasker, a member of the medical staff for 32 years, said, "Reducing inpatient beds after years of expansion felt strange but clearly was the right thing to do." He admitted that the relationship he has with many nurses really helps him practice high-quality, cost-effective medicine. "The ongoing studies for appropriate ways to shorten lengths of stay are one example of how this hospital has faced up to the challenges and responded appropriately," he said.

Dr. Kelly, another longtime member of the medical staff, indicated that the hospital needs to continue to expand outpatient services and provide community outreach to high-risk individuals, especially in the rural area to the north of the city. According to her, the medical staff fully supports WHS's acquisition of select medical practices. "For those physicians, this model removes the burden of managing a practice and gives them direct access to the hospital's EHR," she explained.

Dr. Able, a new member, shared that she sees great possibilities with the PHO, strongly supports the recruitment of family practice physicians from OMC (like herself), and appreciates the support WHS gives to those who want to start a thriving practice. "Although my practice is located in a rural area, I do not feel isolated because of all the support I get. I still have a good relationship with many of the faculty who trained me at OMC Medical School," she added.

Dr. Pelopolis, a veteran at the hospital, was the only physician who offered any critical comments, concerned that WHS continues to be a medical outpost for OMC. "I am most concerned that OMC-contracted physicians—such as Dr. Lincoln—hold leadership positions on our medical staff. Our medical staff has lost the ability to chart its own course." This perspective is shared by a small number of other WHS physicians. However, they realize that if OMC physicians were ineligible for leadership positions, WHS physicians would be in their place and fewer physicians would be able to share the duties of the medicine and surgery departments, making more work for everyone. Dr. Pelopolis, however, has remained adamant about this issue and has written to physicians in these two departments to persuade them to discuss the issue at their next departmental meeting.

Currently, WHS does not employ hospitalists. "We take care of our own," Dr. Taff reasoned. "Maybe someday we will need assistance with inpatient care, but not today." That said, he has been working on a proposal to contract with OHA for 48-hour hospitalist coverage on the weekends. WHS has taken no official position on using hospitalists.

CHALLENGES AND FUTURE PLANS

BEHAVIORAL HEALTH

The OHA board has recommended that OHA develop one or more dedicated units in its affiliate hospitals that specialize in drug- and alcohol-addiction treatment. Once these units are operational, "at least one of the hospitals should also develop a comprehensive inpatient psychiatric facility to serve the entire OHA system," the board said. WHS is one of the affiliates the board is targeting, promising to furnish the hospital with planning parameters if it wishes to assess the feasibility of this project. WHS already has long-standing agreements with Sockalexis Center and Middleboro Community Mental Health Center to provide inpatient emergency psychiatric services, including suicide watch, to WHS patients. Under these agreements, the centers limit emergency psychiatric admissions to 48 hours before the patient must be transferred and cap the total number of inpatient days at 100 per year.

OCCUPATIONAL HEALTH AND OTHER BOARD CONSIDERATIONS

Eric Martin, a member of WHS's board, brought to the board's attention that Physician Care Services (PCS), Inc. may be put up for sale in the near future. According to Martin, the CEO of Carlstead Rayon, PCS provided occupational health services to his employees for many years and, in the process, helped "lower our workers' comp and occupational health costs by at least 15 percent," he said. The company, however, moved its occupational health contract to MIDCARE five years ago.

In another meeting, board chair Daniel Will stated that the board would receive "briefing papers" on the following issues. He asked all members to review these materials for the next meeting's discussion:

- ◆ Should we review the current Affordable Care Act provisions?

- ◆ Should future physician recruitment emphasize primary care or specialty care? Do we need to recruit to replace specific physicians and surgeons?

- ◆ Should we hire a chief information officer and establish an in-house information systems department to support operations and WHS-owned or managed medical practices? What is the future of the hospital's existing consulting and service contracts that address our information systems need?

- ◆ Is there a need and demand for new surgical technologies? Which new technologies should we prioritize?

- ◆ Should the hospital establish an outpatient clinic in the northern rural communities? Where should/could this clinic be located? What services should be provided? What are the associated costs and benefits?

- ◆ What are the ramifications of a rumored 15 to 30 percent increase in OHA affiliation fees?

- ◆ Should the hospital continue its ten-year plan to earn LEED (Leadership in Energy and Environmental Design) certification?

PRIVATE ROOMS

OHA is considering an initiative to brand all affiliated hospitals on the basis of quality and privacy. It had asked each hospital affiliate to indicate its potential bed needs for 2020 and beyond and to undertake a study to determine the financial ramification of making all inpatient medical-surgical beds private (instead of semiprivate). Existing semiprivate rooms can be modified into private rooms for approximately $425,000 per room, and new private rooms (minimum of ten) can be added for approximately $1 million per bed. (These values are expressed in 2019 dollars.) The analysis should assume a 20-year straight-line depreciation approach and no salvage values. OHA can commit up to 70 percent financing at an annual interest rate that does not exceed 4 percent.

OHA POLICY CONCERN

At a recent meeting of the OHA board, affiliates indicated that their supply costs per case-mix adjusted discharge were "higher than they should be" and asked OHA to change its policy of requiring affiliates to secure all supplies from OHA. This topic was included on the agenda for the next meeting.

POTENTIAL LEGISLATIVE CHANGE

This past month, OMC alerted all affiliated hospitals (confidentially) that the Office of the Governor is working with other states on model legislation to limit statewide hospital costs. One model being considered limits annual hospital spending increases to the annual increase in the gross state product. Another option is to decrease hospital Medicaid rates by 3 percent for each of the next five years.

 Tables 5.3 through 5.9 contain the data that may give the WHS board and senior management team insights and ideas for developing new programs, improving clinical quality and performance, expanding into underserved markets, and cutting costs.

On the web at ache.org/books/ Middleboro2

Table 5.1
WHS Hospital
Facility Codes

Adult Cardiology Services	Obstetrics
Adult Diagnostic Catheterization	Occupational Health Services
Airborne-Infection Isolation Room	Oncology Services
Auxiliary Organization	Optical Colonoscopy
Birthing Room–LDR Room–LDRP Room	Orthopedic Services
Cardiac Intensive Care	Outpatient Surgery
Cardiac Rehabilitation	Pain Management Program
Case Management	Patient Education Center
Chemotherapy	Patient Representative Services
Children's Wellness Program	Pediatric Diagnostic Catheterization
Community Health Education	Pediatric Intensive Care Services
Community Outreach	Physical Rehabilitation Outpatient Services
Emergency Department	Positron Emissions Tomography/CT
Endoscopic Intrasound	Primary Care Department
Endoscopic Retrograde	Psychiatric Care
Enrollment Assistance Services	Psychiatric Outpatient Services
Health Fair	Single Photon Emission CT (SPECT)
Health Screening	Sleep Center
Hospital-Based Outpatient Care Center Services	Social Work Services
Inpatient Palliative Care Unit	Support Groups
Linguistic/Translation Services	Tobacco Treatment/Cessation Program
Magnetic Resonance Imaging (MRI)	Trauma Center Certified
Medical-Surgical Intensive Care Services	Ultrasound
Multislice Spiral CT (64 + Slice CT)	Volunteer Services Department
Nutritional Programs	Women's Health Center/Services

Notes: (1) Facility codes as reported to and defined by the American Hospital Association. (2) CT: computed tomography; LDR: labor-delivery-recovery; LDRP: labor-delivery-recovery-postpartum.

Name	Off	Age	Gender	Specialty	Patient Days	Discharges
Department of Medicine, Active Staff						
Able	1	39	2	Family Practice*	604	115
Adelson	1	53	1	Family Practice*	601	120
Downs	1	54	2	Family Practice*	578	121
Dawes	1	44	2	Family Practice*	590	120
Standish	1	49	1	Family Practice*	593	119
Franklin	1	55	1	Family Practice*	423	76
Newton	1	44	2	Family Practice*	456	86
Dodger	1	57	1	Family Practice*	365	71
Best	1	35	2	Family Practice*	340	54
Devishson	2	31	2	Family Practice*	186	43
Doogle	2	36	1	Family Practice*	397	88
Baker	2	38	2	Family Practice	200	44
Evans	2	39	1	Family Practice	197	45
Charkes	2	29	2	Family Practice	187	40
Megg	3	56	1	Family Practice*	302	66
Child	3	49	2	Family Practice*	184	35
Kidd	3	47	1	Family Practice*	256	61
Lady	3	40	2	Family Practice*	278	62
Dadoveci	3	50	1	Family Practice*	287	59
Justin	3	57	2	Family Practice*	288	65
Pelopolis	4	43	1	Family Practice	301	61
Easter	4	68	1	Family Practice	312	66
Fisher	4	40	1	Family Practice	135	28
Kelly	5	51	1	Family Practice	28	6
Hamilton	6	60	1	Family Practice	165	34
Lasker	7	57	1	Family Practice	129	25
Masterson	8	59	2	Family Practice	102	18
Morgan	1	35	1	Internal Medicine	625	121
Lieu	1	54	1	Internal Medicine	498	86
White	1	34	2	Pediatrics*	162	45
Wall	1	37	2	Pediatrics*	31	8
Vicenzio	1	35	1	Pediatrics*	80	20
Hirsh	1	39	2	Pediatrics*	40	11
Snipes	3	45	2	Cardiology	646	105
Zook	1	57	1	Endocrinology	129	24
Hogan	1	50	1	ENT	165	31
Taff	1	43	1	ENT	156	29

Table 5.2
WHS
Medical Staff
Information

*On the web at
ache.org/books/
Middleboro2*

continued

Table 5.2
WHS
Medical Staff
Information
(continued)

On the web at
ache.org/books/
Middleboro2

Name	Off	Age	Gender	Specialty	Patient Days	Discharges
Department of Medicine, Consulting Staff						
Coolidge	3	44	2	ENT	143	31
Miller	3	37	1	Pediatrics	132	25
Kronenberger	3	64	1	ENT	140	31
Polk	3	40	2	OB/GYN	112	20
Isaacson	9	50	1	Cardiology	293	41
Checkic	9	43	2	Rheumatology	134	42
Tafy	9	57	1	Oncology	356	41
Johnson	9	47	1	Cardiology	206	32
Gregson	9	54	1	Internal Medicine	175	32
Warren	9	50	2	OB/GYN	55	12
Werner	9	53	1	Pulmonary Medicine	123	21
Others	9				68	12
Department of Surgery, Active Staff						
Sawyer	1	41	2	General*	659	155
Colon	1	50	1	General*	621	142
Team	1	46	1	General*	241	53
Stein	1	52	1	General*	426	85
Huan	1	37	2	Orthopedic	560	105
Dolittle	1	46	1	Orthopedic	562	124
Hernandez	1	54	1	Orthopedic	426	91
Felix	1	47	2	Urology	303	70
Shaw	1	40	2	OB/GYN*	315	70
Kirby	1	68	2	OB/GYN	44	10
Munson	1	44	2	OB/GYN*	325	79
Kim-Gregoire	1	41	1	OB/GYN*	336	74
Munson	1	47	1	OB/GYN*	341	90
Lewis	1	49	2	OB/GYN*	408	101
Morton	3	55	1	OB/GYN*	372	87
Salt	3	48	1	OB/GYN*	283	73
Department of Surgery, Consulting Staff						
Miller	3	68	1	General	45	7
McKinley	3	65	1	General	38	5
Merrill	9	47	1	General	48	8
Pierce	9	51	2	General	62	10
Skierski	9	54	1	Orthopedic	120	18

continued

Name	Off	Age	Gender	Specialty	Patient Days	Discharges
Nguyen	9	47	2	Orthopedic	83	12
Fremont	9	45	1	Orthopedic	30	4
Fremont	9	45	2	Orthopedic	160	25
Davids	9	50	1	Orthopedic	75	10
Nioxon	9	63	1	Orthopedic	18	3
Grant	9	50	2	Orthopedic	32	4
McGovern	9	53	1	Thoracic	103	14
Gruen	9	50	1	Thoracic	140	20
Dawes	10	56	2	General	106	20
Strimpf	10	54	1	General	124	18
				Total	**20,359**	**4,135**

Pathology and Radiology, Active Staff

Name	Off	Age	Gender	Specialty
Lincoln	1	54	2	Pathology
Ericksen	1	48	2	Radiology
Holland	1	62	1	Radiology
Jippel	1	46	2	Radiology
Yip	1	43	1	Pathology
Stern	1	44	1	Pathology
Rossi	1	34	2	Pathology

Pathology and Radiology, Consulting Staff

Name	Off	Age	Gender	Specialty
Currie	9	58	2	Radiology
Douglas	9	43	2	Radiology
San Remo	9	40	1	Radiology
Sanchez	9	55	1	Pathology
Fillerautz	9	44	1	Pathology
Gathews	9	47	2	Pathology

Anesthesiology, Active Staff

Name	Off	Age	Gender	Specialty
Vllanueva	1	38	2	Anesthesiology
Westerman	1	42	2	Anesthesiology
Chamberlin	1	44	1	Anesthesiology
Wilson	1	54	1	Anesthesiology

Emergency Medicine, Active Staff

Name	Off	Age	Gender	Specialty
Abelson	1	44	1	Emergency
Ferreira	1	51	1	Emergency
Schlossman	1	42	2	Emergency

Table 5.2
WHS Medical Staff Information *(continued)*

On the web at ache.org/books/ Middleboro2

continued

Table 5.2
WHS
Medical Staff
Information
(continued)

On the web at ache.org/books/ Middleboro2

Name	Off	Age	Gender	Specialty	Patient Days	Discharges
Lyons	1	34	1	Emergency		
Calson	1	40	2	Emergency		
Hiller	1	47	1	Emergency		
Sams	1	45	1	Emergency		
Bodansky	1	50	2	Emergency		
Emergency Medicine, Consulting Staff						
Greenberg	9	47	1	Emergency		
Sallowash	9	51	1	Emergency		
Ritco	9	41	1	Emergency		
Fisher	9	60	1	Emergency		

Notes:

Code	Office Location	Gender
1	Middleboro	Male
2	Mifflenville	Female
3	Jasper	
4	Harris City	
5	Statesville	
6	Carterville	
7	Boalsburg	
8	Minortown	
9	Capital City	
10	Other	

* Medical practice owned by WHS and/or OMC.
ENT: ear, nose, throat; OB/GYN: obstetrics/gynecology; Off: office location.

Hospital Service	2019	2018	2017	2016
Pediatrics				
Beds	3	3	3	4
Patient Days	650	687	706	804
Occupancy	59.4%	62.7%	64.5%	55.1%
Maternity				
Beds	7	7	7	9
Patient Days	1,769	1,845	1,950	2,140
Occupancy	69.2%	72.2%	76.3%	65.1%
Medical-Surgical I				
Beds	20	20	20	20
Patient Days	4,748	5,047	6,070	5,578
Occupancy	65.0%	69.1%	83.2%	76.4%
Medical-Surgical II				
Beds	22	22	22	21
Patient Days	5,729	5,367	5,890	5,830
Occupancy	71.3%	66.8%	73.3%	76.1%
Medical-Surgical III				
Beds	24	24	20	20
Patient Days	5,255	5,476	5,378	5,503
Occupancy	60.0%	62.5%	73.7%	75.4%
Intensive Care Unit				
Beds	9	9	12	12
Patient Days	2,208	2,802	2,655	2,282
Occupancy	67.2%	85.3%	60.6%	52.1%
Total Hospital				
Beds	**85**	**85**	**84**	**86**
Patient Days	**20,359**	**21,224**	**22,649**	**22,137**
Occupancy	**65.6%**	**68.4%**	**73.9%**	**70.5%**

Table 5.3
WHS Hospital Inpatient Occupancy by Service

On the web at ache.org/books/ Middleboro2

Table 5.4
WHS Detailed
Utilization
Statistics

*On the web at
ache.org/books/
Middleboro2*

Month	Dis	Patient Days	IP Surgery	OP Surgery	Births	ED Visits	ED Admits	OP Visits
2019								
January	401	1,834	54	307	48	1,098	56	3,962
February	387	1,994	48	267	37	976	48	3,072
March	407	1,860	71	327	61	1,103	55	4,275
April	399	2,078	68	319	60	1,134	51	4,730
May	309	1,327	63	343	52	1,320	69	4,029
June	289	1,359	54	395	41	1,328	63	3,998
July	253	1,359	60	312	47	1,345	68	4,126
August	275	1,405	73	290	48	1,035	50	3,349
September	427	1,916	69	308	47	1,156	51	4,476
October	403	1,856	60	317	49	1,050	44	4,768
November	395	2,304	56	326	44	1,038	57	2,657
December	190	1,067	50	303	52	956	48	3,586
Total	**4,135**	**20,359**	**726**	**3,814**	**586**	**13,539**	**660**	**47,028**
2018								
January	312	1,534	57	305	49	1,962	98	3,956
February	403	1,928	54	301	40	1,064	55	2,728
March	441	2,186	66	317	52	1,058	56	3,668
April	367	2,001	87	488	48	1,040	51	4,387
May	341	1,978	82	322	58	1,120	57	4,704
June	312	1,905	63	325	52	1,110	50	4,826
July	308	1,660	55	266	42	1,118	48	4,128
August	307	1,683	45	282	53	1,268	63	3,938
September	305	1,329	84	365	51	1,269	62	4,256
October	334	1,430	70	345	47	1,255	69	4,570
November	390	2,067	86	318	52	1,278	67	4,761
December	441	1,934	59	219	56	1,259	70	3,673
Total	**4,261**	**21,635**	**808**	**3,853**	**600**	**14,801**	**746**	**49,595**

Notes: (1) Dis: discharges; ED: emergency department; IP: inpatient; OP: outpatient. (2) ED Visits are total ED visits. (3) ED Admits are ED visits that led to an inpatient admission. (4) OP Visits are outpatient visits that exclude ED visits.

	2019	2018	2017
Assets			
Current Assets			
Cash	2,100,452	2,596,223	2,945,231
Short-Term Investments	2,004,383	2,717,342	2,998,345
Accounts Receivable—Gross	30,524,615	28,780,289	26,740,525
Allowances for Uncollectables	6,929,334	6,326,330	6,245,302
Accounts Receivable—Net	23,595,281	22,453,959	20,495,223
Due from Third-Party Payers	612,848	603,448	612,349
Inventories	3,924,336	4,825,330	4,248,562
Prepaid Expenses	123,768	653,119	438,293
Total Current Assets	**32,361,068**	**33,849,421**	**31,738,003**
Noncurrent Assets			
Property, Plant, and Equipment—Gross	109,891,691	111,657,349	114,265,378
Less Accumulated Depreciation	70,763,235	70,763,235	70,763,235
Property, Plant, and Equipment—Net	39,128,456	40,894,114	43,502,143
Other Investments	11,342,554	9,563,252	7,352,993
Total Noncurrent Assets	**82,832,078**	**84,306,787**	**82,593,139**
Liabilities			
Current Liabilities			
Accounts Payable	6,893,556	6,935,796	6,993,564
Accrued Salaries and Wages	893,559	803,273	812,494
Accrued Interest	87,223	93,269	88,343
Other Accrued Expenses	302,363	225,484	266,503
Due to Third-Party Vendors	715,394	519,402	612,453
Long-Term Debt Due Within One Year	6,437,445	6,723,445	6,934,229
Total Current Liabilities	**15,329,540**	**15,300,669**	**15,707,586**
Long-Term Debt	28,453,848	27,445,293	27,815,336
Total Liabilities	**43,783,388**	**42,745,962**	**43,522,922**
Net Assets			
Restricted—Donor	2,136,303	3,883,202	4,134,202
Restricted—Board	9,304,110	14,985,826	18,261,274
Unrestricted	27,608,277	22,691,797	16,674,741
Total Net Assets	**39,048,690**	**41,560,825**	**39,070,217**
Net Assets + Liabilities	**82,832,078**	**84,306,787**	**82,593,139**

Table 5.5
WHS Balance Sheet

On the web at ache.org/books/ Middleboro2

Notes: (1) For fiscal years ending December 31. (2) Numbers are in US dollars.

Table 5.6
WHS Statement of Revenues and Expenses

On the web at ache.org/books/ Middleboro2

	2019	2018	2017
Revenues			
Patient Services Revenue			
Inpatient Net of Allowances and Uncollectables	104,385,637	106,913,798	107,405,940
Outpatient Net of Allowances and Uncollectables	49,100,023	48,023,494	47,223,404
Total	**153,485,660**	**154,937,292**	**154,629,344**
Expenses			
Salaries and Wages	60,345,202	62,494,672	63,693,485
Fringe Benefits	16,445,293	17,347,393	17,324,949
Supplies	40,592,337	38,273,445	37,925,334
Professional Fees	24,399	64,393	67,393
Interest	1,473,995	1,645,202	1,837,252
Depreciation	5,320,554	5,004,364	4,848,263
Amortization	1,656,220	1,756,202	1,824,383
Other	24,286,456	24,208,960	24,384,706
Total	**150,144,456**	**150,794,631**	**151,905,765**
Net Income from Operations	3,341,204	4,142,661	2,723,579
Other Revenues			
Unrestricted Gifts and Bequests	145,386	156,393	132,009
Income from Investments	756,223	793,454	803,295
Miscellaneous Non–Patient Services Revenue	673,667	924,548	902,925
Total	**1,575,276**	**1,874,395**	**1,838,229**
Profit or (Loss)	**4,916,480**	**6,017,056**	**4,561,808**

Notes: (1) Years ending December 31. (2) Numbers are in US dollars.

Diagnosis-Related Group Name	2019	2018	2017	2016
Normal Newborn*	527	532	576	606
Medical Back Problems	402	487	523	480
Vaginal Delivery, No Complication	402	416	470	475
Chest Pain	283	348	387	377
Coronary Atherosclerosis	147	188	154	138
Simple Pneumonia, Pleurisy	145	178	192	168
Other Digestive System Disorders	108	148	139	122
Cesarean Section	102	112	128	130
Major Joint Reattachment of Lower Extremity	80	101	91	89
Cholecystectomy	66	83	70	67
Total Top 10 Discharges (Excluding Births)	**2,262**	**2,593**	**2,730**	**2,652**
Total Hospital Discharges	**4,135**	**4,261**	**4,745**	**4,845**
% Top 10 Discharges (Excluding Births)	**54.70**	**50.66**	**48.43**	**46.42**

Table 5.7
WHS Top Ten DRG Discharges

Note: *Counted as births, not discharges.

Table 5.8
WHS Patient Days by Type and by Payer

Type of PT Day	Total PT Days (%)	Medicare (%)	Medicaid (%)	BC HMO (%)	BC PPO (%)	BC Indem (%)	CS PPO (%)	Comm PPO (%)	Comm Indem (%)	VA + Mil (%)	Other (%)	Self-Pay (%)
Medical	24.5	11.3	3.9	0.0	2.0	1.9	0.5	0.0	2.2	1.4	0.2	1.1
Surgical												
Nonorthopedic	14.4	5.4	2.2	0.2	0.3	1.1	0.3	0.0	3.0	1.0	0.3	0.6
Orthopedic	8.0	2.3	1.1	0.2	0.1	1.3	0.0	0.0	1.1	1.3	0.1	0.5
Obstetric	19.9	0.0	2.7	1.1	6.7	0.0	0.8	0.0	4.2	0.1	0.5	3.8
Newborn	9.0	0.0	2.3	0.9	2.4	0.0	0.2	0.0	2.4	0.0	0.3	0.5
Other Pediatric	1.8	0.0	1.1	0.3	0.0	0.1	0.1	0.0	0.0	0.0	0.0	0.2
ICU/CCU	13.5	5.4	0.7	0.2	0.2	2.4	0.3	0.0	1.6	1.5	0.5	0.7
Psychological/Psychiatric	5.5	2.0	0.2	0.0	0.0	0.0	0.0	0.0	0.0	1.3	0.0	2.0
Substance Abuse												
Detox	1.5	0.0	0.0	0.0	0.0	0.0	0.0	0.0	0.0	1.0	0.0	0.5
Rehab	1.9	0.5	0.0	0.0	0.0	0.3	0.0	0.0	0.2	0.4	0.0	0.5
Total	**100.0**	**26.9**	**14.2**	**2.9**	**11.7**	**7.1**	**2.2**	**0.0**	**14.7**	**8.0**	**1.9**	**10.4**

Note: BC: Blue Cross; Comm: Commercial; CS: Central States; HMO: health maintenance organization; ICU/CCU: intensive care unit/coronary care unit or cardiac ICU; Indem: indemnity; Mil: military; PPO: preferred provider organization; PT: patient.

Category	CMS Core Measure	Benchmark	WHS
Timely and Effective Heart Attack Care	Average number of minutes before outpatients with chest pain or possible heart attack who needed specialized care were transferred to another hospital	58 min	46 min
Timely and Effective Heart Attack Care	Average number of minutes before outpatients with chest pain or possible heart attack got an ECG (electrocardiogram)	7 min	8 min
Timely and Effective Heart Attack Care	Percentage of outpatients with chest pain or possible heart attack who got drugs to break up blood clots within 30 minutes of arrival	59%	45%
Timely and Effective Heart Attack Care	Percentage of outpatients with chest pain who received aspirin within 24 hours of arrival or before transferring from the emergency department	97%	94%
Timely and Effective Heart Attack Care	Percentage of heart attack patients who got drugs to break up blood clots within 30 minutes of arrival	60%	60%
Timely and Effective Heart Attack Care	Percentage of heart attack patients given a procedure to open blocked blood vessels within 90 minutes of arrival	96%	93%
Effective Heart Failure Care	Percentage of heart failure patients given an evaluation of LVS (left ventricular systolic) function	99%	97%
Effective Pneumonia Care	Percentage of pneumonia patients given the most appropriate initial antibiotic(s)	96%	95%
Timely Surgical Care	Percentage of surgery patients who were given an antibiotic at the right time (within 1 hour of surgery) to help prevent infection	99%	95%
Timely Surgical Care	Percentage of surgery patients whose preventive antibiotics were stopped at the right time (within 2 hours after surgery)	98%	97%
Timely Surgical Care	Percentage of patients who got treatment at the right time (within 24 hours before or after surgery) to help prevent blood clots after certain types of surgery	100%	100%
Effective Surgical Care	Percentage of surgery patients taking heart drugs called beta blockers before coming to the hospital who were kept on the beta blockers during the period just before and after surgery	98%	98%
Effective Surgical Care	Percentage of surgery patients who were given the right kind of antibiotic to help prevent infection	99%	96%
Effective Surgical Care	Percentage of surgery patients whose urinary catheters were removed on the first or second day after surgery	98%	96%
Timely Emergency Dept. Care	Average time patients who came to the emergency department with broken bones had to wait before getting pain medication	54 min	44 min
Timely Emergency Dept. Care	Percentage of patients who left the emergency department before being seen	2%	1%
Timely Emergency Dept. Care	Percentage of patients who came to the emergency department with stroke symptoms who received brain scan results within 45 minutes of arrival	66%	60%

Table 5.9
WHS Performance Against CMS Core Measures

continued

Category	CMS Core Measure	Benchmark	WHS
Timely Emergency Dept. Care	Average (median) time patients spent in the emergency department before they were admitted to the hospital as an inpatient	260 min	254 min
Timely Emergency Dept. Care	Average (median) time patients spent in the emergency department before leaving from the visit	89 min	97 min
Timely Emergency Dept. Care	Average time patients spent in the emergency department before leaving from the visit	142 min	124 min
Timely Emergency Dept. Care	Average time patients spent in the emergency department before they were seen by a healthcare professional	26 min	20 min
Preventive Care	Percentage of patients assessed and given influenza vaccination	94%	90%
Preventive Care	Percentage of healthcare workers given influenza vaccination	84%	88%
Effective Children's Asthma Care	Percentage of children and their caregivers who received home management plan-of-care documents while hospitalized for asthma	90%	91%
Effective Stroke Care	Percentage of ischemic stroke patients who got medicine to break up a blood clot within 3 hours after symptoms started	81%	71%
Effective Stroke Care	Percentage of ischemic stroke patients who received medicine known to prevent complications caused by blood clots within 2 days of hospital admission	98%	93%
Effective Stroke Care	Percentage of ischemic or hemorrhagic stroke patients who received treatment to keep blood clots from forming anywhere in the body within 2 days of hospital admission	97%	92%
Effective Stroke Care	Percentage of ischemic stroke patients who received a prescription for medicine known to prevent complications caused by blood clots at discharge	99%	95%
Effective Stroke Care	Percentage of ischemic stroke patients with a type of irregular heartbeat who were given a prescription for a blood thinner at discharge	97%	97%
Effective Stroke Care	Percentage of ischemic stroke patients needing medicine to lower bad cholesterol who were given a prescription for this medicine at discharge	97%	96%
Effective Stroke Care	Percentage of ischemic or hemorrhagic stroke patients or caregivers who received written educational material about stroke care and prevention during the hospital stay	94%	93%
Blood Clot Prevention	Percentage of patients who got treatment to prevent blood clots on the day of or the day after hospital admission or surgery	93%	94%
Blood Clot Prevention	Percentage of patients who got treatment to prevent blood clots on the day of or the day after being admitted to the ICU (intensive care unit)	96%	94%
Blood Clot Prevention	Percentage of patients who developed a blood clot while in the hospital who did not get treatment that could have prevented it	5%	5%

continued

Category	CMS Core Measure	Benchmark	WHS
Blood Clot Treatment	Percentage of patients with blood clots who got recommended treatment, which includes using two different blood thinner medicines at the same time	95%	96%
Blood Clot Treatment	Percentage of patients with blood clots who were treated with an intravenous blood thinner and then were checked to determine if the blood thinner caused unplanned complications	99%	94%
Blood Clot Treatment	Percentage of patients with blood clots who were discharged on a blood thinner medicine and received written instructions about that medicine	90%	86%
Pregnancy and Delivery Care	Percentage of mothers whose deliveries were scheduled too early (1–2 weeks early) when a scheduled delivery was not medically necessary	3%	2%
Use of Medical Imaging	Percentage of outpatients with low back pain who had a magnetic resonance imaging (MRI) scan without trying recommended treatments first, such as physical therapy	40%	40%
Use of Medical Imaging	Percentage of outpatients who had a mammogram, an ultrasound, or an MRI of the breast within 45 days after a screening mammogram	9%	8%
Use of Medical Imaging	Percentage of outpatients who had CT (computed tomography) scans of the chest that were "combination" (double) scans	2%	2%
Use of Medical Imaging	Percentage of outpatients who had CT scans of the abdomen that were "combination" scans	9%	9%
Use of Medical Imaging	Percentage of outpatients who got cardiac imaging stress tests before low-risk outpatient surgery	5%	7%
Use of Medical Imaging	Percentage of outpatients with brain CT scans who got a sinus CT scan at the same time	3%	4%
Surgical Complications	Rate of complications for hip/knee replacement patients	3%	No Difference from National Rate
Surgical Complications	Rate of serious complications (from AHRQ)	< 1%	No Difference from National Rate
Surgical Complications	Death rate among patients with serious treatable complications after surgery	117.5 per 1,000 dis.	No Difference from National Rate
Healthcare-Associated Infections	Rate of central line–associated bloodstream infections (CLABSIs) in ICUs and selected wards	N/A	No Difference from National Rate
Healthcare-Associated Infections	Rate of CLABSIs in ICUs only	N/A	Higher than National Rate

Table 5.9
WHS Performance Against CMS Core Measures *(continued)*

continued

Category	CMS Core Measure	Benchmark	WHS
Healthcare-Associated Infections	Rate of catheter-associated urinary tract infections (CAUTIs) in ICUs and selected wards	N/A	No Difference from National Rate
Healthcare-Associated Infections	Rate of CAUTIs in ICUs only	N/A	No Difference from National Rate
Healthcare-Associated Infections	Rate of surgical-site infections from abdominal hysterectomy	N/A	No Difference from National Rate
Healthcare-Associated Infections	Rate of MRSA (Methicillin-resistant Staphylococcus aureus) blood laboratory identified events (bloodstream infections)	N/A	No Difference from National Rate
Healthcare-Associated Infections	Rate of C. diff (Clostridium difficile) laboratory identified events (intestinal infections)	N/A	No Difference from National Rate
Readmissions and Deaths	Rate of unplanned readmission for COPD (chronic obstructive pulmonary disease) patients	20%	No Difference from National Rate
Readmissions and Deaths	Death rate for COPD patients	8%	No Difference from National Rate
Readmissions and Deaths	Rate of unplanned readmission for heart attack patients	22%	Lower than National Rate
Readmissions and Deaths	Death rate for heart attack patients	12%	No Difference from National Rate
Readmissions and Deaths	Rate of unplanned readmission for heart failure patients	22%	No Difference from National Rate
Readmissions and Deaths	Death rate for heart failure patients	11%	No Difference from National Rate
Readmissions and Deaths	Rate of unplanned readmission for pneumonia patients	17%	No Difference from National Rate

continued

Category	CMS Core Measure	Benchmark	WHS
Readmissions and Deaths	Death rate for pneumonia patients	11%	No Difference from National Rate
Readmissions and Deaths	Rate of unplanned readmission for stroke patients	13%	No Difference from National Rate
Readmissions and Deaths	Death rate for stroke patients	15%	No Difference from National Rate
Readmissions and Deaths	Rate of unplanned readmission for coronary artery bypass graft (CABG) surgery patients	15%	No Difference from National Rate
Readmissions and Deaths	Death rate for CABG surgery patients	3%	No Difference from National Rate
Readmissions and Deaths	Rate of unplanned readmission after hip/knee surgery	5%	No Difference from National Rate
Readmissions and Deaths	Rate of unplanned readmission after discharge from hospital (hospitalwide)	15%	Better than National Rate
Payment and Value of Care	Death rate for heart attack patients	N/A	No Difference from National Rate
Payment and Value of Care	Payment for heart attack patients	N/A	More than National Average
Payment and Value of Care	Death rate for heart failure patients	11%	Less than National Average
Payment and Value of Care	Payment for heart failure patients	N/A	No Difference from National Rate
Payment and Value of Care	Death rate for pneumonia patients	12%	No Difference from National Rate
Payment and Value of Care	Payment for pneumonia patients	N/A	No Difference from National Rate
Patient Survey	Percentage of patients who reported that their doctors "always" communicated well	82%	83%
Patient Survey	Percentage of patients who reported that they "always" received help as soon as they wanted	68%	73%

Table 5.9
WHS
Performance
Against CMS
Core Measures
(continued)

continued

Table 5.9
WHS
Performance
Against CMS
Core Measures
(continued)

Category	CMS Core Measure	Benchmark	WHS
Patient Survey	Percentage of patients who reported that their nurses "always" communicated well	80%	81%
Patient Survey	Percentage of patients who reported that their doctors "always" communicated well	82%	83%
Patient Survey	Percentage of patients who reported that they "always" received help as soon as they wanted	68%	73%
Patient Survey	Percentage of patients who reported that their pain was "always" well controlled	71%	80%
Patient Survey	Percentage of patients who reported that staff "always" explained the medication before giving it to them	65%	74%
Patient Survey	Percentage of patients who reported that their room and bathroom were "always" cleaned	74%	83%

Notes: (1) N/A means not applicable, and either the data are not available or the number of cases is too small for a legitimate conclusion. (2) "Better" means better than national average. (3) "No difference" means no statistical difference exists between the hospital and the national average. (4) AHRQ: Agency for Healthcare Research and Quality; CMS: Centers for Medicare & Medicaid Services.

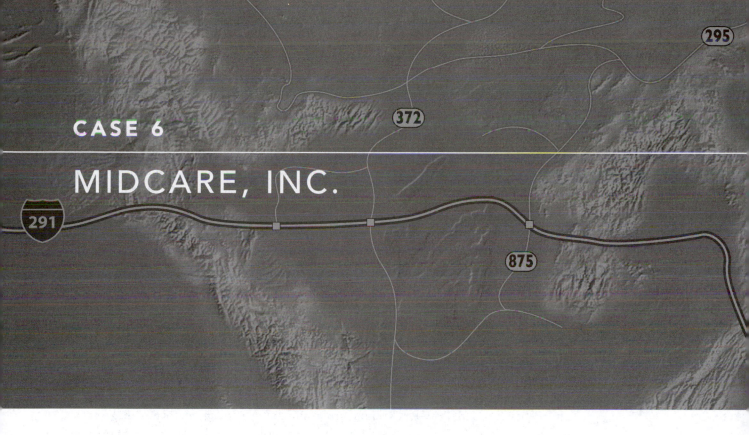

CASE 6

MIDCARE, INC.

Middleboro Medical Center (MIDCARE) was established on January 1, 2015, as "a health system designed to meet the needs of Hillsboro County." This 501(c)(3) nonprofit is composed of a hospital, a physician–hospital organization (PHO), and Health Next. It is also an affiliate of Treeline Health System. The hospital provides diagnostic, outpatient, therapeutic, and emergency medical services and has its own cancer center.

MIDCARE—called Middleboro Community Hospital until 2014—is licensed by the state and approved to operate 300 acute care beds, of which 220 beds are currently staffed as the hospital maintains its significant commitment to ambulatory care. It accepts Medicaid patients, is approved for Blue Cross participation, and is certified for participation in the Medicare program. In addition, it is accredited by The Joint Commission, and its cancer center is accredited by the American College of Surgeons. In fact, The Joint Commission recently granted the hospital a three-year accreditation for consistent compliance with standards. Table 6.1 lists the hospital's current services, as reported to the American Hospital Association.

In 2012, the hospital created the PHO to facilitate the joint (hospital and medical staff) ownership and development of private practices and other collaborative ventures. The PHO has ownership interest in most of the region's medical practices (except for those that belong to

Medical Associates) as well as a local sports and fitness center. In six months, it is scheduled to open two urgent care centers in Middleboro and Mifflenville.

Health Next is a 501(c)(3) that MIDCARE just launched. Although it is still developing its mission and vision statements, it has a clear goal: to benefit the community and improve the population's health. MIDCARE envisions Health Next to be the primary way to coordinate the hospital's community-based services with the public health priorities established by the Hillsboro County Health Department. Health Next's executive director is Ruth Martin, and its board comprises three current MIDCARE board members (Waters, Land, and Meadows) as well as two former board members (Grace Niebauer, a homemaker from Harris City, and Bret Crop, an agricultural business executive from Minortown). Each board member serves a five-year term and has no term limits, making the board self-perpetuating. MIDCARE provides all support services and office space to Health Next.

MIDCARE joined Treeline Health System in 2015. Founded in 1992, Treeline is a cooperative system of 14 tax-exempt community hospitals and regional medical centers located in the tri-state area. It has become one of the stronger regional systems in the United States. Shared services include group purchasing and inventory management, physician and nurse practitioner recruitment, long-term capital borrowing at prime rate plus 0.5 percent, a range of health insurance plans and re-insurance products, a state-of-the-art electronic medical record system, joint liability insurance coverage for physicians and hospitals, and a lease-holding company through which member hospitals can lease capital equipment.

Being a member of Treeline requires MIDCARE to pay annual dues for the services it selects and to appoint one member to the Treeline governing board. Treeline or MIDCARE can cancel this affiliation with 90 days' notice. To become a member, an accredited hospital or medical center must apply and furnish complete financial, quality, and utilization information. Every year, Treeline reviews and comments on the revenues, expenses, and capital budgets of its members. When interviewed, MIDCARE president James Higgens said, "Treeline has helped us in several ways. One good example of this affiliation's value is the reduction of our supply expenses per case-mix-adjusted discharge. This year, the amount was $4,439. Two years ago, it was $5,144. We expect to do even better using Treeline's group purchasing organization for even more of our supplies. Treeline's mean is currently less than $4,000 per case-mix-adjusted hospital discharge." He also indicated that Treeline's assistance with staff recruitment and capital costs and its electronic health record (EHR) has meant money savings for MIDCARE.

HISTORY

PHYSICAL STRUCTURE

Since being erected, the MIDCARE building has been a model of hospital engineering and has garnered community interest. Construction involved demolishing three facilities for the sick to make way for the fully air-conditioned, five-story brick facility on a 68-acre campus. Ample parking surrounds the building. Over the years, increasing service demands have required physical additions to the original structure. Each time a wing or structure was added, the existing space was also modernized. Fund-raising campaigns raised the majority of funds for the additions completed in 1924 and 1946. Federal Hill-Burton monies were used to partially finance the 1962 and 1966 additions. The 2002 construction relied on retained earnings, community philanthropy, and long-term borrowing. A facility-wide modernization program was completed in 2014. This modernization converted a significant number of semiprivate rooms into private rooms and updated the birthing facilities.

In 1960, with the cooperation of Middleboro Trust Company, the hospital established a medical office park on land adjacent to the hospital campus. The hospital alloted space on this land and leased it for 50 years to a condominium association, and then the hospital constructed a three-story building and adjacent parking on the leased land. Following a condominium model, the building was divided into medical suites that were sold only to physicians with active medical staff privileges at the hospital. In 2015, the hospital began purchasing the existing units owned and occupied by physicians, a process that was completed in 2017. At the same time, the hospital constructed a modern medical office building to house ambulatory care clinics and services, physician practices, and high-rise parking. The new building accommodates all the medical practices from the former building but still has ample space for additional occupants. All medical practices in the new building rent their office space.

MIDDLEBORO COMMUNITY HOSPITAL

MIDCARE was originally named Middleboro Community Hospital. The nonprofit hospital opened its doors in 1890 as a short-term, general acute care facility with a 40-bed capacity. Since then, it has slowly grown to its present bed size and has multiplied its offerings with a significant number of outpatient services.

In 1919, the hospital founded a school of nursing. This three-year diploma program was one of the largest in the state and trained many of the nurses who worked at the hospital. In 1985, however, the increasing costs to run the school, the declining interest of local residents, and the increasing popularity of university/college-based nursing programs led the hospital's board of trustees to make the decision to close the school. In 1987, the school officially closed. In 1988, the hospital established a clinical affiliation with State University and area community colleges. Today, the hospital continues to provide clinical rotations for advanced student nurses.

Although basically tranquil in nature, the hospital has experienced volatile periods in its history. First, major disagreements—which started in the 1930s—between area physicians (MDs and DOs) have created two independent systems in Middleboro. For example, DOs—physicians trained in osteopathic medicine—refer patients to other osteopaths (who are often located in Capital City) even though MDs or allopaths who could manage these cases practice in the city and the surrounding areas. Second, ten years ago, the board dismissed the then hospital president, who served in this position for 31 years. The board offered no formal reason for the firing, although the common belief was the board refused the president's request for a multiyear contract. The medical staff fully supported this termination. Nine years ago, the board appointed James Higgens as the new president.

In 2014, the hospital changed its name to Middleboro Medical Center or MIDCARE to signify its transition to a full-service community hospital and regional medical center. Community philanthropy, retained earnings, and long-term borrowing funded the hospital's expansion and modernization. As MIDCARE, the system can "better serve the people of Hillsboro County."

GOVERNANCE

MIDCARE's board of trustees is composed of ten members, each of whom is elected to a four-year term. Elections are held at the board's annual meeting, and nominees for trustee-at-large and trustee officers are presented by the board nominating committee to all hospital incorporators for consideration. Staggered terms of office ensure that no more than three new members are elected annually. Board members may succeed themselves, as there are no limitations on the number of terms an individual can serve on the board. Current board trustees of MIDCARE are as follows; the (number)* indicates the number of years remaining on the current board term:

Michael Rich has been chair for the past 12 years and has served this board for more than 16 years. He is stepping down as chair next year. Peter Steel has been vice chair for 11 years and has served for more than 20 years. His term as vice chair ends this year. All other members, except Elton Giles, have previously served at least one complete term. Melvin Seed has recently given notice that he is unable to serve another term. MIDCARE president Higgens and medical staff president Dr. Frederick Maxwell are ex-officio members.

The standing committees of the board are as follows:

◆ Executive (all board officers)

◆ Long-Range Planning (Steel, Land, Meadows)

◆ Finance (Meadows, Waters, Cornwall, Giles)

◆ Quality Assurance (Drew, Seed, Wheat)

◆ Nominating (Seed, Rich, Land)

The board meets quarterly, and committees meet monthly. Before its annual meeting in March, the board holds a two-day retreat to review the progress toward and to update corporate plans. Once every two years, MIDCARE sponsors each board member to participate in a continuing education program presented by either the American Hospital Association or the State Hospital Association. For the past ten years, the board has retained a consulting firm to assist with its annual self-study. At its next meeting, the board will consider a bylaw change to increase board service to six years.

MANAGEMENT TEAM AND ORGANIZATIONAL STRUCTURE

PRESIDENT

James Higgens holds a bachelor in sociology and a master of hospital administration from a major midwestern university. Prior to becoming president in 2009, he completed a two-year postgraduate residency at Lake Shore Hospital in Chicago and was, for many years, the chief operating officer at Capital City General Hospital in Capital City. He served two years in the US Army Medical Service Corps in Europe.

He is a Fellow in the American College of Healthcare Executives (ACHE) and is currently vice chair of the board of directors of the State Hospital Association. He has authored several professional papers on hospital management and is noted for his ability to interact well with the medical staff and for his understanding of hospital operations. The senior vice presidents report directly to him.

SENIOR VICE PRESIDENT OF FINANCE/CHIEF FINANCIAL OFFICER

John O'Hara, CPA, has held this position for nine years. He is responsible for the Admitting Department and the Business Office, and he is CEO of the PHO. In addition, he provides staff support to the board finance committee and regularly attends all board meetings. His education includes a bachelor in accounting from State University and a master of business administration from an eastern university. A certified public accountant and an active member of the Healthcare Financial Management Association, he has more than 25 years of professional experience, including as vice president of Finance at Seneca Hospital and as assistant controller at two New England hospitals.

Since arriving at MIDCARE, O'Hara has revised and updated many financial practices. On six different occasions, he has received special commendations for excellence from the board, the most recent for upgrading telecommunication services in the hospital at a reduced cost.

When asked what the organization needs in the near future, he mentioned a financial information system that links financial and patient care data (for which he is preparing an RFP—request for proposal—for review of the management team and the board). Also, he thinks "a budgetary process that is based on budgeted units of services instead of FTEs [full-time equivalent employees]" is also necessary.

He negotiates all of the hospital's contracts with physician groups (e.g., radiology professional associations) and, since 2012, has been leading efforts to employ hospitalists and to purchase select medical practices. "We have acquired a number of practices from physicians who are either retiring or leaving to be hospital employees," he said.

O'Hara implements plans that are designed and approved by the president, the management team, and the board. Some of these plans are controversial, such as downsizing inpatient acute care capacity. Current and former employees have blamed him for this decision to terminate or reassign staff. In fact, nurses have signed a petition to hold a unionization election because they fear the implications of the downsizing plan. The nursing staff has voted on unionization before—in 2010—but it resulted in a no vote (57 percent no/43 percent yes). In some employees' perspective, management's termination approach ignores staff seniority and emphasizes "competency and job performance." On at least three occasions, terminated employees had written negative social media posts or comments on the local newspaper's website, insisting that the hospital is looking to retain "only those workers who would work for less."

SENIOR VICE PRESIDENT OF PATIENT CARE SERVICES

This position is newly created but yet to be filled. It will oversee the following patient departments: Anesthesiology, Dietary, Health Education, Laboratory, Nursing, Pharmacy, Physical Therapy, Occupational Therapy, Radiology, Recreation Therapy, Speech Therapy, and Social Services as well as all outpatient departments (including the Emergency Department). "Our intent for this position is to allow greater coordination between and among our inpatient, outpatient, and community-based patient services," Higgens explained. "We expect it to enhance these programs' effectiveness and efficiency." The new senior vice president of Patient Care Services (SVPPCS) is responsible for hiring a direct report—the new vice president of Nursing or chief nursing officier (CNO). The recruitment and selection process for both positions is expected to take nine months. MIDCARE has retained a recruitment firm to identify qualified candidates.

Vice President of Nursing/Chief Nursing Officer

The right person for this position, which is currently vacant, must have a high degree of nursing experience and demonstrated administrative and management talents. The following departments are under this position: Pediatrics, Maternity and Nursery, Medical-Surgical, Intensive Care Unit (ICU) and Coronary Care Unit, Nursing Education and Staff Development, Nursing Quality Assurance, Case Management, Central Sterile Supply, and Operating Rooms.

During the past 15 years, no vice president of Patient Care Services or CNO has lasted for more than five years. Conflicts with the medical staff about patient care practices and with administration about nurse scheduling and staffing levels have led to the most recent resignation from this post. Administration accepted the resignation in stride, telling the board that the former VP could not effectively manage the Nursing Department or communicate administration's policies to the nursing staff. The former VP did not support the decision to reduce the staffing levels in nursing and to replace registered nurses with licensed practical nurses. While she understood the need to lower hospital expenses, she recommended doing so by using smaller nursing units, each with its own manager and support team.

The director of Nursing Education and Staff Development, Gemma Guevara, RN, is currently the acting CNO. She plans to return to her regular duties as soon as the SVPPCS has permanently filled the position. She hopes it will be soon, as she has already expressed her plans to retire in 18 months.

Director of Nursing Education and Staff Development

Guevara has held this position for 20 years. She earned a bachelor in nursing and master in nursing education from State University. Her combined 36 years of experience in nursing and nursing education includes serving in a variety of positions at MIDCARE, such as staff nurse, charge nurse, evening nursing supervisor, and night nursing supervisor. On three different occasions, she has been acting CNO. Well liked and highly regarded by department heads, charge nurses, and head nurses, she knows and gets along well with every nurse at the hospital.

As a direct report of the CNO, Guevara is responsible for ensuring all nurses remain proficient and updated in the nursing practice. Not only does she provide relevant in-hospital seminars and workshops, but she also serves as the liaison between the Nursing Department and the student nurses and administrators from State University School of Nursing.

CMS Core Measures Working Group

The CNO and the chair of the Department of Surgery/medical staff coordinator convene MIDCARE's CMS (Centers for Medicare & Medicaid Services) Core Measures Working Group. Other members of the group are Hazel Webster, RN, director of Nursing Quality Assurance, and Nikki Mathews, RN, director of Case Management. This group examines all CMS quality data and institutes appropriate actions, and it also measures and monitors other specific quality measures.

Nearly two years ago, this group, with help from an outside consultant, developed and implemented a formal quality improvement program to prevent ventilator-associated pneumonia (VAP), catheter-related bloodstream infection (CRBSI), and surgical wound infection (SWI) among hospitalized patients. The program comprises a bundle of services, policies, and procedures that constitute an evidence-based standard of care for each infection. For example, studies indicate that there are 5.3 CRBSI cases in the ICU per 1,000 catheter days and that approximately 18 percent of CRBSIs result in death. Similarly, studies indicate that VAP occurs in up to 15 percent of patients who receive mechanical ventilation. Whenever a bundle of required services, policies, and procedures is not fully executed, the group investigates why, writes a report of its findings, and gives its recommendations to the SVPPCS, who then implements corrections. Frequently, the group must determine whether the failure to adhere to standards or protocols is a system problem or a personnel problem. Since the program was established, the occurrence of VAP, CRBSI, and SWI has declined by at least 65 percent.

VICE PRESIDENT OF MEDICINE/CHIEF MEDICAL OFFICER

Dr. Olivia Stickle was appointed to this position three years ago. She graduated from college and medical school and completed her residency training in internal medicine on the East Coast. After 15 years of clinical practice, she earned a master of health administration from a southern university and became the medical director in a community hospital in another state and then the deputy medical director for Treeline Health System. She joined MIDCARE to manage its hospitalist program and its PHO-owned medical practices. Approximately 20 percent of her time is devoted to being the executive vice president of the PHO. She serves on multiple committees of The Joint Commission, the American Medical Association, and the State Medical Society.

SENIOR VICE PRESIDENT OF OPERATIONS/CHIEF OPERATING OFFICER

Rob Stewart was appointed to this position when it was created several years ago. Prior to that, he was assistant administrator for seven years and then vice president for 15 years for the Professional Services Department, and he completed his graduate program's administrative residency at the hospital. He holds a bachelor and master in health administration from a southern university, is an active member of ACHE, was in the Medical Service Corps of the US Air Force Reserve for six years, and serves on committees of the State Hospital Association. At MIDCARE, he chairs the hospital disaster planning committee and is responsible for the vice president of Human Resources and the assistant vice president of Operations.

VICE PRESIDENT OF HUMAN RESOURCES

Prior to her position, Gloria Bunker was the director of Human Resources for a major bank in Capital City for three years and for a large community hospital in the Midwest for 15 years. Born and raised in Jasper, she has a bachelor in psychology from State University and a master of business administration from a private West Coast university. She is a member of the American Society for Healthcare Human Resources Administration (ASHHRA) and is the former chair of the statewide chapter of ASHHRA in a midwestern state. Since being appointed, she has streamlined the employee evaluation system, retained the services of a national consulting firm to perform extensive wage and salary studies, reviewed and revised all job descriptions, and revised the employee recruitment and outplacement processes. Also, she supervises MIDCARE's volunteer program.

ASSISTANT VICE PRESIDENT OF OPERATIONS

Twenty-eight years ago, Ted Beck graduated from high school and was hired by the hospital as a billing clerk. Since then, he has been accounts receivable manager, director of purchasing, and director of the business office. He was promoted to his current position when the previous assistant vice president retired. Having completed a bachelor in health administration at State University, he enrolled in the university's master of business administration program and became a member of ACHE. For the past three years, MIDCARE employees have voted him "Outstanding Supervisor." At his urging, the hospital sought an affiliation with a national voluntary chain of hospitals, which has enabled the hospital to access joint purchasing services. Currently, he is developing a plan for shared laundry services with area nursing homes.

He is in charge of the following departments: Patient Access, Parking/Security, Engineering and Maintenance, Patient Experience, Housekeeping, Laundry, and Purchasing/Materials Management/Supply Chain Management.

SENIOR VICE PRESIDENT OF INFORMATION SYSTEMS/CHIEF INFORMATION OFFICER

Mabel Watkins was appointed to this position four years ago and was tasked with adopting Treeline's EHR system for use in MIDCARE and all of its owned medical practices. She also oversees all aspects of MIDCARE's information technology (IT) infrastructure, including security. Prior to joining the management team, she was deputy chief information officer for a major medical center in a midwestern city. She earned a bachelor in computer science at State University and a master of business administration at a private eastern university. She has 15 years of experience in hospital IT and is a member of the College of Healthcare Information Management Executives.

According to Watkins, implementation of the Treeline EHR continues to involve all MIDCARE departments and all owned and affiliated medical practices. She also indicated that some of her most difficult challenges include managing the staggering number and types of vendor and service contracts, assessing the value of new technologies, and staying compliant with regulations and best practices for securing protected health information. Her direct reports include the offices of Medical Information and Services, Medical Records, IT Systems Services, IT Grants and Contracts, and IT Systems Security and Telecommunications.

VICE PRESIDENT OF MEDICAL INFORMATION AND SERVICES

Appointed to his position two years ago, Dr. Sindar Manhatten is responsible for MIDCARE's EHR and other information systems that capture, analyze, and report clinical information and data. Although trained in internal medicine, he holds a master of healthcare analytics. Prior to this job, he was chief medical information officer for a regional healthcare system in another state and served three years in Capital City as an EHR consultant to area hospitals and medical centers. He is a recognized expert in CMS's Meaningful Use and guided MIDCARE through the latest stages of this program. He helped establish the protocols so that all owned medical practices are linked to MIDCARE's master EHR. He publishes papers on electronic records regularly and is a noted speaker on system security.

SPECIAL ASSISTANT OF MANAGEMENT

Six months ago, Marie Calley had just earned her master of health and hospital administration from a private eastern university when she was offered the position to work right under the president. In graduate school, she studied with one of the leading experts in the area of hospital strategic planning, but her professional experience is limited to a two-year residency at Coastal Medical Center in a major city on the West Coast. At MIDCARE, she is assigned special projects, performs market and demographic analyses, writes public relations pieces and contributes to publications, assists the senior management team with strategy-related work, and provides administrative support to select committees of the medical staff. She and her husband just moved to Middleboro when he accepted a position with the law firm Giles, Giles & Drew.

INTERNAL REVENUE SERVICE FORM 990 DISCLOSURES

MIDCARE's recent IRS Form 990 indicates its ten highest-paid employees:

Staff Name	Position	Current Salary ($)
James Higgens	President	859,600
John O'Hara	Senior VP, Finance/CFO	513,000
Mabel Watkins	Senior VP, Information Systems/CIO	443,450
Olivia Stickle, MD	VP, Medicine/CMO	422,560
Rob Stewart	Senior VP, Operations/COO	406,500
Sindar Manhatten, MD	VP, Medical Information and Services	301,450
Gemma Guevara	Acting VP, Nursing/CNO	248,500
Marc Shine, MD	Hospitalist	212,445
William Lewis, MD	Hospitalist	198,445
Megan Gupta, MD	Hospitalist	198,320

Total compensation includes benefits, which average 34 percent above salary, as well as performance bonus payments. Emergency, radiology, pathology, and anesthesiology services are provided by contract. Currently, the hospital does not directly employ any physicians in these specialties. Salary data for physicians employed by the PHO are not included here and are reported in the (confidential) annual reports of the PHO.

MEDICAL STAFF AND MEDICAL RESOURCES

There are 179 physicians on the active medical staff and 9 hospitalists on the general medical staff. In 1990, the hospital established a policy that physicians who have "consulting" status on the medical staff must maintain "active" status at Capital City General Hospital, at University Hospital in University Town, or at another hospital. In addition, any appointment to the active or consulting medical staff requires the physician to be board certified and to meet any credentialing requirements. Long ago, waivers were granted for board certification based on 20 or more years of hospital affiliation. The last physician appointed under this waiver policy retired in 2016.

MIDCARE purchases area medical practices and directly employs physicians. Some of these practices are jointly owned by the PHO. In some instances, the acquisition of practices creates larger single-specialty practices. To date, most physicians affiliated with MIDCARE are employed, with the exception of orthopedic surgeons and physicians affiliated with Medical Associates. See table 6.2 for a full list of MIDCARE's medical staff.

On the web at ache.org/books/Middleboro2

The medical departments at MIDCARE are as follows:

- *Department of Anesthesiology.* The hospital maintains a contractual relationship with Anesthesiology Associates of Middleboro Professional Association (PA) to provide all anesthesiology services. Dr. Maxwell is the president of this PA and chair of this department.

- *Department of Emergency Medicine.* The hospital maintains a contractual relationship with Emergency Medical Associates of Middleboro PA to provide emergency services. Dr. Simi Hines is the president of this PA and chair of this department.

- *Department of Family Practice.* This department comprises physicians in private practice. Dr. Joe Apple is the chair of this department.

- *Department of Hospital Medicine.* The hospital employs nine physicians trained in internal medicine to provide in-house, 24/7 care and services as hospitalists. Hospitalists cannot admit nor vote on medical staff resolutions. Hospitalists are managed and supervised by Dr. Stickle, chief medical officer.

- *Department of Internal Medicine.* This department includes private practice physicians in a variety of specialties, including general internal medicine, pediatrics, allergy and immunology, cardiology, gastroenterology, ENT (ear, nose, throat), psychiatry, and oncology and hematology. Dr. Godfrey Hunt is the chair of this department.

- *Department of Pathology.* The hospital maintains a contractual relationship with Pathology Associates of Middleboro PA for all pathology services. Dr. Douglas Lafta is the president of this PA and chair of this department.

- *Department of Radiology.* The hospital maintains a contractual relationship with Radiology Associates of Middleboro PA for all radiology services. Dr. Adam Glorioso is the president of this PA and chair of this department.

- *Department of Surgery.* This department is made up of private practice physicians in a variety of specialties. Dr. Felix Limpey is the chair of this department.

MEDICAL STAFF ORGANIZATION

Dr. Maxwell (Department of Anesthesiology) has been president of the medical staff for two years. The president is elected every two years. No additional compensation is given to elected officers. Dr. Carlos Leatros (Department of Pathology) is vice president. Dr. Limpey (Department of Surgery) is employed part-time by the hospital as the medical staff coordinator. He provides staff support to all medical staff committees. For example, he cochairs the monthly meeting of the CMS Core Measures Working Group.

Standing committees of the medical staff include bylaws, cancer, credentials, critical care education, emergency services, executive, hospitalist practice, medical records, pharmacy and therapeutics, quality assurance, tissue/transfusion, and utilization review. The executive committee of the medical staff meets monthly or as needed, while other committees meet monthly. The entire medical staff meets annually, where the physicians address recredentialing.

Recently, Dr. Raymond Samuels (Department of Pediatrics) wrote to the medical staff officers to express his desire to be considered for president in the next election. Without criticizing the performance of the incumbent, he indicated that the interests of the medical staff are better represented by a physician in private practice than by a physician in a hospital-based practice. His letter suggests that the leadership positions of the medical staff be reserved for physicians with admitting privileges.

CHALLENGES AND OPPORTUNITIES

SPECIAL STUDY OF EMERGENCY DEPARTMENTS

The Department of Health Services Management at State University recently released a report about persons suffering from psychosis or nervous breakdown who are in need of acute mental health services. According to the report, these patients frequently must wait in the emergency department (ED) for extended periods before they can be transferred to appropriate service providers. The state mental hospital in Capital City is the closest facility that accepts involuntary emergency admissions. Local mental health services only provide outpatient treatment. The report states that, in the past year, four such people waited more than three days in the ED before transfer and, for five days, mental health patients awaiting transfer occupied 12 of the 27 beds in the ED. The Department of Health Services Management collected these data as part of a pilot study to determine whether appropriate emergency services are available in communities served by two or more EDs. The study suggests that operational costs in the ED are approximately 18 percent above the operational costs incurred in similar hospitals with similar utilization.

STRATEGY DISCUSSIONS AT THE BOARD RETREAT

Six weeks ago, the board, president, and all senior vice presidents gathered for a two-day strategic review of MIDCARE. The retreat was organized and directed by Rich and Steel, chair and vice chair of the board, respectively. Both had attended an American Hospital Association seminar on strategic options for community hospitals, and both returned asking whether MIDCARE should develop additional off-campus services; acquire and operate additional medical practices; and affiliate with other service providers, including through an asset merger. Attendees of the retreat agreed to not publicly discuss these topics until everyone has had the opportunity "to study the strategic options presented and the most appropriate ways to address them." Also, the board asked management to assess the implications of the Sarbanes-Oxley Act and other relevant laws and regulations on hospital governance. Meeting without the senior managers, the board discussed whether the president's compensation package should include financial incentives linked to the achievement of financial and quality measures. The board agreed to continue this discussion and has asked the State Hospital Association for examples of CEO contracts used at similar hospitals. The retreat conveyed to the entire board the significance of their input into these and other issues.

ELIMINATION OF CERTIFICATE-OF-NEED LAW

Harry Waters, an at-large board trustee and an elected member of the state legislature, has been asked by the governor to introduce legislation that will deregulate the healthcare system and allow the current certificate-of-need (CON) law to lapse at the end of 2022. Waters thinks that, with the governor's endorsement, the bill will pass. He is concerned, however, that deregulation will allow hospitals and other healthcare providers to move into new markets, such as Jasper. He thinks the governor could be convinced to delay abolishing the CON law if he were given compelling reasons. In general, hospital leaders in cities across the state, especially Capital City, strongly support the demise of CON, while leaders of community hospitals in suburban and rural areas want the law retained.

Waters asked board members for their views on this issue and requested Higgens to provide the board with a legal opinion on whether federal antitrust laws and regulations would constrain other hospitals from serving Jasper and other communities traditionally served by MIDCARE. Higgens turned to the hospital counsel—Giles, Giles & Drew— to furnish this opinion within 60 days. The State Hospital Association has reserved any judgment about the CON law until "after the specific legislation has been introduced." Higgens does not think the association will be able to present a unified position given that its constituents have diverging sentiments on this statute. "In a future without CON, antitrust considerations will drive market competition," he said.

Expanded Maternity Services

In 2014, MIDCARE's maternity ward was renovated and its services were upgraded. Today, the hospital offers three types of maternity rooms that "exactly meet our needs and are one of the reasons we are increasing our services to the community," explained Higgens:

1. *Labor-delivery-recovery-postpartum (LDRP) room.* An LDRP room is equipped to accommodate the mother and baby throughout the birthing process and the days afterward, assuming a patient transfer to another unit is not necessary. A designated nurse cares for both mother and baby. The planned length of stay in an LDRP room is 24 to 48 hours after delivery.

2. *Labor-delivery-recovery (LDR) room.* An LDR room is equipped to be used throughout the birthing process and the period of recovery after childbirth. Then, the new mother and baby are transferred to a room and the nursery, respectively. An LDR room may be used by a mother who does not desire LDRP or whose baby needs care in the newborn nursery.

3. *Labor room.* A labor room is equipped to handle an expectant mother in labor, before she is transferred to a delivery room or an operating room for a cesarean section.

In addition, the PHO has brought to the system new physicians and specialties. This addition has expanded expectant or new mothers' choice of obstetricians, gynecologists, pediatricians, and other related providers.

Interview with the President

When asked to assess the current state of MIDCARE, Higgens said, "The past five years have been filled with a great deal of positive change. We continue to accomplish our objectives. We have remodeled our physical facilities and expanded and deepened our reach into our primary markets. Plus, because of our PHO, we have a much tighter and larger network of affiliated physicians who are ready to collaborate with the hospital."

According to Higgens, MIDCARE faces the following challenges in the future: continuing to strengthen finances, long-range planning, creating cooperative ventures with the medical staff, increasing worker productivity, and using the affiliation with Treeline to achieve maximum advantage. He also indicated that Hillsboro County, given its demographic changes and Jasper's proximity to Capital City, might benefit from just one hospital, instead of two.

When asked about long-standing issues in nursing, he stated, "We have reorganized the department and are using a national search firm to find a well-qualified senior vice president for patient care services. Our plan is for this senior vice present to, ultimately, be in charge of all aspects of patient care services in MIDCARE. This should prevent many of the issues we had in the past."

MIDCARE retains Market Solutions, Inc. to perform market analyses and quarterly audits of all guest relations programs and advertising. The contract with Market Solutions is coordinated by Stewart, and Market Solutions staff reports to a committee composed of all the MIDCARE senior vice presidents. "We are very pleased with them," Higgens affirmed. "They provide us insights and resources we previously had no access to nor could develop. This model is leading edge, and other hospitals are considering replicating it."

Higgens named the medical staff and the board as MIDCARE's primary strength. In contrast, he cited the inadequate health insurance coverage of county residents and the low reimbursement rates from state Medicaid and federal Medicare as MIDCARE's primary threats. To cope with these rates, he said, "We have to continue to strive for respectable inpatient occupancy and lower our operational costs throughout the hospital." Although he is aware that a national for-profit firm has recently purchased a hospital just east of Capital City, he sees no consequences for the local market.

"I wish we could forge a meaningful collaboration with Webster Health System to better serve the Jasper market. But antitrust laws and regulations make even such discussions difficult. I do agree that Medical Associates plays a significant role in our market, and we need to be more sensitive to its needs."

Tables 6.3 through 6.9 show how well MIDCARE has performed and how well it has provided for Hillsboro County.

On the web at ache.org/books/ Middleboro2

Adult Cardiac Electrophysiology	Genetic Testing/Counseling
Adult Cardiac Surgery	Geriatric Services
Adult Cardiology Services	Health Fair
Adult Interventional Cardiac Catheterization	Health Research
Airborne Infection Isolation Room	Health Screening
Ambulatory Surgery Center	HIV—AIDS Services
Bariatric/Weight Control Services	Hospital-Based Outpatient Care Center Services
Birthing Room—LDR Room—LDRP Room	
Blood Donor Center	Image Guided Radiation Therapy (IGRT)
Breast Cancer Screening/Mammograms	Immunization Program
Cardiac Intensive Care	Indigent Care Clinic
Cardiac Rehabilitation	Inpatient Palliative Care Unit
Case Management	Intensity-Modulated Radiation Therapy (IMRT)
Chaplaincy/Pastoral Care	
Chemotherapy	Magnetic Resonance Imaging (MRI)
Chiropractic Services	Meals on Wheels
Community Health Education	Medical-Surgical Intensive Care Services
Community Outreach	Mobile Health Services
Complementary and Alternative Medicine Services	Multislice Spiral CT (<64 + Slice CT)
	Multislice Spiral CT (>64 + Slice CT)
Computer-Assisted Orthopedic Surgery (CAOS)	Neurological Services
	Nutritional Programs
Crisis Prevention	Obstetrics
CT Scanner	Occupational Health Services
Dental Services	Oncology Services
Diagnostic Radioisotope Facility	Orthopedic Services
Emergency Department	Outpatient Surgery
Enabling Services	Pain Management Program
Endoscopic Intrasound	Palliative Care Program
Endoscopic Retrograde	Patient-Controlled Analgesia (PCA)
Enrollment Assistance Services	Patient Education Center
Extracorporeal Shock Wave Lithotripter (ESWL)	Patient Representative Services
	Pediatric Intensive Care Services
Fitness Center	Physical Rehabilitation Inpatient Services
Freestanding Outpatient Center	Physical Rehabilitation Outpatient Services
Full-Field Digital Mammography (FFDM)	

continued

Table 6.1
MIDCARE
Hospital
Facility Codes
(continued)

Primary Care Department	Social Work Services
Psychiatric Care	Sports Medicine
Psychiatric Child and Adolescent Services	Support Groups
Psychiatric Consultation/Liaison Services	Teen Outreach Services
Psychiatric Education Services	Tobacco Treatment/Cessation Program
Psychiatric Emergency Services	Trauma Center Certified
Psychiatric Geriatric Services	Ultrasound
Psychiatric Outpatient Services	Urgent Care Center
Psychiatric Partial Hospitalization	Virtual Colonoscopy
Robotic Surgery	Volunteer Services Department
Single Photon Emission CT (SPECT)	Women's Health Center/Services
Sleep Center	Wound Management Services

Notes: (1) Facility codes as reported to and defined by the American Hospital Association. (2) CT: computed tomography; LDR: labor-delivery-recovery; LDRP: labor-delivery-recovery-postpartum.

Table 6.2
MIDCARE
Medical Staff
Information

*On the web at
ache.org/books/
Middleboro2*

Name	Note	Off	Age	Specialty	2019 Patient Days	2019 Discharges
Family Practice, Active Staff						
Apple		6	50	Family Practice	174	38
Banero		8	55	Family Practice	219	50
Fistru		7	58	Family Practice	160	36
Mix		2	45	Family Practice	130	23
Player		5	62	Family Practice	103	21
Internal Medicine, Active Staff						
Barton	MA	1	45	Internal Medicine	745	121
Beata		3	60	Internal Medicine	80	13
Crush		3	58	Internal Medicine	380	49
Cushing		3	62	Internal Medicine	87	12
Davis		3	58	Internal Medicine	203	28
Douglas	MA	1	41	Internal Medicine	790	191
Figher		3	54	Internal Medicine	306	55
Filly		1	58	Internal Medicine*	240	39
Frost	MA	3	41	Internal Medicine	490	105
Grist		3	50	Internal Medicine	140	22
Hippster		1	56	Internal Medicine	250	39
Horse		1	68	Internal Medicine*	544	83
Hunt		8	55	Internal Medicine*	172	28
Jessey		7	60	Internal Medicine	177	20
Justin		1	67	Internal Medicine	310	48
Justin		4	59	Internal Medicine*	84	14
Kessler	MA	1	34	Internal Medicine	658	149
King		3	63	Internal Medicine	64	10
Knach		8	67	Internal Medicine	63	10
Lesko	MA	1	38	Internal Medicine	560	112
Mast		2	41	Internal Medicine	877	116
Master	MA	1	40	Internal Medicine	462	101
Meow		1	60	Internal Medicine*	280	49
Michael		4	45	Internal Medicine	250	43
Nask		5	56	Internal Medicine	203	29
Nostrom		2	57	Internal Medicine	112	17
Ogg		2	39	Internal Medicine	572	85
Paul		2	50	Internal Medicine	126	20
Quinn		6	63	Internal Medicine	156	23
Steel		3	50	Internal Medicine	416	69

continued

Name	Note	Off	Age	Specialty	2019 Patient Days	2019 Discharges
Stocapy		3	57	Internal Medicine	150	22
Trip		6	52	Internal Medicine	263	41
Vogel		5	55	Internal Medicine	103	16
Pediatrics, Active Staff						
Bickford		1	50	Pediatrics*	92	29
Bill		3	59	Pediatrics	52	19
Gavin		1	44	Pediatrics*	54	14
Kettel		3	57	Pediatrics	70	17
Miller		3	40	Pediatrics	103	25
Otter	MA	3	37	Pediatrics	80	20
Pushy		1	50	Pediatrics*	70	17
Quester	MA	3	40	Pediatrics	164	42
Reaper	MA	1	52	Pediatrics	81	25
Samuels	MA	1	47	Pediatrics	114	29
Sloan		1	48	Pediatrics*	94	20
St. James	MA	1	40	Pediatrics	120	45
Turtle		1	58	Pediatrics*	140	34
Unvey	MA	3	56	Pediatrics	145	39
Vesh		1	52	Pediatrics*	42	9
Warren		1	56	Pediatrics*	84	19
Allergy and Immunol-ogy, Active Staff						
Gustave		1	53	Allergy/Immun.*	207	34
Hampshire		3	58	Allergy/Immun.	204	44
Sleek		1	49	Allergy/Immun.*	448	57
Cardiology, Active Staff						
Eastman		1	56	Cardiology*	384	56
Hurst		1	60	Cardiology*	334	49
Rusty		1	60	Cardiology*	180	26
Underwood	MA	1	46	Cardiology	652	145
Victem		1	41	Cardiology*	471	77
Gastroenterology, Active Staff						
Amas		1	60	Gastroenterology	120	22
Autumn	MA	1	44	Gastroenterology	748	155
Eisher		1	55	Gastroenterology*	128	25
Tiger		2	59	Gastroenterology	58	9
Wingate		2	64	Gastroenterology	86	14
Zaller		1	49	Gastroenterology*	1,270	157

Table 6.2
MIDCARE Medical Staff Information *(continued)*

On the web at ache.org/books/ Middleboro2

continued

Table 6.2
MIDCARE
Medical Staff
Information
(continued)

*On the web at
ache.org/books/
Middleboro2*

Name	Note	Off	Age	Specialty	2019 Patient Days	2019 Discharges
Psychiatry, Active Staff						
Actor		1	42	Psychiatry	208	39
Voltaire		1	37	Psychiatry	202	39
Banana		1	50	Psychiatry	202	27
Isher		2	61	Psychiatry	86	10
Freud		1	50	Psychiatry	203	30
Stephens		1	41	Psychiatry	227	34
Jilley		1	39	Psychiatry	260	44
Zeus		2	40	Psychiatry	242	35
Other: Medicine						
Carp		3	54	ENT	300	61
Divan		1	44	Oncology/Hemo*	440	56
Fish		3	49	ENT	280	64
Hatcher		1	53	Oncology/Hemo*	459	82
Schoen		1	39	Oncology/Hemo*	401	77
Smith		1	32	Oncology/Hemo*	290	23
Tunsteb		1	60	ENT	80	18
Weckenson	MA	1	44	ENT	470	110
White		1	63	ENT	68	22
Whittier		1	44	ENT*	353	101
Xerox	MA	1	42	ENT	497	145
Yalper		1	57	ENT*	170	82
Surgery: Orthopedic						
Amberson		1	55	Orthopedic	1,540	210
Dillon		1	64	Orthopedic	1,420	202
Hooper		1	50	Orthopedic	1,253	166
Jones		1	57	Orthopedic	1,376	205
Matthews		1	45	Orthopedic	1,721	211
Questrom	MA	1	39	Orthopedic	1,401	222
Rex		1	57	Orthopedic	1,703	268
Stanley	MA	1	49	Orthopedic	1,507	228
Surgery: General						
Blood		3	56	General	315	55
Cutter		3	63	General	240	40
Hersh	MA	1	40	General	1,200	267
Isherum		1	57	General*	1,245	198
Jackson	MA	1	39	General	734	140
Limpey		1	58	General*	945	127
Munson		1	50	General*	586	85

continued

Name	Note	Off	Age	Specialty	2019 Patient Days	2019 Discharges
Never	MA	1	45	General	870	215
O'Connell	MA	1	49	General	416	104
Putter	MA	1	52	General	601	126
Timas		1	59	General*	1,046	138
Victor		1	57	General*	980	156
Surgery: OB/GYN						
Dustin	MA	1	33	OB/GYN	576	180
Eberle		1	51	OB/GYN*	190	36
Fisher		3	60	OB/GYN*	154	21
Fraser		1	65	OB/GYN*	180	31
Goldstein		3	50	OB/GYN*	220	48
Gost	MA	1	40	OB/GYN	720	197
Stein		3	56	OB/GYN	163	30
Linzetta		3	61	OB/GYN	137	24
Ibby		1	57	OB/GYN*	236	46
Japen		1	56	OB/GYN*	236	48
Lights		1	55	OB/GYN*	186	36
Nester		1	59	OB/GYN*	180	35
Surgery: Other						
Bernal		1	45	Neurosurgery	329	49
Blue		1	46	Eye	150	47
Clock		1	47	Thoracic*	540	82
Crow		1	50	Neurosurgery	334	50
David		1	51	Vascular*	510	77
Eason	MA	1	56	Urology	450	102
Fession		1	44	Bariatric	480	72
Fixer	MA	1	43	Urology	578	97
Frederick		1	47	Vascular*	540	82
Mold		1	45	Urology	350	56
Nerve		1	51	Urology	290	45
Seimer		1	59	Neurosurgery	444	70
Tho		1	42	Plastic	634	97
Underside		1	55	Thoracic*	921	152
Wall		1	58	Plastic	247	41
Yellow		1	44	Thoracic*	540	82

Table 6.2
MIDCARE
Medical Staff
Information
(continued)

*On the web at
ache.org/books/
Middleboro2*

continued

Table 6.2
MIDCARE
Medical Staff
Information
(continued)

*On the web at
ache.org/books/
Middleboro2*

Name	Note	Off	Age	Specialty	2019 Patient Days	2019 Discharges
Department of Medicine, Consulting Staff						
Ange		9	48	Endocrinology	84	8
Carles		9	60	Pulmonary Medicine	28	4
Feada		9	63	Hematology	33	5
Flint		9	56	Oncology	154	12
Kipstein	MA	3	50	Cardiology	201	30
Klock	MA	3	49	OB/GYN	130	14
Lott		9	50	Hematology	112	16
Maeer	MA	3	42	Cardiology	133	18
Malone		9	55	Allergy	31	6
McVoy		9	37	Psychiatry	32	4
Mustard	MA	3	39	OB/GYN	223	50
Parish		9	48	Dermatology	16	3
Rubble		3	54	Oncology	232	31
Thomas		9	51	Psychiatry	74	12
Vitter		9	57	Hematology	52	6
Department of Surgery, Consulting Staff						
Lee	MA	3	40	Orthopedic	56	6
Finn	MA	3	49	Thoracic	39	6
Mike		9	60	Orthopedic	78	9
Picture	MA	3	47	Orthopedic	76	12
Steve	MA	3	47	Thoracic	80	12
Wingate		9	50	Pediatric	60	13
Total					**56,870**	**9,892**
Department of Pathology						
Fisher		1	54	Pathology		
Lafta		1	49	Pathology		
Leatros		1	47	Pathology		
Mautz		1	44	Pathology		
Mixture		1	61	Pathology		
Mushroom		1	42	Pathology		
Nerverto		1	56	Pathology		
Pathos		1	56	Pathology		
Wingate		1	37	Pathology		

continued

Name	Note	Off	Age	Specialty	2019 Patient Days	2019 Discharges
Department of Radiology						
Glorioso		1	52	Radiology		
Picture		1	56	Radiology		
Quadic		1	45	Radiology		
Roetgen		1	61	Radiology		
Sunshine		1	40	Radiology		
Ray		1	45	Radiology		
Hines		1	50	Radiology		
Gershler		1	39	Radiology		
Jinks		1	45	Radiology		
Gotlike		1	52	Radiology		
Ricker		1	34	Radiology		
Smith		1	44	Radiology		
Trippe		1	49	Radiology		
Tracer		1	49	Radiology		
Department of Anesthesiology						
Aaron		1	38	Anesthesiology		
Carter		1	62	Anesthesiology		
Dexter		1	66	Anesthesiology		
Harrington		1	63	Anesthesiology		
Maxwell		1	50	Anesthesiology		
Nelson		1	60	Anesthesiology		
Thomas		1	64	Anesthesiology		
Fisher		1	54	Anesthesiology		
Gass		1	48	Anesthesiology		
Lister		1	61	Anesthesiology		
Mask		1	59	Anesthesiology		
Department of Emergency Medicine						
Casey		1	44	Emergency		
Catle		1	39	Emergency		
Cytesmith		1	60	Emergency		
Goodspeed		1	65	Emergency		
Gotlike		1	52	Emergency		
Hines		1	60	Emergency		
Hotlick		1	58	Emergency		
Ishabi		1	43	Emergency		

Table 6.2

MIDCARE Medical Staff Information *(continued)*

On the web at ache.org/books/ Middleboro2

continued

Table 6.2
MIDCARE
Medical Staff
Information
(continued)

On the web at
ache.org/books/
Middleboro2

Name	Note	Off	Age	Specialty	2019 Patient Days	2019 Discharges
Jinks		1	45	Emergency		
Smooth		1	54	Emergency		
Tobias		1	51	Emergency		
Welby		1	56	Emergency		
Department of Hospital Medicine						
Carlos		1	40	Hospitalist		
Drudge		1	35	Hospitalist		
Frost		1	39	Hospitalist		
Gupta		1	40	Hospitalist		
Lewis		1	50	Hospitalist		
Palmer		1	32	Hospitalist		
Ruderbacker		1	56	Hospitalist		
Shine		1	43	Hospitalist		
Stickle		1	61	Hospitalist		
Vail		1	44	Hospitalist		

Notes:

Code	Office Location
1	Middleboro
2	Mifflenville
3	Jasper
4	Harris City
5	Statesville
6	Carterville
7	Boalsburg
8	Minortown
9	Capital City
10	Other

ENT: ear, nose, throat; MA: Medical Associates; OB/GYN: obstetrics/gynecology; Off: office location.
* Medical practice owned or partially owned by MIDCARE.

Hospital Service	2019	2018	2017	2016
Pediatrics				
Beds	8	8	12	14
Patient Days	1,505	1,634	1,836	1,823
Occupancy	51.5%	56.0%	41.9%	35.7%
Maternity				
Beds	16	16	16	16
Patient Days	4,181	4,024	3,978	3,960
Occupancy	71.6%	68.9%	68.1%	67.8%
Medical-Surgical I				
Beds	48	48	50	50
Patient Days	12,303	11,536	11,034	12,540
Occupancy	70.2%	65.8%	60.5%	68.7%
Medical-Surgical II				
Beds	40	40	50	50
Patient Days	10,249	11,156	11,078	11,004
Occupancy	70.2%	76.4%	60.7%	60.3%
Medical-Surgical III				
Beds	45	45	58	62
Patient Days	11,760	11,692	11,673	11,922
Occupancy	71.6%	71.2%	55.1%	52.7%
Medical-Surgical IV				
Beds	40	43	44	50
Patient Days	10,967	10,995	11,934	11,950
Occupancy	75.1%	70.1%	74.3%	65.5%
ICU/CCU				
Beds	23	20	20	18
Patient Days	5,905	5,328	5,329	5,026
Occupancy	70.3%	73.0%	73.0%	76.5%
Total Hospital				
Beds	220	220	250	260
Patient Days	56,870	56,365	56,862	58,225
Occupancy	70.8%	71.2%	63.2%	62.2%

Table 6.3
MIDCARE
Hospital
Inpatient
Occupancy by
Service

*On the web at
ache.org/books/
Middleboro2*

Note: ICU/CCU: intensive care unit/coronary care unit.

Table 6.4
MIDCARE
Detailed
Utilization
Statistics

*On the web at
ache.org/books/
Middleboro2*

Month	Dis	Patient Days	IP Surgery	OP Surgery	Births	ED Visits	ED Admits	OP Visits
2019								
January	910	4,959	201	370	98	2,534	272	10,558
February	834	4,655	184	304	84	2,245	238	9,973
March	863	5,098	205	272	101	2,757	268	10,567
April	770	5,124	205	344	101	2,245	254	10,445
May	789	5,170	223	309	109	2,110	283	10,254
June	945	5,768	203	351	106	2,203	260	9,856
July	711	4,535	205	367	99	2,083	253	9,635
August	791	4,425	203	360	101	2,068	250	9,356
September	857	4,978	234	463	109	2,205	275	9,835
October	807	4,090	202	426	101	2,003	245	10,023
November	845	4,923	208	409	96	2,209	249	9,956
December	770	3,145	183	403	90	2,027	240	8,245
Total	**9,892**	**56,870**	**2,456**	**4,378**	**1,195**	**26,689**	**3,087**	**118,703**
2018								
January	782	4,718	251	406	99	2,061	270	8,951
February	837	4,848	209	302	90	1,945	265	8,094
March	893	5,149	223	369	110	1,755	289	9,092
April	866	5,000	215	367	109	1,945	365	9,234
May	880	5,320	205	351	110	1,956	310	9,245
June	806	5,112	246	295	91	2,012	270	9,345
July	703	4,734	227	402	103	2,077	280	9,832
August	700	3,650	210	190	90	2,056	263	9,257
September	754	3,967	218	379	94	2,098	289	9,934
October	854	5,025	243	369	101	2,044	240	10,109
November	730	4,775	204	348	103	1,998	279	9,887
December	702	4,067	206	312	90	1,923	288	8,750
Total	**9,507**	**56,365**	**2,657**	**4,090**	**1,190**	**23,870**	**3,408**	**111,730**

Notes: (1) Dis: Discharges; ED: emergency department; IP: inpatient; OP: outpatient. (2) ED Visits are total ED visits. (3) ED Admits are ED visits that led to an inpatient admission. (4) OP Visits are outpatient visits that exclude ED visits.

	2019	2018	2017
Revenues			
Patient Services Revenue			
Inpatient Net of Allowances and Uncollectables	233,405,656	231,961,369	234,812,517
Outpatient Net of Allowances and Uncollectables	137,079,513	133,332,125	127,552,478
Total	**370,485,169**	**365,293,494**	**362,364,995**
Expenses			
Salaries and Wages	141,565,387	142,675,234	144,230,404
Fringe Benefits	36,225,120	37,453,298	37,495,992
Supplies	72,413,334	75,293,440	78,345,020
Professional Fees	8,343,015	6,097,334	4,504,292
Interest	5,200,348	5,876,340	5,945,223
Depreciation	20,674,998	18,345,050	17,334,202
Amortization	35,223,878	32,464,383	30,274,393
Other	37,069,852	30,117,232	20,493,223
Total	**356,715,932**	**348,322,311**	**338,622,749**
Net Income from Operations	13,769,237	16,971,183	23,742,246
Other Revenues			
Unrestricted Gifts and Bequests	1,075,371	1,518,733	827,354
Income from Investments	5,963,757	5,430,203	5,523,494
Miscellaneous Non–Patient Services Revenue	1,029,354	986,284	1,001,482
Total	**8,068,482**	**7,935,220**	**7,352,330**
Profit or (Loss)	**21,837,719**	**24,906,403**	**31,094,576**

Table 6.5
MIDCARE
Statement of
Revenues and
Expenses

*On the web at
ache.org/books/
Middleboro2*

Notes: (1) Years ending December 31. (2) Numbers are in US dollars.

Table 6.6
MIDCARE
Balance Sheet

On the web at
ache.org/books/
Middleboro2

	2019	2018	2017
Assets			
Current Assets			
Cash	10,223,454	23,565,787	24,675,787
Marketable Securities	8,342,848	2,245,363	2,016,334
Accounts Receivable—Gross	80,485,667	82,229,226	81,140,442
Allowances for Uncollectables	15,265,364	13,875,998	12,745,878
Accounts Receivable—Net	65,220,303	68,353,228	68,394,564
Due from Third-Party Payers	2,171,223	2,584,330	2,645,293
Inventories	27,354,995	31,393,446	27,354,995
Prepaid Expenses	7,343,002	5,383,446	3,574,009
Total Current Assets	**120,655,825**	**133,525,600**	**128,660,982**
Noncurrent Assets			
Property, Plant, and Equipment—Gross	663,887,127	623,069,851	608,277,429
Less Accumulated Depreciation	195,392,458	174,717,460	153,042,462
Property, Plant, and Equipment—Net	468,494,669	448,352,391	455,234,967
Other Investments	34,386,223	36,283,446	38,453,998
Total Assets	**623,536,717**	**618,161,437**	**622,349,947**
Liabilities			
Current Liabilities			
Accounts Payable	8,342,030	8,722,303	8,846,283
Accrued Salaries, Wages, and Benefits	3,012,384	3,128,383	3,835,223
Accrued Interest	8,334,959	8,856,383	8,203,451
Other Accrued Expenses	2,554,293	3,485,220	3,748,223
Due to Third-Party Vendors	16,232,773	13,274,303	14,443,929
Long-Term Debt Due Within One Year	20,457,112	18,352,334	16,394,293
Total Current Liabilities	**58,933,551**	**55,818,926**	**55,471,402**
Long-Term Debt	203,035,777	207,968,291	216,605,105
Total Liabilities	**261,969,328**	**263,787,217**	**272,076,507**
Net Assets			
Restricted	2,646,395	17,290,945	34,766,620
Unrestricted	358,920,994	337,083,275	315,506,820
Total Net Assets	**361,567,389**	**354,374,220**	**350,273,440**
Net Assets + Liabilities	**623,536,717**	**618,161,437**	**622,349,947**

Notes: (1) For fiscal years ending December 31. (2) Numbers are in US dollars.

Diagnosis-Related Group (DRG) Name	2019	2018	2017	2016
Normal Newborn*	1,195	1,186	1,082	1,093
Vaginal Delivery, No Complication	1,009	1,007	974	995
Medical Back Problems	770	726	764	655
Cesarean Section	323	351	336	342
Angina Pectoris	400	386	419	454
Other Gastrointestinal	301	314	327	364
Chest Pain	292	290	296	328
Septicemia, Sepsis	205	167	285	265
Pneumonia, Pleurisy	203	165	197	197
Major Joint Operation	112	157	165	175
Total Top 10 Discharges (Excluding Births)	**3,314**	**3,249**	**3,436**	**3,411**
Total Hospital Discharges	**9,872**	**9,507**	**9,256**	**9,372**
% Top 10 Discharges (Excluding Births)	**33.57**	**34.17**	**37.12**	**36.40**

Table 6.7
MIDCARE
Top Ten DRG
Discharges

Note: *Counted as births, not discharges.

Table 6.8
MIDCARE Patient Days by Type and by Payer

Type of PT Day	Total PT Days (%)	Medicare (%)	Medicaid (%)	BC HMO (%)	BC PPO (%)	BC Indem (%)	CS PPO (%)	Comm PPO (%)	Comm Indem (%)	VA + Mil (%)	Other (%)	Self-Pay (%)
Medical	43.1	16.20	2.80	0.20	3.30	0.80	0.70	5.10	10.00	2.00	0.20	1.80
Surgical												
Nonorthopedic	22.1	12.1	2.8	0.1	1.2	0.2	0.1	0.9	1.6	2.1	0.2	0.8
Orthopedic	10.7	3.0	2.7	0.1	0.4	0.2	0.2	0.6	1.6	1.7	0.0	0.2
Obstetric	7.5	0.0	2.0	0.4	1.3	0.1	0.1	0.8	1.7	0.0	0.2	0.9
Newborn	4.3	0.0	1.1	0.2	0.9	0.0	0.0	0.4	1.0	0.0	0.1	0.6
Other Pediatric	3.8	0.0	0.6	0.3	0.7	0.1	0.1	0.0	1.1	0.7	0.0	0.2
ICU/CCU	7.9	5.8	0.2	0.4	0.3	0.0	0.1	0.0	0.7	0.0	0.2	0.2
Psychological/Psychiatric	0.2	0.1	0.0	0.0	0.0	0.0	0.1	0.0	0.0	0.0	0.0	0.0
Substance Abuse												
Detox	0.1	0.0	0.0	0.0	0.0	0.0	0.0	0.0	0.0	0.0	0.0	0.1
Rehab	0.3	0.0	0.0	0.0	0.0	0.0	0.0	0.0	0.0	0.0	0.0	0.3
Total	**100.0**	**37.2**	**12.2**	**1.7**	**8.1**	**1.4**	**1.4**	**7.8**	**17.7**	**6.5**	**0.9**	**5.1**

Note: BC: Blue Cross; Comm: Commercial; CS: Central States; HMO: health maintenance organization; ICU/CCU: intensive care unit/coronary care unit or cardiac ICU; Indem: indemnity; Mil: military; PPO: preferred provider organization; PT: patient; VA: Veterans Administration.

Category	CMS Core Measure	Benchmark	MIDCARE
Timely and Effective Heart Attack Care	Average number of minutes before outpatients with chest pain or possible heart attack who needed specialized care were transferred to another hospital	58 min	42 min
Timely and Effective Heart Attack Care	Average number of minutes before outpatients with chest pain or possible heart attack got an ECG (electrocardiogram)	7 min	7 min
Timely and Effective Heart Attack Care	Percentage of outpatients with chest pain or possible heart attack who got drugs to break up blood clots within 30 minutes of arrival	59%	75%
Timely and Effective Heart Attack Care	Percentage of outpatients with chest pain who received aspirin within 24 hours of arrival or before transferring from the emergency department	97%	97%
Timely and Effective Heart Attack Care	Percentage of heart attack patients who got drugs to break up blood clots within 30 minutes of arrival	60%	57%
Timely and Effective Heart Attack Care	Percentage of heart attack patients given a procedure to open blocked blood vessels within 90 minutes of arrival	96%	96%
Effective Heart Failure Care	Percentage of heart failure patients given an evaluation of LVS (left ventricular systolic) function	99%	99%
Effective Pneumonia Care	Percentage of pneumonia patients given the most appropriate initial antibiotic(s)	96%	100%
Timely Surgical Care	Percentage of surgery patients who were given an antibiotic at the right time (within 1 hour of surgery) to help prevent infection	99%	98%
Timely Surgical Care	Percentage of surgery patients whose preventive antibiotics were stopped at the right time (within 2 hours after surgery)	98%	99%
Timely Surgical Care	Percentage of patients who got treatment at the right time (within 24 hours before or after surgery) to help prevent blood clots after certain types of surgery	100%	100%
Effective Surgical Care	Percentage of surgery patients taking heart drugs called beta blockers before coming to the hospital who were kept on the beta blockers during the period just before and after surgery	98%	98%
Effective Surgical Care	Percentage of surgery patients who were given the right kind of antibiotic to help prevent infection	99%	98%
Effective Surgical Care	Percentage of surgery patients whose urinary catheters were removed on the first or second day after surgery	98%	100%
Timely Emergency Dept. Care	Average time patients who came to the emergency department with broken bones had to wait before getting pain medication	54 min	47 min
Timely Emergency Dept. Care	Percentage of patients who left the emergency department before being seen	2%	1%
Timely Emergency Dept. Care	Percentage of patients who came to the emergency department with stroke symptoms who received brain scan results within 45 minutes of arrival	66%	85%

Table 6.9
MIDCARE
Performance
Against CMS
Core Measures

continued

Table 6.9
MIDCARE
Performance
Against CMS
Core Measures
(continued)

Category	CMS Core Measure	Benchmark	MIDCARE
Timely Emergency Dept. Care	Average median time patients spent in the emergency department before they were admitted to the hospital as an inpatient	260 min	336 min
Timely Emergency Dept. Care	Average (median) time patients spent in the emergency department before leaving from the visit	89 min	130 min
Timely Emergency Dept. Care	Average time patients spent in the emergency department before leaving from the visit	142 min	156 min
Timely Emergency Dept. Care	Average time patients spent in the emergency department before they were seen by a healthcare professional	26 min	35 min
Preventive Care	Percentage of patients assessed and given influenza vaccination	94%	99%
Preventive Care	Percentage of healthcare workers given influenza vaccination	84%	94%
Effective Children's Asthma Care	Percentage of children and their caregivers who received home management plan-of-care documents while hospitalized for asthma	90%	83%
Effective Stroke Care	Percentage of ischemic stroke patients who got medicine to break up a blood clot within 3 hours after symptoms started	81%	75%
Effective Stroke Care	Percentage of ischemic stroke patients who received medicine known to prevent complications caused by blood clots within 2 days of hospital admission	98%	100%
Effective Stroke Care	Percentage of ischemic or hemorrhagic stroke patients who received treatment to keep blood clots from forming anywhere in the body within 2 days of hospital admission	97%	100%
Effective Stroke Care	Percentage of ischemic stroke patients who received a prescription for medicine known to prevent complications caused by blood clots at discharge	99%	100%
Effective Stroke Care	Percentage of ischemic stroke patients with a type of irregular heartbeat who were given a prescription for a blood thinner at discharge	97%	100%
Effective Stroke Care	Percentage of ischemic stroke patients needing medicine to lower bad cholesterol who were given a prescription for this medicine at discharge	97%	99%
Effective Stroke Care	Percentage of ischemic or hemorrhagic stroke patients or caregivers who received written educational material about stroke care and prevention during the hospital stay	94%	83%
Blood Clot Prevention	Percentage of patients who got treatment to prevent blood clots on the day of or day after hospital admission or surgery	93%	99%
Blood Clot Prevention	Percentage of patients who got treatment to prevent blood clots on the day of or the day after being admitted to the ICU (intensive care unit)	96%	100%
Blood Clot Prevention	Percentage of patients who developed a blood clot while in the hospital who did not get treatment that could have prevented it	5%	3%

continued

Category	CMS Core Measure	Benchmark	MIDCARE
Blood Clot Treatment	Percentage of patients with blood clots who got recommended treatment, which includes using two different blood thinner medicines at the same time	95%	96%
Blood Clot Treatment	Percentage of patients with blood clots who were treated with an intravenous blood thinner and then were checked to determine if the blood thinner caused unplanned complications	99%	94%
Blood Clot Treatment	Percentage of patients with blood clots who were discharged on a blood thinner medicine and received written instructions about that medicine	90%	86%
Pregnancy and Delivery Care	Percentage of mothers whose deliveries were scheduled too early (1–2 weeks early) when a scheduled delivery was not medically necessary	3%	2%
Use of Medical Imaging	Percentage of outpatients with low back pain who had a magnetic resonance imaging (MRI) scan without trying recommended treatments first, such as physical therapy	40%	24%
Use of Medical Imaging	Percentage of outpatients who had a mammogram, an ultrasound, or an MRI of the breast within 45 days after a screening mammogram	9%	8%
Use of Medical Imaging	Percentage of outpatients who had CT (computed tomography) scans of the chest that were "combination" (double) scans	2%	2%
Use of Medical Imaging	Percentage of outpatient CT scans of the abdomen that were "combination" scans	9%	9%
Use of Medical Imaging	Percentage of outpatients who got cardiac imaging stress tests before low-risk outpatient surgery	5%	4%
Use of Medical Imaging	Percentage of outpatients with brain CT scans who got a sinus CT scan at the same time	3%	4%
Surgical Complications	Rate of complications for hip/knee replacement patients	3%	No Difference from National Rate
Surgical Complications	Rate of serious complications (from AHRQ)	<1%	No Difference from National Rate
Surgical Complications	Death rate among patients with serious treatable complications after surgery	117.5 per 1,000 dis.	No Difference from National Rate
Healthcare-Associated Infections	Rate of central line–associated bloodstream infections (CLABSIs) in ICUs and selected wards	N/A	No Difference from National Rate
Healthcare-Associated Infections	Rate of CLABSIs in ICUs only	N/A	No Difference from National Rate

Table 6.9
MIDCARE
Performance
Against CMS
Core Measures
(continued)

continued

Category	CMS Core Measure	Benchmark	MIDCARE
Healthcare-Associated Infections	Rate of catheter-associated urinary tract infections (CAUTIs) in ICUs and selected wards	N/A	No Difference from National Rate
Healthcare-Associated Infections	Rate of CAUTIs in ICUs only	N/A	No Difference from National Rate
Healthcare-Associated Infections	Rate of surgical-site infections from abdominal hysterectomy	N/A	No Difference from National Rate
Healthcare-Associated Infections	Rate of MRSA (Methicillin-resistant Staphylococcus aureus) blood laboratory identified events (blood-stream infections)	N/A	No Difference from National Rate
Healthcare-Associated Infections	Rate of C. diff (Clostridium difficile) laboratory identified events (intestinal infections)	N/A	No Difference from National Rate
Readmissions and Deaths	Rate of unplanned readmission for COPD (chronic obstructive pulmonary disease) patients	20%	No Difference from National Rate
Readmissions and Deaths	Death rate for COPD patients	8%	No Difference from National Rate
Readmissions and Deaths	Rate of unplanned readmission for heart attack patients	22%	No Difference from National Rate
Readmissions and Deaths	Death rate for heart attack patients	12%	No Difference from National Rate
Readmissions and Deaths	Rate of unplanned readmission for heart failure patients	22%	No Difference from National Rate
Readmissions and Deaths	Death rate for heart failure patients	11%	No Difference from National Rate
Readmissions and Deaths	Rate of unplanned readmission for pneumonia patients	17%	No Difference from National Rate

continued

Category	CMS Core Measure	Benchmark	MIDCARE
Readmissions and Deaths	Death rate for pneumonia patients	11%	No Difference from National Rate
Readmissions and Deaths	Rate of unplanned readmission for stroke patients	13%	No Difference from National Rate
Readmissions and Deaths	Death rate for stroke patients	15%	No Difference from National Rate
Readmissions and Deaths	Rate of unplanned readmission for coronary artery bypass graft (CABG) surgery patients	15%	No Difference from National Rate
Readmissions and Deaths	Death rate for CABG surgery patients	3%	No Difference from National Rate
Readmissions and Deaths	Rate of unplanned readmission after hip/knee surgery	5%	No Difference from National Rate
Readmissions and Deaths	Rate of unplanned readmission after discharge from hospital (hospitalwide)	15%	Better than National Rate
Payment and Value of Care	Payment for heart failure patients	N/A	More than National Average
Payment and Value of Care	Payment for pneumonia patients	N/A	More than National Average
Payment and Value of Care	Death rate for heart attack patients	N/A	No Difference from National Rate
Payment and Value of Care	Payment for heart attack patients	N/A	More than National Average
Payment and Value of Care	Death rate for heart failure patients	11%	Less than National Average
Payment and Value of Care	Payment for heart failure patients	$15,223	No Difference from National Rate
Payment and Value of Care	Death rate for pneumonia patients	12%	No Difference from National Rate
Payment and Value of Care	Payment for pneumonia patients	$14, 294	No Difference from National Rate
Patient Survey	Percentage of patients who reported that their nurses "always" communicated well	80%	83%

Table 6.9
MIDCARE
Performance
Against CMS
Core Measures
(continued)

continued

Table 6.9
MIDCARE
Performance
Against CMS
Core Measures
(continued)

Category	CMS Core Measure	Benchmark	MIDCARE
Patient Survey	Percentage of patients who reported that their doctors "always" communicated well	82%	89%
Patient Survey	Percentage of patients who reported that they "always" received help as soon as they wanted	68%	82%
Patient Survey	Percentage of patients who reported that their pain was "always" well controlled	71%	80%
Patient Survey	Percentage of patients who reported that staff "always" explained the medication before giving it to them	65%	78%
Patient Survey	Percentage of patients who reported that their room and bathroom were "always" cleaned	74%	94%

Notes: (1) N/A means not applicable and either the data are not available or the number of cases is too small for a legitimate conclusion. (2) "Better" means better than national average. (3) "No difference" means no statistical difference exists between the hospital and the national average. (4) AHRQ: Agency for Healthcare Research and Quality; CMS: Centers for Medicare & Medicaid Services.

CASE 7

MEDICAL ASSOCIATES

Medical Associates is a for-profit multispecialty medical group. It operates two facilities—one is in Middleboro (which opened in 1995 and is approximately three miles from MIDCARE), and the other is in Jasper (which opened in 2002 on the eastern edge of town and is now adjacent to the new interstate). In 2017, Medical Associates added a 24/7 convenient care center—called Medical Associates Express—to its Jasper location.

All Medical Associates physicians maintain active staff privileges at an accredited hospital and consulting staff privileges at other hospitals. These physicians provide services in the following specialties: cardiology, ENT (ear, nose, throat), family medicine, gastroenterology, general surgery, internal medicine, obstetrics/gynecology, orthopedic surgery, pediatrics, urgent and convenient care, and urology. Currently, 23 physicians staff the facility in Middleboro, and many of these 23 maintain active staff privileges at MIDCARE and consulting staff privileges at Capital City General Hospital. At the Jasper facility, 17 physicians provide medical services, and some of these 17 maintain active staff privileges at MIDCARE or at Capital City General Hospital as well as consulting staff privileges at other hospitals in Hillsboro County. Ambulatory surgical services are available at the Jasper facility, and Medical Associates physicians in Middleboro provide ambulatory surgery at MIDCARE.

Medical Associates is organized as a for-profit, professional corporation. Each of its shareholders has rights to distributed earnings based on a predetermined formula approved by the board of directors. The total number of shares equals the number of shareholder physicians. For example, a new physician is recruited and hired on a three-year contract that provides a fixed salary and benefits. At the end of three years, the physician is either offered the opportunity to join Medical Associates as a shareholder or is terminated. If asked to join, the physician must purchase one share in the practice. If terminated, the physician leaves and the group repurchases the physician's share. According to the bylaws of Medical Associates, the buy-in and severance rate is "equal to the total equity of the corporation divided by the number of partner physicians." This formula can be changed by a two-thirds vote of the partner physicians.

All physicians affiliated with Medical Associates sign a contractual covenant that, should they or the group terminate the relationship, they cannot practice within a 30-mile radius of Middleboro for two years without paying compensatory damages equal to the compensation they received from the group for the previous two years. In 1978, the covenant was tested in state court and found to be legal. Since that time, no former Medical Associate physician has disputed it.

HISTORY

Medical Associates was founded in 1951 as a single-specialty medical practice in Middleboro. Under the leadership of Dr. James R. Fairchild, a board-certified internist, it slowly expanded in size and, in 1963, added other specialties. It has provided specialty and sub-specialty medical and surgical care since 1972.

Dr. Fairchild was an early proponent of multispecialty medical care. For almost 15 years, he chaired the committee on multispecialty medical practice of the State Medical Society. He received special awards from the American Medical Association for writing articles that examined the value of multispecialty medicine in rural areas. For many years, he personally recruited all new physicians. Trained in internal medicine at a midwestern medical school, he completed his residency training at a large midwestern medical center known for its innovative approaches to serving rural areas using a large multispecialty group. As he later expressed in his articles and many speeches, "multispecialty medical practices truly serve the patient's interests of high quality, convenience, and reasonable costs." In 1972, under his leadership, Medical Associates required all affiliated physicians to be board certified within three years, a decision that was controversial at the time. Throughout his career with Medical Associates, he served as its president and medical director. He also supervised all professional and administrative staff until 1972, when he hired a full-time executive manager.

On the occasion of his retirement in 1988, the Jasper facility was renamed Fairchild Medical Center. Although retired, Dr. Fairchild still attends the annual meetings of the board as an "interested observer." He has been a long-term critic of the two hospitals in Middleboro—namely, MIDCARE and Webster Health System. When he retired, he blamed "the lack of innovation in medical care in our community on the self-interested behaviors and approaches each hospital has followed for decades. The problem is our hospitals do not listen to the practicing physician who knows best the needs of the patients."

In 1972, Medical Associates hired its first DO, a physician trained in osteopathic medicine. Dr. Maynard Kricnicki, who subsequently became a partner, practiced in Jasper but used the hospital resources in Capital City. According to Dr. Fairchild, the late Dr. Kricnicki was "one of our finest primary care physicians before primary care became the rage. He practiced successfully with the group for many years. Osteopathic Medical Center even built and dedicated a memorial to him and his enormous contributions."

Over the past 15 years, all of the original Medical Associates physicians have either retired or left Hillsboro County. Many physicians have joined the group in the past ten years, most of whom did so immediately after completing a residency in their medical specialty.

OPERATIONS AND SERVICES

THE FACILITIES

Each of the two Medical Associates facilities is a modern, one-story building with ample parking and room for expansion. The Middleboro facility is 48,500 square feet, T-shaped, and sits on a 9.75-acre campus. It opened in 1995 and was modernized and expanded in 2002 and 2012. It was featured in a 2013 article in the national trade publication *Medical Group News*.

The Jasper facility is 42,590 square feet, H-shaped, and sits on a 25-acre campus. The building is divided into 25 medical suites. When Medical Associates purchased this land in 1990, it also acquired a 30-year option on a 225-acre undeveloped parcel adjacent to the facility, an option Dr. Fairchild lobbied to get approved. This option, which cost $35,000, establishes a purchase price not to exceed "the average prevailing rate plus 10 percent for undeveloped farmland in Hillsboro County as established by independent appraisal." The land is now adjacent to the interstate highway that will soon open in Jasper.

Both the Jasper and Middleboro facilities share a centralized appointment and patient registration system. Existing and new patients who prefer to use the Medical Associates website can register online, which generates a "medical portal" through which they can access their own health records and test results, schedule or change an appointment, contact their physician, and so on. Patients may also use the group's toll-free telephone number to conduct such business.

The Middleboro facility has a centralized waiting area and, like the Jasper facility, is divided into 25 medical suites. Physician suites (each with two to four examination rooms) are assigned by medical specialty. Family medicine and pediatrics are located in the east and west wings, and surgery is located in the south wing. The center of the facility houses the common waiting area and patient accounts. All other departments are located in the basement. The Jasper facility also has a centralized waiting area. Family medicine and pediatrics are located in the front wing, while surgery is located in the rear wing with medical records, imaging, and laboratory. All physician suites have three examination rooms. While both facilities have their own medical records, imaging, and laboratory, the Middleboro facility provides all other services (e.g., patient accounts) using telecommunications and computer systems.

Each facility is equipped with a comprehensive array of imaging technologies (such as ultrasound, X-ray, computed tomography [CT], and magnetic resonance imaging [MRI]) and drawing stations (leased from and calibrated by Wythe Laboratories in Capital City) for basic blood chemistries and urinalyses done in-house. Wythe Laboratories is under contract to administer and process medical tests for all patients at both facilities. Medical Associates also contracts with Radiology Partners in Capital City to read and interpret all diagnostic images. All X-ray, MRI, and CT images are transmitted electronically to Radiology Partners, which reads them and submits a report to the facility electronically. Under the existing agreement, Medical Associates owns and operates its own imaging equipment and employs the needed technicians. Other contracted services at both facilities include snow removal and grounds maintenance, janitorial, and laundry.

The operating hours at each facility are the same: open 8 a.m. to 6 p.m., Mondays through Saturdays; closed Sundays and on all federal holidays. All telephone inquiries before midnight are handled by a registered nurse; after midnight but before 7 a.m., inquiries are handled by an answering service, which contacts on-call physicians as needed. In 2015, Medical Associates extended its office hours to 9 p.m. on two evenings per week.

On January 15, 2014, Medical Associates opened an ambulatory surgical service in the lower level of the Jasper facility. Outpatient surgery is provided five days per week, and most surgeries are scheduled between 7:30 a.m. and 3:00 p.m. Two fully equipped surgical suites are available, accompanied by waiting and recovery areas. Mary Knoph, RN, is the director of Ambulatory Surgery Services and reports to the chair of the Department of Surgery.

STAFF COMPENSATION AND BENEFITS

All full-time employees work a 40-hour week and qualify for a full benefits package, which includes two weeks' vacation and family coverage in a comprehensive health and dental insurance plan. Sick days are earned at the rate of one per month, with a maximum bank of 30 days. Medical Associates maintains a 401(k) retirement plan for all employees but does not contribute to any employee's plan. Part-time employees are hired at an hourly rate and receive no voluntary benefits or vacation days. Any part-time employee who is scheduled to work more than 948 hours in a calendar year may purchase the employee health insurance plan by paying the prorated difference between the percentage of time worked and the total annual premium.

All physicians are provided with comprehensive benefits, including fully paid medical liability insurance and five days of continuing medical education. Staff physicians are hired for a fixed two-year salary, negotiated at the time of hiring, and qualify for four weeks of paid vacation per year. Shareholding physicians are compensated using a predetermined formula based on the revenues they generate (the net revenue Medical Associates receives for the services provided by the physician) offset by their expenses (the physician's share of all direct and indirect costs associated with her practice). During the fiscal year, each physician is compensated monthly, according to an estimated difference between revenues and expenses. At the end of the fiscal year, the physician is given the difference between total funds previously drawn and his total share of corporate earnings as determined by the formula. To qualify for 100 percent of the share, the physician must work 230 days in a fiscal year. The total draw is reduced on a straight percentage basis for each day under the 230 days. Physicians who work more than 230 days share on a pro rata basis.

PATIENT INSURANCE AND THIRD-PARTY PAYER REIMBURSEMENT

Medical Associates provides services on a fee-for-service basis and has a long-standing policy of accepting "any insurance plan presented to us by patients." As such, it has a contractual relationship with area health maintenance organizations (HMOs) as well as preferred provider organizations (PPOs), including Statewide Blue Shield, Central State Good Health Plan, and two commercial HMOs/PPOs. Medical Associates also maintains a contractual relationship with managed care plans offered by Blue Shield and commercial insurers.

Prices charged at both facilities are exactly the same. All patients are provided a detailed bill or account statement. Patients covered by most insurance plans are billed only for any outstanding balances not paid by their insurer (which receives the bill first and directly from Medical Associates). Patients covered by indemnity or other forms of insurance are required to pay (by cash, check, or credit card) and are provided a bill to send to their insurance carrier for reimbursement. Wythe Laboratories, Radiology Partners, and other independent providers bill separately for services they rendered.

Medicare accounts for approximately 35 percent of Medical Associates's total gross revenue, while Medicaid accounts for approximately 15 percent. The other 50 percent of total gross revenue comes primarily from commercial/private insurance.

MEDICAL ASSOCIATES EXPRESS, INC.

On July 1, 2017, Medical Associates opened Medical Associates Express, housed in a 5,000-square-foot building across from the parking lot of the Jasper facility. Called Express for short, it is a convenient care or walk-in clinic that is open 24/7 per week, including on all holidays. It has four examination and treatment rooms, a basic X-ray service, and a reception area. It is a wholly owned subsidiary corporation, and its employees are not employees of Medical Associates. It pays a fee to Medical Associates to provide system support (for billing and reimbursement, use of the electronic health record [EHR], and information systems maintenance, among others) and services as the building's owner and landlord.

Medical Associates leases space in the building to other healthcare organizations, including Sockalexis Center, a behavioral health and counseling services provider. Adjacent to the Express suite is a regional drawing station owned and operated by Wythe Laboratories. The station is staffed by Wythe employees (e.g., phlebotomists) and is open for business from 7 a.m. to 11 p.m. on weekdays and from 7 a.m. to 7 p.m. on weekends. A med-evacuation helicopter pad is located on this side of the campus as well. Medical Associates donated the pad space to the Town of Jasper, whose emergency medical system is responsible for the pad's operation and upkeep. From this location, the average flying time to Capital City General Hospital is 18 minutes.

Express has a three-member board of directors who are elected for a three-year term by Medical Associates' board of directors. Two of the three Express board members must be members of the Medical Associates board. Cynthia Worley, the executive manager of Medical Associates, also serves as the president of Express. Dr. Clyde Eason serves as Express's medical director and is responsible for all clinical appointments, clinical protocols, and case review.

Advanced registered nurse practitioners, physician assistants, and medical assistants provide the services. Generally, nurse practitioners are available from 7 a.m. to 11 p.m., and physician assistants cover the overnight shift from 11 p.m. to 7 a.m. Medical assistants work on all shifts, and receptionists are at the front desk from 7 a.m. to 11 p.m. The clinical staff can consult, as needed, with Medical Associates physicians, who are available on a rotating on-call basis. One innovative feature of the Medical Associates–Express linkage is that if an Express nurse practitioner, for example, referred a patient to Medical Associates, the patient is not charged for the Express visit. Thus far, utilization has met and exceeded expectations. The average utilization is 4 patients per hour, and daily utilization ranges from 2 to 14 per hour.

Express does not treat broken bones; puncture wounds; injuries requiring sutures; injuries involving the eyes, face, or groin; back injuries; injuries from motor vehicle accidents; or workers' compensation injuries (or provide evaluations for such). It does offer care for minor illnesses (e.g., cold, flu, and allergy symptoms; sore and strep throat), minor injuries (e.g., mild burns, small cuts that need stitches, sprains and strains), joint pain, and temporary skin conditions (e.g., Athlete's foot, shingles, rashes). It can perform suture and staple removal, screening and testing (e.g., for high cholesterol, diabetes, high blood pressure), and vaccinations (e.g., flu shot, pneumonia shot, children's immunization and booster shot, HPV prevention injection). Birth control prescriptions as well as urinary tract and bladder infection treatments are available for women. Every service has a specific price, and the Express website lists these prices as well as the current waiting times for procedures.

GOVERNANCE

A seven-member elected board of directors represents shareholder interests. Each director serves a three-year term, and the terms are staggered so that no more than three new members are elected annually. No term limits exist. The full board meets monthly and hosts its annual meeting in December, during which the members whose terms are not expiring elect new directors, with each shareholder having one vote. All shareholders are invited to the annual meeting. Continuing board members serve as a nominating committee and formally recommend a slate of candidates. New board members take office on January 1 of the following year. Once the new board members have been elected, the entire new board then elects its president, vice president, secretary, and treasurer. Following is a list of the board of directors (effective January 1, 2020):

Medical Associates Board of Directors

Members, Department	Term Expires
Raymond Samuels, Pediatrics, *President*	2020
Jules Putter, Surgery—General, *Vice President*	2021
Kevin Kipstein, Cardiology, *Secretary*	2022
Douglas Fixer, Urology, *Treasurer*	2022
Sarah Lee, Surgery—Orthopedic, *At-Large*	2020
Mark Stanley, Surgery—Orthopedic, *At-Large*	2021
Ursula Unvey, Pediatrics, *At-Large*	2020

Between the board's monthly meetings, the standing committees meet. Any five board members can request a special meeting of the board by providing written notice to the president.

The board has four standing committees and uses ad hoc committees as needed. Standing committees make recommendations to the full board. Standing committees include the audit, clinical standard and quality, finance, and management committees.

AUDIT COMMITTEE

This committee is chaired by the board's treasurer and is composed of two other board members. It oversees the preparation for Medical Associates's annual financial audit by an independent accounting firm. It is responsible for implementing all recommendations in the auditor's management letter. Every three years, the committee recommends to the board the individual or firm that should perform the audit. Current members of this committee are Dr. Fixer (chair), Dr. Stanley, and Worley (ex officio member).

CLINICAL STANDARD AND QUALITY COMMITTEE

This committee is chaired by the board's vice president and includes one other board member and the medical director (ex officio, unless also an elected member of the board). It annually reviews Medical Associates's medical quality assurance plan and systems to monitor and manage quality. It also reviews the medical credentials of any new physician. Every third year, it recommends to the board who should be appointed (or reappointed) as medical director. This committee oversees Medical Associates's Meaningful Use program and medical information system launched in 2012. This committee also addresses all questions concerning the credentials and fitness of physicians. Current members of this committee are Dr. Putter (chair), Dr. Unvey, and Dr. Eason (ex officio member, medical director).

FINANCE COMMITTEE

This committee meets monthly to review Medical Associates's financial statements and to make recommendations to the full board. It also reviews the budget created by the executive manager and recommends this budget to the board for ratification. Medical Associates's fiscal year begins on January 1 and ends on December 31. In the December meeting, the board generally approves the budget for the upcoming fiscal year. Current members of this committee are Dr. Kipstein (chair), Dr. Lee, and Worley.

MANAGEMENT COMMITTEE

The board's president chairs this committee. Other members include the medical director, the chair of each medical department, one other board member, and the executive manager. This committee meets monthly to review Medical Associates's operations, including the budget performance, and to address management problems and issues. Current members of this committee are Dr. Samuels (board president and committee chair), Dr. Kipstein, Dr. Eason, Dr. Putter (chair of the Department of Surgery), Dr. Thomas Underwood (chair of the Department of Medicine), and Worley.

MEDICAL DEPARTMENTS AND ORGANIZATIONAL STRUCTURE

Medical Associates's medical director is appointed for a three-year term by the board. In accordance with the group's bylaws, "the medical director cannot be the board's president or vice president." The medical director oversees the development and implementation of the medical quality assurance plan, medical care protocols, and (with participating insurance plans) the formulary. The medical director must approve all new or revised contracts involving ancillary services, such as imaging and laboratory services, before the president can sign the contract. Increasingly, the medical director is responsible for all relations and contracts with managed care plans. As compensation, the medical director receives an extra 20 percent of his or her practice-based compensation.

Dr. Eason has been the medical director at Medical Associates for the past seven years. He is a graduate of an eastern medical school, completed advanced education in his medical specialty at a major midwestern medical center, and holds a master of public health in occupational medicine. He is board certified in his internal medicine subspecialty and in occupational health. Born in Middleboro, Dr. Eason returned to town after completing his medical education. He has been affiliated with Medical Associates for 15 years and is married to a member of the Fairchild family.

Medical Associates has two departments: medicine and surgery. Each department chair is elected annually in December by the physician shareholders assigned to the specific department. A chair receives a 12 percent stipend in addition to any practice-based compensation. A chair is responsible for convening monthly medical staff meetings and representing the medical department on the management committee. In addition, a chair serves as the supervisor for all clinical and administrative staff assigned to the medical department, such as registered nurses, medical assistants, and receptionists.

Dr. Putter is the chair of the Department of Surgery. He has held this position for the past seven years, but he has been affiliated with Medical Associates since the group recruited him 20 years ago. On three previous occasions, he served on the board of directors—and twice as board president. He is a graduate of a western medical school and completed a degree in advanced medical education in general surgery at a major midwestern teaching hospital.

Dr. Underwood has just been elected as chair of the Department of Medicine. He is a graduate of a southern medical school and completed his advanced medical education at teaching hospitals in the Midwest and on the East Coast. Previously, he was chair of the board's ad hoc committee on long-range planning and medical recruitment.

The medical director resolves any disputes, while the chief of a medical department determines the work schedules of department physicians. All physicians rotate on-call duties and Saturdays. In the past, physicians typically worked one Saturday every six weeks.

ADMINISTRATION

Cynthia Worley is the executive manager at Medical Associates. She reports to the board president and is responsible for all nonmedical operations, including patient accounts, communications, building maintenance and grounds, materials management, medical records, information systems, imaging, laboratory services, and all nonclinical staff. She also serves as the controller for the corporation. A graduate from an eastern university and holder of a master of business administration and master of health services administration, she was appointed to her position when her predecessor retired. Prior to joining Medical Associates, she was the associate vice president of a midwestern medical center with responsibility for the acquisition and management of all medical practices and was the associate director of administration at a 65-physician group in a neighboring state. She is an active member of the Medical Group Management Association. Born and raised in Capital City, she still has family across Hillsboro County.

Worley maintains an office in the Middleboro facility and travels to the Jasper facility at least once a week. All employees not assigned to a specific physician or to Ambulatory Surgery (e.g., registered nurses, medical assistants) report directly to her. These employees include Ella Smythe (director of Patient Accounts and Business Operations), Christine Clark (director of Human Resources), Spencer Mangrove (bookkeeper), Hank Hammer (director of Maintenance), Shreya Batterjee (director of Medical Records), Alice Byte (director of Management Information System), Faith Kitchen (manager of Imaging Services, Middleboro), Warren Kidder (manager of Imaging Services, Jasper), Robin Swisher (manager of Laboratory Services, Middleboro), and Helena Morgan (manager of Laboratory Services, Jasper).

SUCCESSES, CHALLENGES, AND PLANS

COMPLIANCE WITH MEANINGFUL USE

When asked to name her most significant accomplishment since joining Medical Associates, Worley cited Medical Associates's state-of-the-art EHR that could—if desired—be linked to the EHR of any hospital in the area. She indicated that defining the system parameters, getting board approval for the most crucial elements, overseeing the installation, and then field-testing the finished system were some of the most complex tasks she has undertaken in her career. "I understand now why my predecessor decided to retire instead of roll out such a system" she joked. "Achieving compliance with all stage 2 criteria of CMS's Meaningful Use program was a lengthy, arduous process but a significant accomplishment." The EHR at Medical Associates is able to process all medication orders, generate and transmit prescriptions electronically, record demographics, record vital signs, record smoking status, report ambulatory clinical quality measures, incorporate clinical lab results, and provide immunization data. The system also provides clinical summaries and educational resources to patients and is the basis of Medical Associates's expanded website and patient information system.

AMBULATORY SURGERY SERVICE AT THE MIDDLEBORO FACILITY

Medical Associates has achieved its targeted utilization and financial projections for the ambulatory surgical service at the Jasper facility. It may now be time to consider a similar service at the Middleboro facility. The renovation and expansion of the space will cost approximately $550,000, and approximately $350,000 of that amount will be used for equipment. Current prices are approximately $100 per square foot for renovation and $250 per square foot for new construction. The lower level of the Middleboro facility has sufficient space for an ambulatory surgical service similar to that in Jasper. Existing mechanical systems and parking are also sufficient to support this service.

Medical Associates faces a 3.5 percent cost of capital. The anticipated salvage value of these new fixed assets will be $350,000 after five years. To do this project, the group needs to recruit at least two general surgeons or ENT (ear, nose, throat) physicians for the Jasper facility to free up the Middleboro physicians to work in the ambulatory surgical service. Recruitment is underway. Based on preliminary estimates, this project's operational revenue is expected to exceed total expenses for each of the first five years. Medical Associates estimates that this service, using the standard RVU (relative value unit) system used in hospitals, will generate 1.1 surgical procedures per case.

"We have a track record and the plan to expand ambulatory survey into the Middleboro market," Worley said. "It should be a win–win service for Medical Associates and the community. We understand the concern expressed by MIDCARE and are waiting for their response to the idea of a joint venture."

FEASIBILITY OF A CARDIAC HOSPITAL

Recently, Medical Associates and Cardiology Hospitals of America (CHA) announced a joint feasibility study to construct a cardiac hospital in Jasper that will serve Hillsboro County and its surrounding communities. Under the feasibility agreement, Medical Associates can financially participate and be a significant (but minority) owner in this proprietary hospital. In announcing the study, Dr. Herman Goodfellow, president of CHA, stated that this project should have little or no discernible impact on neighboring general hospitals: "CHA hospitals bring the newest technologies to a community—technologies that general hospitals may not be able to afford or support; our number one goal is to address heart disease. We don't have a number two goal." A formal feasibility report is expected in three months.

The Jasper Industrial Development Authority (JIDA) estimated that this new hospital could be a top-ten employer within five years of opening and has tentatively agreed to lease land in the Jasper Industrial Park to CHA. In addition, JIDA indicated that the new hospital will generate a significant amount of tax revenue. Dr. Goodfellow stated in his press briefing that the hospital will serve residents of Hillsboro County as well as Capital City and University Town, and he said the hospital will invite appropriate affiliations with physicians in these areas.

Board president Dr. Samuels said that Medical Associates could either donate or lease land for the project, but the group will want this hospital's physicians to be affiliated with Medical Associates. He acknowledged the challenges associated with the current certificate-of-need (CON) law, but believed that Medical Associates and CHA, together, could secure either a legislative or gubernatorial special exemption. "Another option might be to undertake the project when the CON law lapses this year," he mused. "I have requested that the State Medical Society advocate for CON to lapse as scheduled."

EXECUTION OF THE LAND OPTION

The 30-year option on the parcel adjacent to the Jasper facility must be fully executed in the near future. In 2015, Medical Associates partially executed the option by acquiring and then selling 50 acres. Under Worley's leadership, this partial execution secured working capital for Medical Associates and contributed to its strategic position. The land option established a purchase price not to exceed "the average prevailing rate plus 10 percent for undeveloped farm land in Hillsboro County." In 2015, the purchase price was $2,800 per acre. In the next few years, this price is estimated to be $3,000 per acre.

Undeveloped land that Medical Associates acquires via the land option will be taxed at the rate of $400 per acre per year with a 5 percent increase per year. The remaining 175-acre parcel, once acquired, could immediately be subdivided. The 25 acres along the anticipated new highway could be sold for $30,000 per acre. The remaining land would then be owned and retained by Medical Associates for potential expansion or subsequent sale, or it could be sold at the prevailing rate. A local real estate developer has indicated that his corporation is interested in buying the entire 175-acre parcel for $1 million. Medical Associates has been advised that any financial action it takes should not raise its long-term debt to a net asset ratio higher than 27.5 percent. The hurdle rate is 6 percent, and the group can borrow funds at 3.5 percent. Medical Associates needs to develop a business plan regarding this land option.

REVIEW OF THE MEDICAL APPOINTMENT SYSTEM

National studies suggest that, on average, pediatricians devote 92 percent of their time to ambulatory appointments and OB/GYN physicians devote 70 percent. Currently, Medical Associates's appointment system uses 15-minute slots in pediatrics (four per hour) and 20 minutes in OB/GYN (three per hour). The mean service rate as determined by a special study is 5.0 per hour in pediatrics and 4.5 per hour in OB/GYN. Medical Associates is concerned that demand will quickly outpace its ability to serve these patients, so an independent review of its current systems and capacities is needed.

REGISTERED NURSES VERSUS MEDICAL ASSISTANTS

Five years ago, Medical Associates began to change its staffing by hiring medical assistants (MAs) instead of relying solely on registered nurses (RNs). Currently, all physicians in primary care service are assigned one RN or MA to assist with patient care, and every two physicians in surgery are assigned one RN. RNs who retire or resign have been replaced with MAs. On five recent occasions, when an RN assigned to a senior staff physician left, the senior physician demanded that the RN be replaced by another RN already assigned to a junior staff physician (a nonshareholder) and that a new MA be hired for that physician. This ad hoc practice of job switching has caused internal turmoil between the senior and junior physicians and has led to the subsequent resignation of two RNs who did not want to be reassigned. In 2010, one staff physician resigned from Medical Associates and cited this practice as the primary reason for deciding to relocate his office.

Trying to resolve this issue has led to many discussions. Confusion exists around whom staff should report to and who has the authority to change job assignments. Some employees believe they report to the physician for or with whom they actually work, and others say the reassignment authority lies with the chair of the medical department, the executive manager, or the board of directors. At the last three board meetings, this issue was discussed but not resolved. Dr. Doris Dustin (OB/GYN) has recently filed a formal complaint with the board concerning the upcoming reassignment of her nurse to Dr. Quinton Reaper (Pediatrics).

FINANCIAL RESTRUCTURING

At a recent board retreat, a consultant recommended that Medical Associates retain more of its annual earnings before sharing them with the shareholders. He specifically recommended increasing the overhead cost to include at least an additional 6 percent contribution to net assets. This suggestion was controversial. Some physicians wanted to avoid being taxed twice—first on corporate profits and then on individual income. As one physician noted, "If we don't make a large corporate profit, we minimize our corporate taxes."

Medical Associates's partial execution of the land option in 2015 significantly improved its balance sheet and provided capital for service expansion (e.g., Medical Associates Express) and enhancement (e.g., Meaningful Use–compliant EHR). "We need to retain a higher percentage of our annual earnings to be able to access development capital," Worley said about the consultant's recommendation. "The land option has already provided us the capital to turn the corner and become a much more prominent and strategic player. It is my responsibility to educate the partners that our individual and collective financial interests are served by finding innovative ways to expand our net assets."

OTHER CONCERNS AND PLANS

The clinical standards and quality committee recently recommended adding at least two primary care physicians to the Jasper facility. This recommendation has reopened the issue of whether Medical Associates should recruit physicians trained in family practice or physicians trained in general internal medicine, OB/GYN, or pediatrics. Dr. Putter, chair of the committee and the Department of Surgery, submitted a compelling argument in favor of family practice physicians, but he was directly challenged by Dr. Underwood, chair of the Department of Medicine. Dr. Putter has indicated that his committee remains gridlocked on this issue and cannot proceed with recruiting until it is resolved.

In addition, the committee informed the board that Medical Associates needs one or two professional analysts on staff if it is to fulfill the expectations associated with medical outcome studies requested by HMO clients and Blue Shield. Dr. Eason has reported that he devotes approximately 20 percent of his time to fulfilling requests for this type of information and that he needs professional assistance to relieve him of this burden. The board has yet to act on this information. The budget for 2020, however, was approved without the additional staff requested by Dr. Eason.

Patient referrals between physicians have always occurred within Medical Associates. The ambulatory surgical service in the Jasper facility, however, is beginning to stress the surgeons based at the Middleboro facility, who are now expected to perform certain outpatient surgeries in Jasper. As stated by Dr. Harvey Hersh, a general surgeon in the Middleboro facility, "I am spending too much windshield time traveling back and forth between the two facilities and seeing my patients in MIDCARE. Something needs to be done. My time is too valuable to spend in my car." Dr. Eason met with the surgeons to explain that a certain level of inconvenience is necessary in the short run until this service is established. The Middleboro surgeons accepted Dr. Eason's promise that the problem would be resolved in the next three to six months, perhaps by using locum tenens surgeons.

Jeffrey Whittier, regional vice president of Clearwater Medical Systems, a publicly traded corporation that owns and operates physician offices and groups, has recently contacted Medical Associates to determine whether it is for sale. Whittier indicated that Clearwater "would be interested in furnishing an offer if Medical Associates would seriously consider it." Dr. Samuels has indicated that the group will reply to his inquiry after the next meeting of the board. Meanwhile, OHA Ventures in Capital City has also expressed to Medical Associates that it would like the opportunity to develop a proposal for the purchase of either the Jasper group or the entire Jasper facility, which would then be leased back to Medical Associates at a specific long-term rate.

At the past board meeting, the board instructed Dr. Eason to secure additional consultants to help the board develop an appropriate strategy for responding to the creation of accountable care organizations within the area. The board also agreed to use CPT (current procedural terminology) codes 98966 and 98969 for qualifying non–face-to-face services. In accordance with American Medical Association recommendations, the patient must originate the phone call or e-mail and must be an established patient of Medical Associates, along with other conditions. Medical Associates plans to inform its patients within six months whether their insurance plans reimburse for these types of services (according to the rules providers must follow to use these specific CPT codes for reimbursement) and how to use such services.

Last year, Medical Associates agreed to participate in the second-opinion program of the Smith Brothers Clinic, a nationally recognized medical center known for its diagnostic expertise. Under this program, Medical Associates physicians and patients can visit a Smith Brothers Clinic to receive a second opinion at no charge. In return, physicians refer their patients, as needed, directly to the clinic. Medical Associates just began participating in a similar program for cardiology cases by the Cuyahoga Clinic, another highly regarded national healthcare organization. As a result of its participation in these relationships, Medical Associates is able to advertise that it is a clinical affiliate of both highly respected clinical networks. Worley explained that "these arrangements are part of Medical Associates's plan to brand our services and provide additional value to our patients. We plan to consider additional opportunities." The board has requested Worley to conduct an evaluation of these agreements and present her findings at the next annual meeting.

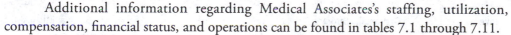

On the web at ache.org/books/ Middleboro2

Additional information regarding Medical Associates's staffing, utilization, compensation, financial status, and operations can be found in tables 7.1 through 7.11.

Table 7.1
Medical
Associates
Affiliated
Physicians

*On the web at
ache.org/books/
Middleboro2*

Name	Specialty	Age	Facility	Gender	Active	Consulting
Autumn	Gastroenterology	44	M	1	MIDCARE	CCG
Barton	Internal Medicine	45	M	1	MIDCARE	CCG
Chan	Pediatrics	37	J	2	CCG	MIDCARE
Coolidge	ENT	44	J	2	CCG	OMC, WHS
Darwali	OB/GYN	39	J	1	CCG	MIDCARE
Douglas	Internal Medicine	41	M	1	MIDCARE	CCG
Dustin	OB/GYN	33	M	2	MIDCARE	CCG
Eason	Internal Medicine	56	M	1	MIDCARE	CCG
Finn	General Surgery	47	J	2	CCG	MIDCARE
Fixer	Urology	43	M	1	MIDCARE	CCG
Flores	General Surgery	45	M	1	MIDCARE	CCG
Frost	Internal Medicine	41	J	2	MIDCARE	CCG
Goldwater	Orthopedic Surgery	44	J	1	CCG	WHS, OMC
Gost	OB/GYN	45	M	1	MIDCARE	CCG
Hersh	General Surgery	40	M	1	MIDCARE	CCG
Jackson	General Surgery	39	M	2	MIDCARE	CCG
Kessler	Internal Medicine	34	M	2	MIDCARE	CCG
Kipstein	Cardiology	50	J	1	CCG	MIDCARE
Klock	OB/GYN	49	J	2	CCG	MIDCARE
Lee	Orthopedic Surgery	40	J	2	CCG	MIDCARE
Lesko	Internal Medicine	38	M	1	MIDCARE	CCG
Maeer	Cardiology	42	J	2	CCG	MIDCARE
Master	Internal Medicine	40	M	1	MIDCARE	CCG
O'Connell	General Surgery	49	M	2	MIDCARE	CCG
Otter	Pediatrics	37	J	2	CCG	MIDCARE
Qin	Orthopedic Surgery	47	J	1	CCG	MIDCARE
Polk	OB/GYN	40	J	2	OMC	WHS
Putter	General Surgery	62	M	1	MIDCARE	CCG
Qestrom	Orthopedic Surgery	39	M	1	MIDCARE	CCG
Quester	Pediatrics	40	J	2	MIDCARE	CCG
Reaper	Pediatrics	59	M	1	MIDCARE	CCG
Samuels	Pediatrics	47	M	1	MIDCARE	CCG
St. James	Pediatrics	40	M	2	MIDCARE	CCG
Stanley	Orthopedic Surgery	49	M	1	MIDCARE	CCG
Steve	Orthopedic Surgery	47	J	1	CCG	MIDCARE
Underwood	Cardiology	46	M	1	MIDCARE	CCG
Unvey	Pediatrics	56	J	2	MIDCARE	CCG

Continued

Name	Specialty	Age	Facility	Gender	Active	Consulting
Walberger	ENT	42	M	2	MIDCARE	CCG
Washington	Internal Medicine	43	J	2	CCG	WHS
Weckensen	ENT	44	M	1	MIDCARE	CCG

Notes: (1) As of December 31, 2019. (2) Facility: J–Jasper, M–Middleboro. (3) Gender: 1–Male, 2–Female. (4) Active: Active staff privileges by hospital. (5) Consulting: Consulting staff privileges by hospital. (6) CCG: Capital City General Hospital; MIDCARE: Middleboro Medical Center; OMC: Osteopathic Medical Center; WHS: Webster Health System. (7) ENT: ear, nose, throat; OB/GYN: obstetrics/gynecology.

Table 7.1

Medical Associates Affiliated Physicians *(continued)*

On the web at ache.org/books/ Middleboro2

Name	Specialty	2019			2018			2017		
		Appts	PT Days	Dis	Appts	PT Days	Dis	Appts	PT Days	Dis
Department of Medicine										
St. James	Pediatrics	5,521	120	45	5,432	135	40	5,234	178	59
Samuels	Pediatrics	5,167	114	29	5,234	123	30	5,005	126	32
Reaper	Pediatrics	5,234	99	25	5,134	102	24	4,687	98	32
Gost	OB/GYN	4,319	720	177	4,138	734	164	4,023	793	170
Dustin	OB/GYN	4,625	650	193	4,456	645	187	4,044	696	190
Autumn	Gastro	2,789	755	156	2,705	745	144	2,656	801	131
Underwood	Cardio	4,456	677	133	4,178	606	105	4,277	545	109
Master	Int Med	3,623	492	102	4,263	501	102	2,330	535	135
Lesko	Int Med	4,034	560	102	4,083	525	98	4,405	555	99
Kessler	Int Med	4,256	712	161	2,033	204	45	0	0	0
Douglas	Int Med	4,340	820	210	4,256	834	187	4,456	902	167
Barton	Int Med	4,206	850	177	4,256	654	152	4,124	756	165
Subtotal		**52,570**	**6,569**	**1,510**	**50,168**	**5,808**	**1,278**	**45,241**	**5,985**	**1,289**
Department of Surgery										
Flores	General	2,546	870	215	2,206	830	204	2,345	854	207
Putter	General	912	630	126	1,112	720	160	1,345	779	199
O'Connell	General	1,456	416	104	1,045	418	103	867	436	109
Jackson	General	1,843	792	167	1,678	722	134	1,767	812	99
Hersh	General	1,245	1,200	267	1,045	1,103	245	1,956	1,223	265
Walberger	ENT	2,845	504	131	2,840	512	134	3,405	529	143
Weckensen	ENT	2,945	483	104	2,834	477	99	2,341	490	105
Stanley	Ortho	1,766	1,544	279	1,862	1,647	298	2,645	1,767	202

Table 7.2

Medical Associates Utilization Statistics for Middleboro Facility

On the web at ache.org/books/ Middleboro2

continued

Table 7.2
Medical
Associates
Utilization
Statistics for
Middleboro
Facility
(continued)

On the web at
ache.org/books/
Middleboro2

Name	Specialty	2019			2018			2017		
		Appts	PT Days	Dis	Appts	PT Days	Dis	Appts	PT Days	Dis
Qestrom	Ortho	1,799	1,433	220	1,566	1,153	208	2,675	1,254	267
Fixer	Urology	2,403	578	143	2,202	598	142	2,005	612	157
Eason	Int Med	1,645	457	101	1,470	459	101	1,034	499	101
Subtotal		**21,405**	**8,907**	**1,857**	**19,860**	**8,639**	**1,828**	**22,385**	**9,255**	**1,854**
Total		**73,975**	**15,476**	**3,367**	**70,028**	**14,447**	**3,106**	**67,626**	**15,240**	**3,143**

Notes: (1) Appts: appointments; Dis: discharges (all hospitals); PT Days: patient days (all hospitals).
(2) ENT: ear, nose, throat; OB/GYN: obstetrics/gynecology.

Table 7.3
Medical
Associates
Utilization
Statistics for
Jasper Facility

On the web at
ache.org/books/
Middleboro2

Name	Specialty	2019			2018			2017		
		Appts	PT Days	Dis	Appts	PT Days	Dis	Appts	PT Days	Dis
Department of Medicine										
Chan	Pediatrics	4,604	212	78	3,324	276	90	4,125	303	90
Unvey	Pediatrics	4,767	234	66	4,654	267	69	4,209	291	81
Otter	Pediatrics	4,523	206	51	4,045	224	57	4,509	205	45
Quester	Pediatrics	4,033	312	75	3,978	356	76	3,956	334	79
Polk	OB/GYN	3,651	650	140	3,612	984	202	3,487	982	215
Klock	OB/GYN	3,749	607	135	3,256	1,115	256	3,356	1,138	267
Darwali	OB/GYN	4,317	908	245	4,450	1,102	315	4,245	1,298	335
Washington	Int Med	3,745	712	156	2,867	505	101	2,456	536	146
Frost	Int Med	4,980	700	176	3,156	646	120	2,077	495	103
Kipstein	Cardiology	4,126	612	145	3,682	700	156	3,933	596	133
Maeer	Cardiology	4,682	698	167	4,356	512	102	4,631	878	175
Subtotal		**47,177**	**5,851**	**1,434**	**41,380**	**6,687**	**1,544**	**40,984**	**7,056**	**1,669**
Department of Surgery										
Finn	General	1,587	806	165	1,601	1,206	245	700	830	203
Steve	Ortho	1,266	612	134	1,534	733	167	793	723	154
Lee	Ortho	2,156	885	231	1,935	893	287	1,689	1,104	303
Qin	Ortho	1,920	957	245	1,756	1,234	298	2,156	1,556	366
Coolidge	ENT	3,369	345	123	3,278	806	323	1,433	345	143
Goldwater	Ortho	2,877	1,134	278	2,645	1,376	325	2,034	1,589	387
Subtotal		**13,175**	**4,739**	**1,176**	**12,749**	**6,248**	**1,645**	**8,805**	**6,147**	**1,556**
Total		**60,352**	**10,590**	**2,610**	**54,129**	**12,935**	**3,189**	**49,789**	**13,203**	**3,225**

Notes: (1) Appts: appointments; Dis: discharges (all hospitals); PT Days: patient days (all hospitals).
(2) ENT: ear, nose, throat; OB/GYN: obstetrics/gynecology.

	Patient Visits	
	2019	**2018**
January	2,976	0
February	2,890	0
March	3,348	0
April	2,880	0
May	2,901	0
June	2,736	0
July	2,381	480
August	2,827	912
September	2,304	1,355
October	2,456	1,205
November	2,880	1,956
December	3,124	2,455
Total Visits	**33,703**	**8,363**
Weekdays		
7 a.m.–3 p.m.	23,885	6,566
3 p.m.–11 p.m.	5,971	1,149
11 p.m.–7 a.m.	3,317	492
Subtotal	**33,173**	**8,207**
Weekends		
7 a.m.–3 p.m.	313	86
3 p.m.–11 p.m.	111	31
11 p.m.–7 a.m.	106	39
Subtotal	**530**	**156**
Total Visits	**33,703**	**8,363**

Table 7.4
Medical Associates Express Utilization

Table 7.5
Medical
Associates
Hospital
Utilization by
Location and
Department

Department	Location	Discharges		Patient Days	
		All	HC	All	HC
Medicine	Middleboro	1,510	1,489	6,559	6,459
Surgery	Middleboro	1,857	1,816	8,907	8,689
Subtotal		**3,367**	**3,305**	**15,466**	**15,148**
Medicine	Jasper	1,910	795	7,693	2,812
Surgery	Jasper	700	193	2,897	391
Subtotal		**2,610**	**988**	**10,590**	**3,203**
Total		**5,977**	**4,293**	**26,056**	**18,351**

Notes: (1) For 12-month period ending December 31, 2019. (2) All: all hospitals; HC: hospitals in Hillsboro County (MIDCARE and WHS).

Table 7.6
Medical
Associates
Staff Physicians

Physician Name	Specialty	Facility	2019 Salary ($US)	Contract Expiration Date
K. Kessler	Internal Medicine	Middleboro	203,000	7/1/20
E. Frost	Internal Medicine	Jasper	206,000	3/1/21
L. Coolidge	ENT	Jasper	226,450	7/1/21

Notes: (1) As of December 31, 2019. (2) Staff physicians are hired on a three-year contract.

	2019	2018	2017
Revenues			
Patient Revenue—Gross	59,234,686	56,784,560	55,254,303
Allowance	10,206,445	8,934,229	8,010,292
Bad Debt	560,223	519,476	498,207
Net Patient Services Revenue	48,468,018	47,330,855	46,745,804
Other Revenue			
Management Fees	250,000	75,000	0
Real Estate Rentals	300,000	164,229	0
Other	8,070	3,026	7,456
Total Other	558,070	242,255	7,456
Total Revenue	**49,026,088**	**47,573,110**	**46,753,260**
Expenses			
Physician Compensation	18,334,234	18,038,448	17,959,345
Other Professional Services	19,445,292	19,100,334	18,454,202
General Services	3,245,696	3,296,383	2,956,303
Fiscal Services	2,745,102	2,610,449	2,438,283
Interest	4,332	7,256	56,343
Depreciation	1,841,231	1,997,170	2,361,678
Total Operating Expenses	**45,615,887**	**45,050,040**	**44,226,154**
Pretax Income (Loss)	3,410,201	2,523,070	2,527,106
Taxes	1,295,876	958,767	960,300
Profit or (Loss)	**2,114,325**	**1,564,303**	**1,566,806**

Table 7.7
Medical Associates Statement of Revenues and Expenses

On the web at ache.org/books/ Middleboro2

Notes: (1) Years ending December 31. (2) Numbers are in US dollars.

Table 7.8
Medical
Associates
Balance Sheet

*On the web at
ache.org/books/
Middleboro2*

	2019	2018	2017
Assets			
Current Assets			
Cash and Marketable Securities	1,752,484	1,656,393	1,667,252
Accounts Receivable—Gross	8,026,443	7,523,214	7,342,645
Allowances for Uncollectables	−927,353	−689,303	−612,039
Accounts Receivable—Net	7,099,090	6,833,911	6,730,606
Due from Third-Party Payers	156,343	134,998	167,454
Inventory	339,129	343,102	315,383
Prepaid Expenses	54,848	97,220	61,202
Total Current Assets	**9,401,894**	**9,065,624**	**8,941,897**
Noncurrent Assets		162,763	150,250
Property, Plant, and Equipment—Gross		663,887,127	608,277,429
Less Accumulated Depreciation	11,084,473	9,243,242	7,246,072
Property, Plant, and Equipment—Net	56,207,980	55,960,198	47,947,373
Other Investments	1,917,234	2,120,940	2,087,230
Total Assets	**67,527,108**	**67,146,762**	**58,976,500**
Liabilities			
Current Liabilities			
Accounts Payable	1,933,429	1,882,494	1,701,905
Accrued Salaries and Wages	1,837,240	1,801,282	1,735,240
Accrued Interest	180,238	200,345	210,876
Other Accrued Expenses	137,450	154,203	150,239
Accrued Vacation Days	92,867	90,124	84,236
Due to Third-Party Vendors	198,335	100,000	81,564
Long-Term Debt Due in 1 Year	52,040	59,234	62,191
Total Current Liabilities	**4,431,599**	**4,287,682**	**4,026,251**
Long-Term Debt	103,228	234,282	2,453,889
Total Liabilities	**4,534,827**	**4,521,964**	**6,480,140**
Net Assets	62,992,281	62,624,798	52,496,360
Net Assets + Total Liabilities	**67,527,108**	**67,146,762**	**58,976,500**

Notes: (1) For fiscal years ending December 31. (2) Numbers are in US dollars.

	2019	2018
Revenues	2,976	0
Patient Services—Gross	3,124,350	794,485
Allowances and Discounts	−4,268	−1,055
Deductions for Bad Debt	−1,055	−345
Patient Services—Net	3,129,673	793,085
Expenses	2,381	480
Salaries and Wages	1,970,920	885,230
Benefits	512,439	221,308
Management Fee	250,000	75,000
Advertising	56,300	55,020
Computer Support	12,000	2,000
Insurance	18,850	8,500
Laundry and Housekeeping	6,390	2,195
Legal/Audit	1,850	1,850
Medical Supplies	14,923	5,483
Office Supplies	10,449	5,005
Printing and Postage	5,400	1,745
Facility and Equipment Rent	250,000	94,223
Repairs and Maintenance	1,267	342
Internet and Telephone	6,320	3,160
Interest	3,222	1,004
Depreciation	5,800	4,245
Total Expenses	3,126,130	1,366,310
Income (Loss) Before Taxes	3,543	−573,225
Federal and State Taxes*	709	0
Income (Loss) After Taxes	2,834	−573,225

Notes: (1) Years ending December 31. (2) Numbers are in US dollars. (3) *Includes carryforward tax credits.

Table 7.9
Medical Associates Express Statement of Revenues and Operations

On the web at ache.org/books/Middleboro2

Table 7.10
Medical
Associates
Express Balance
Sheet

On the web at
ache.org/books/
Middleboro2

	2019	2018
Assets		
Current Assets		
Cash	41,440	32,040
Cash Equivalents	245,163	240,783
Accounts Receivable	4,523	2,045
Inventory	36,801	15,330
Prepaid Expenses	825	325
Total Current Assets	**287,312**	**258,483**
Investments	162,763	150,250
Property and Equipment		
Equipment and Leasehold Improvements—Gross	123,556	104,200
Less Accumulated Depreciation	10,045	4,245
Equipment and Leasehold Improvements—Net	113,511	99,955
Total Assets	**563,586**	**508,688**
Liabilities		
Current Liabilities		
Accounts Payable	120,440	65,330
Accrued Expenses	49,337	50,283
Total Current Liabilities	**169,777**	**115,613**
Notes Payable	64,200	66,300
Total Liabilities	**233,977**	**181,913**
Net Assets		
Common Stock Authorized and Issued*	900,000	900,000
Cumulative Operating Gain/Loss After Taxes	−570,391	−573,225
Total Net Assets	**329,609**	**326,775**
Net Assets + Liabilities	**563,586**	**508,688**

Notes: (1) *Common Stock at $10,000 par value per share, 90 shares authorized. (2) For fiscal years ending December 31. (3) Numbers are in US dollars.

Month	Total Cases	Types of Cases		
		ENT	Ortho	Other
January	283	47	123	113
February	257	57	101	99
March	276	94	109	73
April	254	71	94	89
May	263	52	129	82
June	214	56	74	84
July	265	68	108	89
August	221	42	86	93
September	216	40	73	103
October	279	56	109	114
November	287	58	129	100
December	257	60	114	83
Total	**3,072**	**701**	**1,249**	**1,122**

Table 7.11
Medical Associates Ambulatory Surgical Services Procedures

Notes: (1) For 12-month period ending December 31, 2019. (2) ENT: ear, nose, throat; Ortho: orthopedic.

JASPER GARDENS

Jasper Gardens is a tax-paying, Medicare- and Medicaid-certified nursing home with a license to operate 110 beds. Currently, it operates and staffs 106 beds in both private and semiprivate rooms. It is fully approved to provide skilled nursing and rehabilitation services covered by Medicare, and most of its residents and patients are covered by Medicaid. Physical, occupational, recreational, and speech therapy are offered on-site. Respiratory therapy is also available from a contracted provider. Area citizens may receive rehabilitation services on an outpatient basis, using either Medicare Part B or commercial insurance to pay for the associated charges. Jasper Gardens accepts all forms of payment.

Situated on 100 acres of land adjacent to the soon-to-be-completed new highway—approximately one mile from the planned Jasper–East exit and five miles east of the center of Jasper—the facility is a one-story modern building with ample parking and significant room for expansion. It is owned and operated by Jefferson Partners.

JEFFERSON PARTNERS, LLC

Jefferson Partners owns and operates nursing homes, assisted living facilities, retirement living communities, and adult day care centers in the greater Capital City area and other communities throughout the state. It is a private-equity partnership of investors, none of whom is involved in the day-to-day management of the corporation. It holds quarterly board meetings, and the board's executive committee meets monthly with the senior management team to review operations and issues.

Jefferson Partners has two operating divisions: Management and Property. The Management division provides centralized administrative services—such as payroll, legal, financial management, and group purchasing—to facilities for a fee. The Property division buys the buildings and land and then leases them to wholly owned subsidiary corporations, which actually run and manage the individual operations such as Jasper Gardens. As such, Jasper Gardens is merely leasing its current property.

The senior management team of Jefferson Partners includes Ralph Jefferson, president and CEO; Wanda Charles, RN, vice president of Operations; Norman Fellows, director of Corporate Development and Acquisitions; and Gayle Wyman, chief financial officer. This team approves the annual budget for each facility. Charles meets monthly with facility administrators to monitor operations and to address problems and issues. Jefferson Partners maintains a central office with a small staff in Capital City.

Jefferson Partners has filed a preliminary zoning and planning application for a continuing care retirement community (CCRC). The campus of Jasper Gardens is one of three potential sites identified in this application; the other two are on the grounds of two other nursing homes outside of Hillsboro County. The preliminary application indicates the corporation's interest in building an assisted living facility with 88 single- and double-occupancy units as well as 50 adult single-family homes. These facilities will be on the same campus, forming the CCRC. The projected operational date for this project is three years after it is approved.

HISTORY

Mary and John Decker founded Jasper Gardens Nursing Home in 1960. It was housed in a former resort that accommodated 45 residents in semiprivate rooms. In the 1970s, the facility was expanded to accommodate 70 residents and was licensed by Medicaid and Medicare. In 1980, the Deckers sold the facility to the Armstrong family, who built four new wings of patient rooms, each with 12 semiprivate rooms. On each expansion, the state awarded a certificate of need (CON). Construction between 1981 and 1983 converted the original resort house into administrative offices and common areas.

Between 1990 and 1995, Jasper Gardens was modified into its current configuration of five wings and a central building for administrative services. The resort house was demolished and replaced with a new structure, and a new wing was added to the existing four. Jefferson Partners acquired the facility in 1995 and has continually invested in updating it. Today, the facility is modern, spacious, and tastefully decorated to emphasize a warm, comfortable environment for its residents.

Until 1992, the state CON law regulated any nursing home expansions that cost more than $500,000. Today, that threshold is the same for both nursing homes and acute care facilities. Also in 1992, the state ceased allowing any nursing home to expand its bed capacity by 5 percent each year without a CON, regardless of cost. Capital costs are capped and used to determine state Medicaid rates for nursing homes; they constitute less than 5 percent to a rate calculation. Currently, there is a moratorium on CON applications for skilled nursing facility and intermediate care facility beds because of pending changes to the state CON law. However, the governor has granted permission to increase the number of beds in a nursing home if the total number of nursing home beds within a county remains unchanged.

When it was originally founded, Jasper Gardens was in a relatively rural environment. Today, the area has become suburban, marked by a number of new housing subdivisions, chain stores and restaurants, and a shopping mall about a quarter of a mile away. The area is expected to grow and develop even more with the opening of the new interstate highway between Jasper and Capital City.

In 2007, Resident Community Councils were introduced in Jasper Gardens. These councils enable residents to express their wishes and preferences, big and small. Jasper Gardens's brochure stresses this and other resident-centered features:

Jasper Gardens residents have a choice regarding how they want to live. We promise to listen to and strive to accommodate wishes and preferences so that we can fulfill them every day. They may wish to experience our Fine Dining program, which creates an inviting, restaurant-like atmosphere with fine china, polished silverware, tablecloths and cloth napkins, personal assistance from our attentive staff, and—of course—fresh and well-balanced meals. They may opt to dine at local restaurants occassionally or regularly by themselves or with a group of friends. Or they may prefer to bring food back to their rooms to enjoy in private.

We honor residents' requests regarding bathing or showering times, days, and frequency. Our staff—each of whom is assigned to a resident—are happy to accommodate such requests and incorporate them, when possible, into the resident's daily care and routine.

Jasper Gardens opens our doors to social functions, meetings, celebrations, and other events hosted and organized by community members. We encourage our residents to partake in activities that are open to everyone, but only if they choose to do so.

These efforts have resulted in Jasper Gardens being recognized as a regional leader in empowering residents and creating a home-like atmosphere. For the past four years, it has been a semi-finalist for the statewide Quality-of-Life Award bestowed by the governor to a nursing home that consistently demonstrates its commitment to resident independence, choice, and well-being.

SERVICES AND OPERATIONS

Jasper Gardens classifies its patients and residents as follows: The term *resident* is used when the individual's average length of stay (ALOS) is more than three months, whereas the term *patient* is used when the individual's ALOS is fewer than 100 days. Similarly, it classifies many of its services as either *intermediate care* or *skilled care*. Intermediate care services emphasize long-term residential services. The ALOS for intermediate care is approximately 2.8 years and has been increasing. The average age of residents is approximately 87 years and has slowly been increasing. Some residents in the intermediate care category have the ability to pay for care when they are initially admitted. However, after "spending down" their available personal resources, these residents have to rely on Medicaid to finance their care. Over the past five years, the average spend-down period for residents has dropped from 26 months to 19 months. A few patients in this category are covered by private nursing home insurance or insurance provided by the Veterans Administration.

Skilled care services emphasize short-term treatment. These patients are in the nursing home for post-hospital rehabilitation, for example. Those older than 65 years rely on Medicare as their primary insurance and thus make use of physical, occupational, and speech therapy services. Those not eligible for Medicare typically rely on a private health insurance plan. The ALOS for Medicare patients has been decreasing over the past five years.

Registered nurses (RNs), licensed practical nurses (LPNs), licensed nursing assistants (LNAs), and medication nursing assistants (MNAs) deliver the services. A part-time registered dietitian supervises all matters related to food and nutrition. Social work services are offered during the admissions process and on an inpatient basis. Pharmacy services are coordinated with DRUGCO, Inc., a pharmacy under contract with Jefferson Partners.

The medical director is James A. Child, DO, who is board certified in family practice and gerontology and operates a practice in Jasper with Drs. Freda Evans and David Contreras, who provide backup, on-call services as needed. All three physicians have active and consulting staff privileges at Osteopathic Medical Center in Capital City. Dr. Child devotes approximately a half day per week to his patients in Jasper Gardens.

Four of the five wings in the building have nine semiprivate rooms and two private rooms, for a total of eight private rooms. The fifth wing has 13 semiprivate rooms and houses the Rehabilitation Services department. Each wing has a nursing station, a shower room, and a small library. Wireless Internet connection (Wi-Fi) is available throughout the facility. The beauty salon and barbershop are located in the central commons area.

Most patients enter Jasper Gardens after discharge from area hospitals. Primary referral sources include the hospitals located in Middleboro and Capital City.

MANAGEMENT TEAM AND ORGANIZATIONAL STRUCTURE

Jasper Gardens has a flat management structure. Members of its senior management team report to the administrator, who in turn reports to the vice president of Operations for Jefferson Partners. The senior management team meets to review the budget reports furnished by Jefferson Partners. Each of the senior managers supervises and directs multiple departments and staff.

ADMINISTRATOR

Jayne Winters, NHA, is the licensed administrator of Jasper Gardens. Upon graduating with a bachelor in health services management from an eastern university in 2006, she entered an Administrator in Training (AIT) program at a Jefferson Partners facility in Capital City. Upon completion of the AIT program, she earned her state license and was appointed as assistant administrator at Jefferson Partners's largest nursing home/assisted living and congregate living (apartment) facility in Capital City. She was appointed administrator of Jasper Gardens in 2010. She is active in the State Association of Long-Term Care Administrators and lives in Jasper.

With the help of her administrative assistant Chloe Hyde, Winters handles all aspects of personnel and human resources functions, including advertising job vacancies, screening applicants (e.g., background checks), and administering compensation and benefit policies. Wage and salary rates are set during the annual budgeting process, and changes to the rates require the approval of Jefferson Partners. She is also responsible for all marketing activities, including producing advertisements, brochures, and in-person or online/social media promotions. Her employment contract does include certain incentives and penalties that are tied to quality of care and financial performance.

Winters relies on a "dashboard report" to stay abreast of the management issues in the facility. This weekly report includes the following information for the latest week, month, and quarter as well as year to date:

- Revenue and expense budget performance

- Payroll information (budgeted versus actual hours, dollars, and overtime)

- Patient census by payer

- Admissions and discharges

- Therapy revenue, expenses, and hours

- Employee health insurance claims submitted

In addition, she monitors the following primary quality indicators:

- Facility-acquired pressure ulcers

- Falls

- Injuries

- Weight loss

- Reportable events

- Acute discharges

Challenges and Successes

Over the past 18 months, some employees have filed formal grievances related to "unfair interpretations" of sick leave policies, merit pay adjustments, and rates paid to part-time workers who work on national holidays. During this same period, three employees were discharged for failure to perform stated duties. One of Winters's first actions as administrator was the dismissal of three employees for nepotism, a dismissal still remembered by many staff members who deemed it inappropriate because the employees were hired before a formal policy on nepotism was instituted. Recently, she dismissed two more employees for poor attendance and work performance.

When interviewed, Winters admitted that Medicaid pricing has continued to force the facility to reconsider its staffing levels and, in some instances, reduce staff. Like other nursing homes, Jasper Gardens works within very modest annual financial margins, so even small staffing increases could easily evaporate its modest profits. However, "patient acuity and levels of need have increased significantly," she said. "More and more of our older residents are exhibiting behavioral problems and seem to need more and more care. Our staffing level, though, has remained about the same."

A union has never represented the hourly staff. Winters and her management team have heard rumors that a local union in Capital City was sending out cards to the hourly staff to determine their interest in being represented by a union. If a sufficient number of cards are returned to the union, then the union will petition the state labor board for permission to hold an election and form a bargaining unit at the facility.

Some residents use electric wheelchairs and mobility carts to get around inside the nursing home and to frequent the small park on campus. Medicare purchases these carts for any mobility-impaired individual who is aged 65 years or older. In the past 18 months, two crashes occurred inside the facility that injured three residents. Because the sidewalks outside Jasper Gardens are wide, a few residents use their wheelchairs and carts to go to the nearby shopping mall. To leave the campus, a resident must secure permission from the supervising nurse and take a cell phone furnished by the nursing home. Legal counsel is reviewing this practice to ensure that it is compliant with current laws and regulations. Two different families have requested that the residents be prohibited from using the carts outside the property. Current policies do not allow for such restrictions unless they are based on appropriate legal (e.g., power of attorney) or medical orders. Recently, one resident started walking to the mall, became disoriented on the way there, got lost, and had to be brought back to the facility by the police. This is the fifth such incident within the past six months.

In the past two years, Jasper Gardens has received a deficiency-free survey—Level B—from the state survey team. This score, Winters explained, is a notable improvement over the conditions at the facility when she arrived. Prior to 2010, the facility was consistently found to operate at Level E or Level F, which indicated widespread potential to cause more than minimal harm to patients and residents. She credited these positive surveys to her dedicated staff, changes in some job responsibilities, and a solid team effort.

Four years ago, the facility hired a certified therapeutic recreation specialist to staff its Recreation Services department. The first specialist was so well received that more specialists were hired. Today, Jasper Gardens's Recreation Services department is known as one of the best in the state.

Three years ago, workers' compensation rates at the facility soared, doubling the number of workplace injury claims from years past. The most common injury reported was lower back strain as a result of assisting or lifting residents and patients from their beds. In response, Jefferson Partners instituted a new policy and ordered new equipment designed to minimize injury and help staff protect themselves while assisting residents. Since then, no employee has reported back injuries.

Asked to comment on this assortment of issues, Winters said,

I am very pleased with the progress we have made. The facility looks good, the staff is very dedicated, and the owners are comfortable with our profit margins. We have been challenged to get our personnel system in better shape, but we continue to work on improvements and have always been responsive to the needs of our workers. I sincerely hope that we do not unionize, although we fully support our employees' rights in this area. Jefferson Partners wants us to keep developing this facility, especially with the opening of the interstate highway. This road will significantly cut down on the travel time between Jasper and Capital City and will open up opportunities for us to attract consumers who did not consider us in the past because of our location. We also have the space and the infrastructure on our campus for Jefferson Partners's proposed senior-living apartments and an assisted living facility.

DIRECTOR OF PATIENT SERVICES

Michele Regan, RN, was appointed director of Patient Services in 2009. She holds a bachelor in nursing and a master in geriatric nursing from State University and has more than 20 years of professional experience in long-term care nursing. In 2004, she joined the nursing staff at Jasper Gardens as the day-shift charge nurse. Her responsibilities as director include managing the two day-shift (7 a.m.–3 p.m.) charge nurses—each of whom leads the caregivers for approximately half of the patients and residents—as well as the evening (3 p.m.–11 p.m.) and night (11 p.m.–7 a.m.) nursing supervisors. In addition, she oversees the Rehabilitation (physical therapy [PT], occupational therapy [OT], and speech therapy [ST]), Dietary, and Recreation Services departments as well as coordinates all pharmaceutical services.

When interviewed, Regan indicated that Jasper Gardens rarely has problems with hiring qualified RNs and LPNs, although it experiences the expected workforce turnover; she added that she would like to hire more MNAs. One problem with staffing has always been scheduling, as she explained:

> We seem to be in a Catch-22. In the past, we relied on floating full-time staff to cover shifts as needed, but we recently started hiring part-time workers to save money. Scheduling them to work a few extra hours to cover a shift occasionally has been very difficult and disappointing, though. This move may have saved us some money, but it is costing us something else. The critical complaint from part-timers has been not having sick leave, something that is very important to those who have to tend to their sick children.

Regan manages the facility's drug formulary, with guidance from Dr. Child, and ensures that adequate pharmacy stock is maintained and that effective inventory safeguards are in place. She is also responsible for ordering and inventorying all medical supplies. Medical supplies are purchased using contracts negotiated and administrated by Jefferson Partners.

When asked what changes she would like to see implemented, she offered this:

Our current policy concerning residents being hospitalized and then returning may need to be reconsidered. The policy is that we will not keep a bed open for a resident who is admitted to a hospital unless the resident pays for the bed during the hospitalization or absence. Unless paid, we will refill the bed after 24 hours. We also have a 10-day limit on how long any bed may be unoccupied even if the per diem charges are being paid. This policy can cause problems for our residents, even though it might be a required business practice. We really try to accommodate our residents, but frequently we can't. Another change I'd like to see is to dedicate one wing to residents with Alzheimer's and dementia, an idea that has been discussed with the owners. Having a separate wing for these residents would allow us to expand the range of patient care services we can offer.

Director of Admissions and Social Services

Betsy Hemp has been the director of Admissions and Social Services since 1999. She holds a bachelor and master in social work from a West Coast university and has more than 15 years of experience. Prior to this job, she held a similar position at a nursing home in Capital City.

Hemp meets with all prospective residents and their families, assists potential and current residents in applying and qualifying for Medicaid, periodically leads the team that reviews the medical and social needs of all residents, and files reports as needed. Each resident maintains a modest cash account to support certain expenses or purchases (e.g., beauty shop). She manages this account, in keeping with federal and state regulations, and periodically files the needed reports. Aside from working with the discharge teams at MIDCARE, Webster Health System, and Capital City hospitals, she also has regular contact with Hillsboro Health and other home health agencies in Capital City. When interviewed, she offered the following general comments:

Overall, I enjoy working here. Jasper Gardens is not unique, but we have a dedicated staff that makes us special. Our resident population is getting older, and our recent admissions have required significantly more therapy and services than what I've seen in the past. Changes in Medicaid eligibility make aspects of my job demanding. For example, I spend a great deal of time completing the Minimum Data Set on residents to be admitted and I spend a great deal of time filing reports on our current residents. This place really does reflect the community we serve. Most of our residents come from Jasper, although we're hoping the new interstate brings us some "out of towners" from Capital City. We are fortunate that a significant number of our residents have family and friends who still come to visit them. We seem to have more visitors than other nursing homes do.

DIRECTOR OF PLANT OPERATIONS

As the director of Plant Operations, Connor Doyle is responsible for all aspects of the building and grounds, including maintenance, laundry, and housekeeping services. His staff maintains and operates the van that transports residents to appointments, shopping trips, and other outings. A military veteran, he has served in this role since 2006 and, before that, was the associate director of facilities at another nursing home in Capital City. Under his leadership, Jasper Gardens has received no negative reports or citations and has passed all inspections, including fire safety. In 2011, he led the installation of new on-site generators, enabling the facility to function "off the electric grid" for a minimum of 12 days. This installation completed a plan to make the nursing home energy independent to ensure the safety of all residents.

Based on Doyle's recommendation, Jasper Gardens established a new policy that all residents who want to use motorized wheelchairs and carts must complete driving lessons from a trained instructor and earn an operator's license issued by the facility. Doyle offered insights into his job:

Those electric carts—some call them scooters—cause some tricky problems. Most can't be stored inside the facility because of building regulations regarding recharging. We have had to build a storage space for them in another building, and we bring them in and out as the residents want them. Sometimes, my staff feel like we are running a valet parking service. I have thought about suggesting they should be banned, especially inside the facility because they can mark or mar the floors and walls. But those scooters do help those residents who can no longer walk but want to remain mobile.

As far as this facility is concerned, I am very proud of how the Plant Operations team has made and continues to make this old facility clean, well-lit, and look attractive. And safe—let's not forget safe! Now that we are energy independent, I sleep better at night. All of the employees understand and comply with our need to periodically have fire and emergency drills. This has helped a great deal, as we don't hear any grumblings when we have to move a lot of people in and out of the wings in an orderly fashion. One of my many duties is security. We wear badges. We are trained to question any visitors, vendors, or strangers on the property. We have alarm systems and multiple security checks in place. But my staff and I get called if any of those things don't go as planned. I do question whether we can and should remain as open as we are now. Residents can potentially leave any time they want, and outsiders can enter multiple doors from 7 a.m. to 8 p.m., before the building is "locked" for the night. This may be an issue that needs attention.

Senior Administrative Assistant and Bookkeeper

Bonnie Keana is the senior administrative assistant and bookkeeper. She is responsible for preparing the payroll and supervising the posting of the financial journal and the general ledger. Jefferson Partners provides budget status reports every week and interim financial statements monthly based on information she prepares. She is also in charge of local purchasing, and she supervises the reception staff.

Management Meetings

Every Tuesday morning, Winters, Regan, and Hemp meet and review the status of all patients. Data include quality measures used by the Medicare Quality Improvement Organization and Centers for Medicare & Medicaid Services (CMS) as well as other data reported to Jefferson Partners. Once a month, this trio invites others (including the medical director and members of Jasper Gardens's continuous quality improvement committee) to review all data to determine which patients/CMS items need attention, why, and the treatment and prevention approaches being used. Every Friday morning, this same group—along with Doyle and Keana—meets as the management team and reviews the most recent dashboard report and budget status report as well as discusses other issues that need management's attention.

Concerns and Opportunities

Personnel and Union Activity

Winters and Regan indicated that access to qualified professional staff has not been a major problem. In fact, they have been able to hire highly qualified professionals who have generally stayed with the facility for a long time. Over the years, however, wages for some jobs have not kept pace with wages in the regional market. This trend is directly traceable to the Medicaid rates paid by the state. Over the past ten years, state Medicaid rates have fallen from being the tenth highest to the eighth lowest in the country.

Four years ago, union organizers from Capital City mailed cards to the hourly employees of Jasper Gardens. This effort did not yield a sufficient number of responses, which would signal organizers to move ahead with a staff petition to form a bargaining unit. Two years ago, an external consultant hired by Jefferson Partners conducted a staff survey. In this survey, employees expressed three primary job concerns: (1) wages were below market norms, (2) benefits were administered unfairly, and (3) job expectations were unclear. As a response, Jefferson Partners authorized some wage increases and committed to following a standardized system of benefits for all employees. This system is promised to be included in an expanded employee manual, but the manual has not yet been published. To date, no real progress has been made in the development of a comprehensive personnel manual. In addition, Jefferson Partners instructed Winters to review and update all job descriptions and to enhance the annual evaluation process. Merit pay was introduced last year, but it has met with mixed reviews and results. Four years ago, the personnel system was ad hoc and poorly defined, and it still exhibits a number of shortcomings today. For example, a number of employees remain confused about what specific benefits they are eligible for and how they can use those benefits.

REHABILITATION SERVICES UTILIZATION

Rehabilitation services (e.g., PT, OT, ST) are available to both Jasper Gardens residents and members of the community. Most users of these services have Medicare Part B or private insurance. Outpatient utilization continues to be modest. Currently, individuals in need of ambulatory rehabilitation services typically visit a local solo provider or travel to a group practice in either Capital City or Middleboro. Jefferson Partners has asked Jasper Gardens to propose a plan to address this potential outpatient market, as part of the facility's draft budget for next year.

Jefferson Partners estimates, on the basis of statewide statistics, that annual service inpatient and outpatient demands (in relative value units) should be approximately 9,000 units in PT, 8,500 units in OT, and 700 units in ST. Space is available to meet the needs of more patients. Workers' comp provides an annual limit of up to 24 PT or OT visits per year per injury. Regan, the supervisor of the Rehabilitation Services department, splits her time between her administrative duties and clinical duties (providing PT), although Jefferson Partners has established that a target of 90 percent of available staff time in a rehabilitation unit must be devoted to patient care. Institutional profitability has increasingly become dependent on the success of the skilled nursing unit and outpatient rehabilitation service. Medicaid reimbursement rates for intermediate care have made achieving institutional profitability difficult.

ADMISSION POLICY

Jefferson Partners requires everyone who applies to be a patient or resident at Jasper Gardens to undergo a background check as a condition of admission. Compliance with this requirement ensures that no individual with a felony conviction as a sexual predator or offender will be admitted. The admission staff explains this policy to all applicants and inquirers. Jefferson Partners has implemented this policy at all of its facilities; however, it is under legal review at two of the corporation's nursing homes.

SPECIAL PROGRAMS AND NEW INITIATIVES

Inpatient Hospice Care

Capital City VNA and Hospice has approached Jefferson Partners with a proposal to establish a Medicare-certified inpatient hospice at Jasper Gardens. Under this contractual agreement, Jasper Gardens would designate private rooms in the facility for inpatient hospice patients. Capital City VNA and Hospice would provide the care and management. Its medical director would supervise and direct the cases, and its nurses would provide 24/7 care with support and extra coverage from Jasper Gardens nurses, as needed. This hospice would be open to Medicare-eligible citizens of Jasper and beyond.

Jasper Gardens is able to enter into this contract because it is within the Medicare regulations for skilled nursing facilities. It could provide staffing and direct patient services, and it could dedicate a wing with private rooms and areas for friends and family. Capital City VNA and Hospice would pay Jasper Gardens (as a subcontractor) a price (to be negotiated) per patient day. Direct service costs would be approximately $75 per day for the requested services. The Pharmacy Service department at Jasper Gardens would supply the needed drugs and durable medical equipment at cost, and Capital City VNA and Hospice would pay the pharmacy directly for this cost. The initial estimate is that Jasper Gardens could add a new wing with four to eight private rooms at approximately $150,000 per private room (minimum of four).

Assisted Living Facility and Retirement Housing

In 2015, the state applied for and received a Home and Community-Based Services (HCBS) waiver from the federal government. The HCBS waiver allows the state to use Medicaid funds to provide qualifying participants with services and support that enable those participants to remain living in their own (or a family member's) home instead of moving into a nursing home. With this move, the state has created a safety net for providers of long-term care services.

Part of Jefferson Partners's strategic plan is to establish more services on the Jasper Gardens campus—such as an assisted living facility, senior apartments, and retirement housing that make up the CCRC option mentioned earlier—to use up the land it currently owns in a location that is attractive because of its proximity to the new interstate highway. This plan would designate Winters as the campus CEO, who would oversee all the facilities. Jasper Gardens's employees would augment the staffing at the new facilities as needed.

Jefferson Partners is currently determining cost estimates for building these facilities and is preparing a conceptual plan for its architects within six months. Using construction costs in the greater Jasper area, the assisted living facility may cost approximately $350 per square foot and the senior apartments and retirement housing may cost around $250 per square foot. Previously, the Jasper Planning Board indicated that zoning would make these facilities a "natural addition" to the Jasper Gardens campus. The taxes imposed on this campus would help the town defray the costs of developing infrastructures (e.g., roads, water and sewer lines), which it began three years ago.

A number of interrelated questions about this project have to be answered:

1. What model for independent living units (e.g., detached housing, townhomes, congregate-style facility) should be constructed, and what entrance model should be employed? In some markets, Jefferson Partners uses a simple rental model: Residents pay a monthly rent for their independent housing unit; they pay extra for additional services, such as intermediate care or transportation. In one market, Jefferson Partners uses an equity model: Residents pay an upfront fee to own their housing unit. Preliminary research has suggested that several equity arrangements are employed across the country, and all of them involve a monthly fee in addition to an upfront entrance fee.

2. How much should the monthly and/or upfront fees be, and should these fees be fixed (subject to inflation increases) at a certain level or be refundable? Setting the fee parameters accurately is essential.

3. What should be the target size for each facility, and what are the associated costs for each? Jefferson Partners has indicated that it will complete the market and financial feasibility study for the project later this year.

4. What is the average length of rental in an assisted living facility? Some studies suggest that, on average, residents stay for 5.4 years (with a standard deviation of 2.3 years).

5. Which groups of people should these facilities be marketed to? National studies suggest that these types of facilities are attractive to specific segments of the population.

6. Will there be "local participation" (meaning a tax abatement) from the Town of Jasper? In its planning and zoning application for the CCRC, Jefferson Partners indicated such financial relief is essential to the success of this project.

Information Systems Development

Jefferson Partners has recently signed a new contract with Nursing Home Systems to install the latest version of a comprehensive electronic health record (EHR). Like other EHRs, this system is an integrated medical record with order-entry capabilities for supplies, tests, and all other clinical activities. Jefferson Partners requires each of its facilities that accepts Medicare or Medicaid to adopt this EHR. This installation takes advantage of the Wi-Fi already running throughout Jasper Gardens.

Osteopathic Medical Center (OMC) in Capital City invited Jasper Gardens to participate in its telehealth program. In this program, a Jasper Gardens patient or resident is evaluated, diagnosed, educated, treated, and monitored by an attending physician at OMC using telecommunications means and self-taken health data. The system enables the patient or resident to consult with or "see" a physician without having to travel to that physician (unless necessary). Per Jefferson Partners's policy, a patient or resident who is transferred to a hospital or leaves loses his bed in Jasper Gardens after 24 hours. OMC did not indicate the cost of this telehealth program.

Alzheimer's and Dementia Wing

Acting on staff's suggestion, Jefferson Partners has requested Winters and Regan to assess the need and demand for a wing dedicated to patients with Alzheimer's disease and patients suffering from dementia. This assessment should include whether the wing must be secured or unsecured, what staffing level must be in place, what care or services must be provided, and what other space options must be considered. This analysis must be completed before any decision can be made concerning additional construction on the site.

Mountain View Recovery, Inc.

Mountain View Recovery, a national chain of drug rehabilitation centers, contacted Jefferson Partners to determine its interest in selling 15 to 20 acres of land adjacent to Jasper Gardens. The chain—a publicly held corporation that runs 37 facilities—is planning on building and operating a 50-bed inpatient and outpatient center with 30-, 45-, 60-, and 90-day rehabilitation programs and luxury accommodation. A full range of therapies and services would be provided to adult clients addicted to cocaine, codeine, crack, heroin, marijuana, methamphetamines, oxycodone, Xanax, and prescription painkillers. It would not accept Medicaid or Medicare.

To acquire the land, Mountain View Recovery would pay Jefferson Partners with stock in the corporation. It also expressed interest in purchasing select support services (e.g., laundry, facility maintenance) from Jasper Gardens or Jefferson Partners. It asked that its inquiry and plans be kept confidential between the two organizations. Charles has scheduled a visit with Winters to discuss this potential venture. According to Charles, the board of Jefferson Partners is very interested in pursuing this proposal.

Additional information regarding Jasper Gardens's patient population, staffing, financial status, and operations can be found in tables 8.1 through 8.7.

On the web at ache.org/books/ Middleboro2

	2019	2018	2017	2016
Type of Primary Insurance				
Skilled Care				
Medicare	24	22	24	30
Commercial	1	2	0	1
Subtotal	25	24	24	31
Intermediate Care				
Medicaid	55	53	52	48
Veterans Administration	6	4	2	1
Private Insurance	1	0	0	1
Self-Pay	12	14	21	19
Subtotal	74	71	75	69
Total Filled Beds	99	95	99	100
Total Number of Beds	106	106	106	106
Facility Occupancy	93.4%	89.6%	93.4%	94.3%

Table 8.1
Jasper Gardens Patient Census by Type of Insurance

Note: Years ending December 31.

Table 8.2
Jasper Gardens
Resident
Information

*On the web at
ache.org/books/
Middleboro2*

Number	Age	Gender	Months	Comm	Ins	Ref	S or I
1	99	2	81.0	9	2	4	I
2	99	2	88.0	5	2	2	I
3	98	2	32.0	9	2	3	I
4	97	2	75.0	9	2	2	I
5	96	1	41.0	1	2	3	I
6	96	2	30.0	3	2	4	I
7	94	2	21.0	1	2	2	I
8	94	2	27.0	3	2	2	I
9	93	2	76.0	5	2	1	I
10	93	2	17.0	3	2	4	I
11	93	2	34.0	2	2	5	I
12	93	1	25.0	3	2	2	I
13	92	2	31.0	1	2	3	I
14	92	2	20.0	3	2	5	I
15	92	2	73.0	9	2	1	I
16	91	2	84.0	5	2	1	I
17	90	2	72.0	5	2	2	I
18	90	2	56.0	5	2	2	I
19	90	2	24.0	5	2	1	I
20	90	2	30.0	9	2	3	I
21	90	1	23.0	1	2	6	I
22	90	2	19.0	3	2	2	I
23	90	2	19.0	3	2	6	I
24	90	2	39.0	3	2	1	I
25	90	1	48.0	3	2	1	I
26	89	2	23.0	9	2	4	I
27	89	2	24.0	3	2	2	I
28	89	1	38.0	3	2	1	I
29	89	2	22.0	3	2	6	I
30	89	1	60.0	3	2	1	I
31	89	2	4.0	2	2	5	I
32	89	2	30.0	9	2	3	I
33	88	2	38.0	3	2	2	I
34	88	1	30.0	3	2	2	I
35	88	2	5.0	3	2	5	I
36	88	2	24.0	9	2	6	I
37	88	2	26.0	9	2	5	I
38	88	1	35.0	3	2	1	I

continued

Number	Age	Gender	Months	Comm	Ins	Ref	S or I
39	87	2	30.0	5	2	1	I
40	87	2	21.0	9	2	6	I
41	87	2	30.0	3	2	2	I
42	87	2	8.0	10	2	6	I
43	87	2	9.0	1	2	5	I
44	86	2	30.0	3	2	3	I
45	86	2	35.0	3	2	1	I
46	34	1	34.0	3	2	6	I
47	86	2	26.0	3	2	3	I
48	85	1	23.0	3	2	3	I
49	85	2	33.0	2	2	6	I
50	85	1	7.0	4	6	6	I
51	84	1	20.0	6	2	5	I
52	84	2	37.0	3	2	1	I
53	84	1	32.0	3	2	5	I
54	84	2	31.0	3	2	1	I
55	83	1	8.0	3	2	5	I
56	83	1	13.0	3	2	5	I
57	72	2	23.0	9	3	4	I
58	56	1	45.0	9	3	5	I
59	64	1	38.0	9	3	4	I
60	89	2	69.0	3	3	5	I
61	71	2	11.0	3	6	1	I
62	68	2	8.0	3	6	2	I
63	66	1	9.0	3	6	5	I
64	63	1	2.5	3	4	2	I
65	63	1	2.0	3	6	2	I
66	62	2	3.0	3	3	1	I
67	61	2	9.0	3	6	5	I
68	60	1	7.0	3	6	3	I
69	59	1	0.5	1	3	2	I
70	59	2	3.0	3	6	1	I
71	59	2	10.0	1	6	1	I
72	58	1	7.0	3	6	1	I
73	56	2	10.0	3	6	2	I
74	28	2	12.0	2	6	1	I
75	90	2	1.0	5	1	4	S
76	89	1	8.0	5	1	6	S
77	88	2	2.0	3	1	1	S
78	88	2	1.0	5	1	2	S

Table 8.2

Jasper Gardens
Resident
Information
(continued)

*On the web at
ache.org/books/
Middleboro2*

continued

Table 8.2
Jasper Gardens
Resident
Information
(continued)

*On the web at
ache.org/books/
Middleboro2*

Number	Age	Gender	Months	Comm	Ins	Ref	S or I
79	85	2	2.0	3	1	2	S
80	82	1	0.4	2	1	2	S
81	82	2	0.8	9	1	2	S
82	80	2	0.9	5	1	1	S
83	80	2	0.2	5	1	4	S
84	80	1	1.5	3	1	1	S
85	80	1	0.5	5	1	6	S
86	78	2	0.3	1	1	5	S
87	78	1	1.0	3	1	2	S
88	77	2	0.2	3	1	1	S
89	73	2	2.0	3	1	1	S
90	71	2	0.8	3	1	4	S
91	70	2	0.9	5	1	4	S
92	70	2	0.5	3	1	4	S
93	69	2	1.0	3	1	1	S
94	68	2	0.5	3	1	2	S
95	68	2	2.0	3	1	3	S
96	67	1	0.5	3	1	2	S
97	66	2	2.3	3	1	6	S
98	65	2	0.5	3	1	4	S
99	83	2	0.5	3	4	2	S

Notes: (1) As of December 31, 2019. (2) Number: patient ID number. (3) Gender: 1—Male; 2—Female. (4) Comm: community of origin. (5) Ins: insurance. (6) Ref: hospital referred to. (7) S: skilled care; I: intermediate care.

Code	Community	Insurance	Referral Center
1	Middleboro	Medicare	MIDCARE
2	Mifflenville	Medicaid	Webster Health System
3	Jasper	VA	Osteopathic Medical Center
4	Harris City	Commercial	Other Capital City Hospital
5	Statesville	Other Private	From Home
6	Carterville	Self-Pay	Other
7	Boalsburg		
8	Minortown		
9	Capital City		
10	Other		

Table 8.3
Jasper Gardens Staffing (Full-Time Equivalent [FTE])

	2019	2018	2017	2016
Administration				
Administrator	1.0	1.0	1.0	1.0
Director of Admissions	1.0	1.0	1.0	1.0
Nurses with Admin Duties	2.0	1.5	1.0	1.0
Admin Assistant/Bookkeeper	0.8	0.8	0.8	0.8
Receptionist	2.0	2.3	2.2	2.0
Admin Clerks	1.5	1.5	1.5	1.0
Medical Records Tech	0.5	0.5	0.5	0.5
Other	4.0	4.0	3.0	2.0
Subtotal	**11.8**	**11.6**	**10.0**	**8.3**
Patient Services				
Director	1.0	1.0	1.0	1.0
Medical Director	0.1	0.1	0.1	0.1
Dentist	0.1	0.1	0.1	0.1
Registered Nurses	13.4	13.8	14.0	14.0
Licensed Nursing Assistants	32.1	30.1	27.3	26.3
Licensed Practical Nurses	8.9	9.0	9.3	9.3
Medication Nursing Assistants	4.0	4.3	4.0	3.0
Assistant Director, Rehab	0.7	0.7	0.5	0.5
Physical Therapists	2.3	2.3	2.5	1.5
Physical Therapy Assistant	0.3	0.5	0.4	0.4
Occupational Therapist	1.5	1.0	1.0	1.0
COTA	0.5	0.8	0.8	0.8
Speech Therapist	0.3	0.4	0.4	0.4
Mental Health Aide	0.4	0.3	0.3	0.0
Assistant Director, Dietary	1.2	1.2	1.0	1.0
Dietitian	0.6	0.6	0.6	0.6
Food Services Personnel	15.9	16.3	16.5	17.5
Assistant Director, Recreation	0.3	0.3	0.2	0.2
CTRS	1.5	1.2	1.3	0.8
Subtotal	**85.1**	**84.0**	**81.3**	**78.5**
Plant Operations				
Director	0.4	0.4	0.4	0.4
Housekeeping Personnel	7.4	7.5	7.0	6.5
Maintenance Staff	0.6	0.6	0.6	0.6
Subtotal	**8.4**	**8.5**	**8.0**	**7.5**
Total Staff	**105.3**	**104.1**	**99.3**	**94.3**

Notes: (1) 1 FTE worker is paid for 2,080 hours per year. (2) For benefits, full-time is defined as 80 percent time or higher. (3) 100 percent time salaried workers work 1,896 hours per year. (4) COTA: certified occupational therapy assistant; CTRS: certified therapeutic recreation specialist.

	2019	2018	2017	2016
Patient Days				
Skilled: Medicare	4,730	5,430	5,833	6,723
Skilled: Other	560	518	534	510
ICF: Medicaid	18,975	18,656	18,668	16,752
ICF: Self-Pay	4,320	6,040	7,245	6,802
ICF: VA	2,142	1,440	720	355
ICF: Private Insurance	365	45	75	365
Total	**31,092**	**32,129**	**33,075**	**31,507**
Annual Occupancy				
SNF: 31 beds	46.8%	52.6%	56.3%	63.9%
ICF: 75 Beds	94.3%	95.6%	97.6%	88.7%
Overall: 106 Beds	80.4%	83.0%	85.5%	81.4%
Resident Deaths	20	18	25	22
Rehab Services in RVUs: Inpatient and Outpatient				
PT Treatments	9,322	9,537	9,725	9,971
OT Treatments	7,270	7,023	6,530	6,938
ST Treatments	202	208	256	205
Total	**16,794**	**16,768**	**16,511**	**17,114**

Notes: (1) 1 RVU is 15-minute service unit. (2) ICF: intermediate care facility; OT: occupational therapy; PT: physical therapy; RVU: relative value unit; SNF: skilled nursing facility; ST: speech therapy; VA: Veterans Administration.

	2019	2018	2017	2016
Revenues				
Room and Board				
Skilled Care				
Medicare—A	2,604,238	2,602,587	2,806,022	3,031,569
Commercial	502,334	534,229	501,449	496,230
Intermediate Care				
Medicaid	4,156,604	4,198,356	4,195,291	3,993,282
Self-Pay	1,734,377	1,839,202	1,920,445	2,134,203
Veterans Administration	781,830	892,334	523,669	430,228
Private Insurance	140,525	154,330	163,220	173,240
Subtotal	**9,919,908**	**10,221,038**	**10,110,096**	**10,258,752**
Ancillary Revenue				
Skilled Care				
Medicare—A and B	1,005,235	867,334	813,226	901,347
Commercial and Other	38,675	39,294	42,393	44,356
Intermediate Care				
Medicaid	19,547	14,292	13,258	16,393
Other	14,457	10,350	8,945	8,236
Subtotal	**1,077,914**	**931,270**	**877,822**	**970,332**
Other Revenue				
Interest	18,417	13,292	15,202	16,729
Miscellaneous	3,683	3,125	5,403	6,230
Subtotal	**22,100**	**16,417**	**20,605**	**22,959**
Total Gross Revenue	**11,019,922**	**11,168,725**	**11,008,523**	**11,252,043**
Deductions				
Less Provider Tax	347,560	343,501	313,996	302,547
Less Contractual Allowances	3,001,232	3,100,238	2,935,330	3,002,116
Total Net Revenue	**7,671,130**	**7,724,986**	**7,759,197**	**7,947,380**
Expenses				
Personnel				
Salaries and Wages	3,342,123	3,317,938	3,421,804	3,485,520
Benefits—All	956,838	995,381	1,094,977	1,219,932
Subtotal	**4,298,961**	**4,313,319**	**4,516,781**	**4,705,452**
Admin and General				
Equipment	132,445	102,445	110,338	85,233
Accounting Fees	60,000	60,000	70,000	80,000
Telephone	33,799	34,292	35,292	35,920
Insurance—General	30,319	29,200	29,500	34,290

Table 8.5
Jasper Gardens
Statement of
Operations

*On the web at
ache.org/books/
Middleboro2*

continued

Table 8.5
Jasper Gardens
Statement of
Operations
(continued)

*On the web at
ache.org/books/
Middleboro2*

	2019	2018	2017	2016
Payroll Services	18,228	18,200	18,400	16,393
MIS Management	16,415	16,000	16,000	15,300
Dues and Licenses	13,054	14,303	13,500	17,202
Office Supplies	10,424	8,939	7,830	5,920
Postage	9,379	9,100	9,320	8,983
Legal	8,000	12,503	17,394	12,302
Auto	7,893	7,893	7,893	7,893
Marketing and Advertising	6,000	6,000	5,780	5,500
Misc Bank Charges	3,800	2,000	2,560	2,830
Admin Equipment Rental	4,785	5,640	5,500	4,950
Other Professional Fees	8,979	3,502	3,012	2,640
Printing and Publishing	1,489	1,648	1,102	1,100
Subtotal	**365,009**	**331,665**	**353,421**	**336,456**
Other Operating Expenses				
Maintenance Supplies	24,010	22,310	22,740	21,640
Maintenance Repairs	50,880	34,272	23,784	24,450
Utilities—All	319,234	240,120	250,123	250,282
Oxygen Services	30,175	18,393	17,202	14,383
Food	365,220	254,499	255,206	244,351
General Supplies	202,364	190,303	173,445	178,202
Laboratory Services	28,511	32,404	28,400	23,450
Pharmacy Services	207,494	215,450	212,004	215,202
Imaging Services	11,003	13,204	15,202	11,023
Medical Equipment Rental	64,897	64,897	64,897	60,200
Capital Lease	850,000	950,000	900,000	900,000
Depreciation—All	204,783	205,294	210,494	211,474
Bad Debt	6,600	6,000	5,325	5,270
Subtotal	**2,365,171**	**2,247,146**	**2,178,822**	**2,159,927**
Non-Operating Expenses				
Management Fee	625,000	800,000	700,000	725,000
Subtotal	**625,000**	**800,000**	**700,000**	**725,000**
Total Expenses	**7,654,141**	**7,692,130**	**7,749,024**	**7,926,835**
Total Net Revenue	**7,671,130**	**7,724,986**	**7,759,197**	**7,947,380**
Pretax Profit or (Loss)	16,989	32,856	10,173	20,545
All Taxes	5,776	11,171	3,459	6,985
Net Profit—After Tax	**11,213**	**21,685**	**6,714**	**13,560**

Notes: (1) Years ending December 31. (2) Numbers are in US dollars. (3) MIS: management information system.

	2019	2018	2017	2016
Assets				
Current				
Cash	1,734,272	1,035,449	994,224	1,005,228
Patient Trust Cash	22,919	24,900	23,491	21,403
Subtotal	**1,757,191**	**1,060,349**	**1,017,715**	**1,026,631**
Accounts Receivable—Net	1,437,220	1,456,292	1,569,252	1,790,239
Inventory	56,404	60,340	62,360	49,372
Prepaid Expenses	150,694	145,202	137,223	139,335
Subtotal	**3,401,509**	**2,722,183**	**2,786,550**	**3,005,577**
Property, Plant, and Equipment (PPE)				
Building and Land Improvements	814,300	795,756	690,202	680,272
Fixed and Leasehold Equipment	740,112	655,223	665,223	623,443
Furniture and Other Equipment	1,082,011	995,292	990,385	994,283
Automobile	7,227	14,454	21,681	28,908
Gross PPE	**2,643,650**	**2,460,725**	**2,367,491**	**2,326,906**
Less Accumulated Depreciation	2,220,606	2,015,823	1,810,529	1,600,235
Net PPE	**423,044**	**444,902**	**556,962**	**726,671**
Other Assets				
Security Deposits	11,565	9,450	10,474	12,570
Total Assets	**3,836,118**	**3,176,535**	**3,353,986**	**3,744,818**
Liabilities				
Current				
Accounts Payable	1,033,424	945,223	967,349	845,223
Accrued Expenses	435,640	485,223	490,338	395,225
Patient Trust Liability	22,919	24,900	23,491	21,403
Accrued Interest	9,371	9,145	8,628	8,120
Subtotal	**1,501,354**	**1,464,491**	**1,489,806**	**1,269,971**
Long Term				
Deferred Lease Obligations	41,464	34,229	28,045	50,229
Notes Payable	74,260	62,450	56,330	40,375
Line of Credit	100,950	100,450	150,784	150,387
Subtotal	**216,674**	**197,129**	**235,159**	**240,991**
Total Liabilities	**1,718,028**	**1,661,620**	**1,724,965**	**1,510,962**
Net Assets	**2,118,090**	**1,514,915**	**1,629,021**	**2,233,856**
Net Assets + Liabilities	**3,836,118**	**3,176,535**	**3,353,986**	**3,744,818**

Table 8.6
Jasper Gardens Balance Sheet

On the web at ache.org/books/ Middleboro2

Notes: (1) Years ending December 31. (2) Numbers are in US dollars.

Measure	Jasper Gardens	State Average
General Information		
Overall rating	Average	
Health inspections	Average	
Staffing	Average	
Quality measures	Below Average	
Automatic sprinkler systems in all required areas	Yes	
Health and Safety		
Overall rating	Average	
Health inspections	Average	
Total number of health deficiencies	1	2.6
Number of complaints	0	0–21
Fire safety: number of fire deficiencies	0	0–10
Staffing		
Overall rating	Average	
RN staff only	Above Average	
Total number of licensed staff hours per resident day	1 hr 41 min	1 hr 30 min
RN hours per resident per day	1 hr 6 min	53 min
LPN/LVN hours per resident day	37 min	45 min
CNA hours per resident per day	32 min	20 min
Physical therapy staff hours per resident per day	4 min	5 min
Quality Measures		
Overall rating	Below Average	
Quality measures	Below Average	
Quality: Short-Stay Residents		
Percentage of short-stay residents who self-report moderate to severe pain	18.3	21.4
Percentage of short-stay residents with pressure ulcers that are new or worsened	1.9	2.3
Percentage of short-stay residents assessed and appropriately given the seasonal influenza vaccine	91.2	90.0

continued

Measure	Jasper Gardens	State Average
Percentage of short-stay residents assessed and appropriately given the pneumococcal vaccine	95.1	87.3
Percentage of short-stay residents who newly received an antipsychotic medication	1.6	2.4
Quality: Long-Stay Residents		
Percentage of long-stay residents experiencing one or more falls with major injury	5.5	4.0
Percentage of long-stay residents with a urinary tract infection	9.3	4.4
Percentage of long-stay residents who self-report moderate to severe pain	7.0	9.9
Percentage of long-stay, high-risk residents with pressure ulcers	9.1	3.8
Percentage of long-stay, low-risk residents who lose control of their bowels or bladder	42.1	46.3
Percentage of long-stay residents who have/had a catheter inserted and left in their bladder	6.1	3.2
Percentage of long-stay residents who were physically restrained	0.8	0.5
Percentage of long-stay residents whose needs for help with daily activities has increased	16.2	19.3
Percentage of long-stay residents who lose too much weight	9.3	7.0
Percentage of long-stay residents who have depressive symptoms	10.8	6.5
Percentage of long-stay residents assessed and appropriately given the seasonal influenza vaccine	98.5	98.1
Percentage of long-stay residents assessed and appropriately given the pneumococcal vaccine	31.3	97.9
Percentage of long-stay residents who received an antipsychotic medication	20.2	17.1
Penalties		
Federal fines in the last three years	0.0	
Federal payment denials in the last three years	0.0	

Table 8.7
Jasper Gardens Performance Against CMS Quality Measures

Notes: (1) As of December 31, 2019. (2) CMS: Centers for Medicare & Medicaid Services; CNA: certified nursing assistant; LPN/LVN: licensed practical nurse/licensed vocational nurse; RN: registered nurse.

HILLSBORO COUNTY HEALTH DEPARTMENT

E stablished in 1946, the Hillsboro County Health Department (HCHD) is a municipal department in the county's government that receives all of its funding from the county and from federal and state grants. HCHD is accountable to the Hillsboro County Commissioners. HCHD's mission and vision (revised and approved in 2012) are as follows:

Mission: To improve the health of individuals, families, and the community through disease prevention, health promotion, and programs to mitigate environmental threats to health and well-being.

Vision: We want Hillsboro County to be as healthy as the other communities in our state and region. To accomplish this, we improve access to quality healthcare services and maintain an environment free of threats to the public's health.

The following are HCHD's functional responsibilities:

◆ Collect, disseminate, and monitor health status information as part of its effort to identify physical and environmental health issues.

◆ Assess the accessibility, effectiveness, and quality of select health services.

◆ Serve as the county's public health advocate. As such, HCHD defines public health priorities and needs and relies on evidence-based practice to promote, prevent, and improve physical, mental, and environmental health and well-being. Services are provided directly to the public or, using grants, to area health agencies in an effort to carry out the core functions of public health and the essential public health services as defined by the state and the Centers for Disease Control and Prevention.

◆ Study and report health problems and hazards using epidemiology.

◆ Enforce laws and regulations that protect physical, mental, and environmental health and that ensure safety.

◆ Oversee Manorhaven, a 110-bed long-term care facility. Located in Middleboro, Manorhaven is owned and operated by the county. Financially, it is independent of the HCHD, but it uses select administrative services (e.g., payroll, human resources) provided by the county. This facility is a distinct line item in the county budget because it is both a revenue and an expense. Its administrator is appointed by the Hillsboro County Commissioners, following the recommendation of the HCHD director, and reports directly to the HCHD director.

HILLSBORO COUNTY BOARD OF HEALTH

The Hillsboro County Board of Health—a member of the National Association of Local Boards of Health—is an independent board appointed by the Hillsboro County Commissioners. It was created by statute to identify public health issues and concerns as well as provide programmatic advice and policy guidance to HCHD. Its 12 members serve five-year terms each and can be reappointed; following is the current roster of members:

Hillsboro County Board of Health

Members	Term Expires
Doris Felix, DO, *Chair*	
Surgeon, Webster Health System	2021
Micah Foxx, DO, *Vice Chair*	
Occupational health physician, Physician Care Services	2020
Milo Fudge	
School nurse, Middleboro High School	2021
Gemma Guevara, RN	
Director, Nursing Education and Staff Development, MIDCARE	2021
Edith Masterman	
Retired	2020
Catherine Newfields, RN	
Chief operating officer, Hillsboro Health	2021
Raymond Samuels, MD	
Pediatrician, Medical Associates	2020
Helen Vosper, RN	
Retired	2021
TBD	
Community representative	Vacant
TBD	
Community representative	Vacant
John Snow, *Secretary, Ex Officio*	
Director, HCHD	
Paige Magnet, DO, *Ex Officio*	
Health officer/Medical examiner, HCHD	

The *2019 Annual Report* published by the Board of Health includes the recently revised state guidelines for physical activity in K–12 public schools. The board is considering using these recommendations to assist community leaders to establish locally supported "Action for Healthy Kids" programs. At least three members of the board advocate for these guidelines to be adopted as a public health priority for the next five years.

MANAGEMENT TEAM AND ORGANIZATIONAL STRUCTURE

OFFICE OF THE DIRECTOR

Annually, the Hillsboro County Commissioners, on the basis of the Board of Health's recommendation, make a merit-based political appointment to fill the director of HCHD position. For the past 11 years, the commissioners have appointed John Snow, who has been employed by the department for 17 years. He holds a bachelor in biology from State University and a master of public health from a leading midwestern university.

As director, Snow is responsible for safeguarding the health of the residents of Hillsboro County and for enforcing all state and local health regulations, including fining violators. He is on state and national task forces on developing a competent public health workforce for the next several decades, serves as the vice president of the State Public Health Association (and frequently attends the annual meeting of the American Public Health Association), is the leading spokesperson for public health in nonmetropolitan areas in the state, and has frequently testified before the Committee on Public Health sponsored by the governor and endorsed by the state legislature. In addition, he is responsible for executing Health Impact Assessments in accordance with the guidelines of the Centers for Disease Control and Prevention as well as the World Health Organization. Over the past three years, HCHD has conducted assessments of municipal transportation systems and land use.

When interviewed, Snow indicated that he is concerned that the public health challenges and agenda in Hillsboro County continue to grow but the funding sources continue to shrink. He affirmed the need to cut the county's appropriation for public health, but he worried that "some of our larger grants may actually be cancelled in the next one to three years." HCHD has had to reduce the work hours of some employees, but overall it has not had to dismiss any workers. "Any reduction to our workforce has been based on attrition related to retirement or voluntary action," he explained. Six years ago, the State Department of Public Health employed a professional liaison in Washington, DC, to monitor and inform the state and its counties of available federal grants related to their public health missions. Counties will need to contribute funds to this effort when the liaison's contract is renewed after 2019. "This Washington liaison service has led to our public health needs being first in the nation when grant funding is made available," Snow said.

Another area of concern is the drug addiction epidemic and lack of prevention and treatment programs in the county. He said, "The recent report by the Hillsboro County Police Chiefs Association documents our issue with drug abuse and opioid addiction, especially in the smaller communities. We need to act quickly. As many parts of our country and state have done, we may have overlooked a significant public health issue for far too many years." He has included this issue on the agenda of the next meeting of the Board of Health.

Yet another of Snow's concerns is the aging of his department personnel. "Within five years, more than one-third of our workers will be eligible for retirement," he stated. "It has always been difficult for government offices to attract qualified workers, especially in the area of environmental health services. We anticipate it will be just as hard to replace retiring employees with trained individuals just starting their career."

Other challenges stem from the department's unique relationship with Manorhaven. Manorhaven has a separate budget that is approved by the Hillsboro County Commissioners. By county regulation, however, HCHD is responsible for any financial losses the facility incurs. Fifteen years ago, for example, HCHD had to cover an $84,000 shortfall in the facility's budget. The regulation was established in 1984, following the recommendations of a blue-ribbon commission to increase the efficiency of local and county governments. Today, state Medicaid reimbursement rates have become so low that Manorhaven faces an uncertain future. To maintain oversight, Snow meets quarterly with the facility's management team to review its finances. There has been speculation that he has met with the county's attorney to discuss the potential sale of Manorhaven.

When asked about plans for accountable care organizations (ACOs), Snow indicated that the department is fully prepared to work with one or more ACOs that share its mission to improve the health of the citizens of Hillsboro County. In addition, HCHD has been communicating with Webster Health System (WHS) and MIDCARE to collaborate on creating the community health needs assessment. He noted that "it has been a major challenge getting the two hospitals to agree with each other on much of anything. But this assessment is something we all have to do." WHS has participated in HCHD projects in the past, however. Five years ago, using Federal Demonstration Partnership grant money and space donated by the local towns involved, the department—along with WHS and other organizations—sponsored the opening of two rural health primary clinics in Carterville and Harris City. Each clinic is a 501(c)(3) facility with a local board of directors. Today, both Rural Clinics, Inc. locations serve patients from 10 a.m.–3 p.m., Monday through Saturday.

Snow gives credit to HCHD's website for significantly extending the reach and enhancing the reputation of the department. He thinks the department's continued online presence will eventually lessen—if not eliminate—the need for printed annual reports and consumer information sheets. He added, "Other health departments have had a lot of success with social media, which is something we need to copy. We're a little behind the digital times, but we're quickly catching up."

HCHD's senior management team meets every two weeks to review plans and accomplishments. At this meeting, budget variances are discussed and plans are reviewed for the next 30 to 60 days. Before developing a budget request, which is submitted to and approved by the Hillsboro County Commissioners, team members meet with their counterparts in the State Department of Public Health to best estimate state support for county public health programs.

ADMINISTRATIVE SERVICES DIVISION

This division provides management, financial, and administrative support—including grant review and oversight—to the entire department. It is responsible for preparing and managing the budget and staffing plans. As director of the division, Jimmy Pagget retains the part-time services of Dr. Paige Magnet as Hillsboro County's health officer and medical examiner. Pagget has held this position for 27 years; prior to this appointment, he was a senior analyst for the State Department of Revenue Administration.

By statute, each incorporated city and town in Hillsboro County must designate a health officer to coordinate local services and needs with the HCHD. Every quarter, Dr. Magnet meets with each of the designated health officers. The current health officers are as follows (the * indicates that the person receives from the city or town a stipend of $1,000 per year to cover his or her time and expenses):

City or Town	Name	Position
Boalsburg	Simon Fistru*	Physician, General Practice
Carterville	Gus Burns	Deputy Chief, Carterville Fire and EMS
Harris City	Audra Adams*	Physician, General Practice
Jasper	Nathan Spark	Chief, Jasper Volunteer Fire Department
Middleboro	Bruce Sullivan	Director, Public Works
Mifflenville	Benny Fufe*	Deputy Mayor
Minortown	Ivan Kelly*	Physician, General Practice
Statesville	Billie Clark-Adams	Nurse, retired

In his interview, Pagget emphasized Snow's perspectives on the department's budget: "While I am grateful that a significant portion of our financial support comes from grants and contracts, they create a vulnerability and potential volatility. Without this support, we could not fulfill our mission." He mentioned that the State Public Employees Union recently signed a five-year contract with salary increases of 2 to 3 percent per year but no increases in benefit coverage. Beginning next year, the state's contribution for health and dental insurance will be frozen at its current rate, and employees will be required to contribute to the cost of their own health insurance. Employees who opt out of the health insurance benefit will receive $4,000. An additional week of vacation will be granted to employees with more than 20 years of service. The state and union continue to discuss employee pensions. Currently, workers do not contribute to the state retirement plan, which is an unfunded liability. The county identifies this as a significant issue.

The Administrative Services division is responsible for distributing all grants and contracts. For grants that allow indirect cost recovery, HCHD has a 3 percent negotiated indirect cost rate with the Environmental Protection Agency (EPA) and the US Department of Health & Human Services. HCHD receives no indirect reimbursement from state grants and private foundations. When the department awards grants and contracts, it makes no allowances for indirect costs; only direct costs are covered.

Currently, HCHD's budget allocates money for facility maintenance and utilities. When an HCHD division is located in a privately owned facility, the department is not responsible for building rental or lease expenses. These costs are covered directly in the facility budget of the county. Each HCHD division has an equipment budget that covers the acquisition and maintenance of all office equipment, including computer hardware and software. A departmentwide committee, chaired by Pagget, prioritizes and coordinates the acquisition of all equipment. The supplies budget covers office supplies and work-related travel.

Environmental Health Division

Sally Brownell, the director of this division, holds a master of science in environmental health from State University and is a registered environmental health specialist. She joined the department 18 months ago, having served in a similar position in a western state. She is a member of Hillsboro County's HAZMAT (hazardous material) team.

The division is in charge of the following programs or services: arboviral program, campgrounds (licensure and inspection), emergency preparedness, food service sanitation (licensure and inspection), health facility inspection, lead paint abatement, mosquito and tick control, public swimming pools, rabies control, radon control, safe drinking water, and private sewage treatment. In addition, the division maintains multiple contractual relationships with independent and state public health laboratories to provide public health laboratory services. The State Department of Environmental Services performs air-quality surveillance.

Brownell said, "Each year's budget requires us to adjust to our level of support. For example, the division has had to prioritize its inspections. Our current policy is that if an establishment that engages in food preparation has passed inspection without any conditions for four consecutive years, the department can (if needed) waive the fifth year inspection."

She noted other environment-related areas of concerns. First, the lead paint abatement program did fewer home inspections this year because of a change in leadership that affected staff coverage. Old houses, especially in the northern part of the county, need increased attention given their age and the likelihood that they contain lead-based paint. The resettlement in the community of refugees and immigrants who have limited English proficiency also contributes to the issue given the difficulty of communicating lead-abatement strategies to this population. When secondary prevention measures are implemented, children regularly present with elevated blood lead levels. If not addressed, these elevated blood lead levels can eventually stunt children's cognitive development and school performance, leading to increased social costs. Unless the division can better demonstrate to the state the need for this program, it may be curtailed or eliminated.

Second, a bedbug infestation is menacing the lower-income districts of the county. This environmental issue may be attributed to absentee landlords, poor-quality living conditions, social determinants of health, and cultural and language differences that impede communication. This division educates the occupants of these infested units about preventive measures and connects them with social service agencies that can provide replacement furniture.

Third, since DDT spraying was banned 40 or so years ago, mosquito control has remained an issue. State funding has ceased for mosquito surveillance in the county. As a result, the division has resorted to enlisting community volunteers. It is a cost-effective approach to conducting surveillance for the presence of mosquito-borne diseases, such as West Nile virus and Eastern equine encephalitis.

Fourth, the EPA has identified one hazardous waste site in the county. In the 1950s and 1960s, the JM Asbestos Company inadvertently contaminated the soil, groundwater, and the Swift River that runs through the county. The extent of the environmental contamination and the resultant health effects on the employees and their families—as well as local residents who lived within a five-mile radius and those who fished downstream from the plant—qualified this site to be declared a Superfund site. This division is currently working with the EPA and the Agency for Toxic Substances and Disease Registry (ATSDR) to conduct a public health assessment. Recently, at HCHD's request, the ATSDR provided a health consultation to identify and assess the site owned by Carlstead Rayon. Preliminary studies indicate that Carlstead Rayon will be designated a hazardous waste site. In response, Carlstead Rayon has threatened to abandon its plant and leave the county if such a declaration is made.

Thus far in her tenure, Brownell has testified before the state legislature regarding the following bills:

◆   HB 2701 would eliminate water fluoridation. This bill is being amended to require a warning to property owners served by the municipal water system that their water supply is fluoridated. This warning would be included in the quarterly water bill.

◆   HB 2405 would allow communities to impose a moratorium on refugee resettlement in the county.

COMMUNITY HEALTH AND HEALTH PROMOTION DIVISION

Russell Martin has been the director of this division for nine years. His credentials include a master of public health from a leading midwestern university and more than ten years of experience in a similar position with the State Department of Public Health. He serves on the regional and state Emergency Preparedness Task Force. He is scheduled to retire in the next two years.

The division contracts with healthcare providers in the area to address the following community health needs: vision screening, hearing screening, tobacco control, school health (including oral health), substance abuse prevention, and adult health promotion. In addition, it runs an adult health program as well as an osteoporosis prevention and screening program. It frequently cosponsors initiatives with the local chapter of AARP, Red Cross, and Rural Clinics, Inc. It holds clinics and screenings in facilities across the county, including at Manorhaven, as well as health promotion seminars, workshops, and fairs in every public school in the county. Three times a year, it—with funding from one or more corporate sponsors—organizes a 5K road race to promote an active lifestyle and call attention to the dangers of obesity.

The tobacco control program includes enforcing the state and county regulation that prohibits smoking in public spaces and in any licensed establishments such as restaurants, bars, coffee shops, and stores. It offers smoking cessation classes quarterly and tobacco-free literature at numerous health fairs throughout the county.

The oral health program is run by two dental hygienists who travel by van to six elementary schools during the school year. The hygienists conduct oral screenings for dental caries, perform cleanings, and apply dental sealants. Once a week, they are joined by two volunteer dentists, who perform minor procedures such as extractions. The Kiwanis Club donated the dental van. The van is currently in need of major repairs, and a replacement van will cost approximately $300,000.

Six months ago, the Jasper Regional Educational Cooperative approached the HCHD to provide staffing and services to the Jasper school system. The school board would transfer all school health funding to HCHD for a five-year renewable contract. This plan is currently under review.

Martin indicated that grant funds might be available to expand health promotions, especially in the area of health behavior, such as a hand-washing campaign in schools and healthcare facilities.

Snow has recently asked Martin to draft a response to an open letter published in the *Middleboro Sentinel.* The letter called for school officials to ban sugary drinks and to adopt a "healthy vending" policy in all public schools. The leader of a county coalition of concerned parents and nurses signed the letter.

DISEASE PREVENTION DIVISION

For 27 years, Candice McCory, RN, has been the director of this division. She holds a bachelor in nursing and an advanced certificate in epidemiology from State University. As needed, she fills in for Snow as the deputy director of HCHD.

The division provides direct services and contracts with healthcare agencies in the area to fulfill prevention-related services, such as breast and cervical cancer screening; communicable disease control, including case investigations; family planning education and services; healthy eating; HIV/AIDS counseling and testing; immunization planning and clinics; sexually transmitted disease (STD) diagnosis and treatment referral; and a women, infants, and children (WIC) program.

When interviewed, McCory indicated her division "has the highest level of professionalism and productivity. I am especially proud of our workers and what we have accomplished with limited resources." She also mentioned that her division managed a countywide immunization and dental health program, saying, "We are especially fortunate that so many area dentists volunteer their time to provide indigent dental care, especially in the rural parts of our county." She expressed concern over rural women: "Women's health is a significant issue in this county, especially in our very rural communities. Needs and issues just aren't identified, or they are not addressed. In response to this concern, we now either hold or sponsor family planning clinics throughout the county frequently, in conjunction with programs and services provided under the WIC program. Our attempts to organize women's health outreach programs with hospitals and other providers have had limited success. Of all the area providers, Hillsboro Health has been the most responsive to our needs."

Recently, state funding for STD screening, including HIV/AIDS counseling, was cut. As a result, the Public Health Specialist I position was eliminated. Prior to the termination of this position, the standardized mortality ratio for HIV/AIDS in the county was greater than 1.0.

Last month, Snow asked McCory to develop recommendations and a budget for expanding the adult immunization services provided by HCHD. Given that flu shots are available in local pharmacies, HCHD may no longer have to provide this service and instead focus its resources on other immunizations, such as shots for shingles for senior citizens.

ISSUES AND CONCERNS

The statewide Task Force on Public Health, composed of business and civic leaders, that the governor tasked with examining whether regional rather than county-specific health departments are more economical has come back with recommendations. Under the task force's tentative plan, regional health departments that cover between 1 and 1.5 million lives would be organized under the direct control of the State Department of Public Health. Individual counties would be billed for their share of the cost. The statewide chapter of Hillsboro County Commissioners has opposed this plan because it removes local control but requires local taxes to support statewide programs.

Brownell, Martin, and McCory have formally requested the HCHD to reconsider its current organizational structure. They have asked that consultants be hired to address three questions:

1. Should the department be organized into three divisions? If so, what should be each division's primary responsibilities? If not, how should it be organized?

2. Should the Administrative Services Division be separate, or should it be folded into the Office of the Director or the program-oriented divisions? (

3. What services and programs can and should the department contract to other health agencies, such as WHS, MIDCARE, and Hillsboro Health?

Snow has promised to discuss these questions with the Hillsboro County Commissioners and report to the directors whether financial support for consultants will be made available in the department's annual budget request.

A recent editorial in the *Middleboro Sentinel* questioned whether HCHD is prepared to address public health issues such as a flu epidemic. Also, the State Board of Health has recommended that small county departments, such as the HCHD, must either expand their services or contract with other local healthcare agencies to create regional health departments. HCHD is currently considering the issues and alternatives.

The HCHD is responsible for implementing the statewide Home and Community-Based Services (HCBS) waiver under section 1915(c). The HCBS waiver allows Medicaid to cover the expenses of community-based homes for special populations (e.g., persons with mental health issues or developmental disabilities) and to screen all Medicaid-eligible patients before they are admitted to a residential long-term care facility. Under the current plan, any individual who is Medicaid eligible and can be cared for at home will be denied admission into a nursing home. In the past five years, the state has twice been found to be in violation of the 1999 US Supreme Court decision in the case *Olmstead v. L.C.*

Tables 9.4 through 9.6 provide detailed financial information for HCHD. These data indicate that approximately 40 percent of the resources used to support public health

*On the web at
ache.org/books/
Middleboro2*

programs in Hillsboro County are from grants and contracts. "This makes us especially vulnerable to changes in funding at the federal, state, and local levels," Snow said. "Unless our county's economy improves, the county will not approve increasing expenditures for public health."

After returning from a meeting by the National Public Health Performance Standards Program, Snow indicated that the HCHD should become more engaged with this program. He has asked the senior management staff to examine whether the HCHD should seek national accreditation and whether the HCHD meets or can meet the national standards for a local health department. "It appears that the marginal benefits associated with accreditation far exceed its marginal costs," Snow reasoned.

Representatives from the fire, police, and ambulance services make up the leadership of the county Emergency Preparedness Task Force. The 24-member task force is obligated annually to provide the Hillsboro County Commissioners with (1) a status report that describes the county's readiness to address large-scale emergencies and (2) recommendations for action. The county still has not achieved communication-system integration among all first responders in the county. Snow continues to suggest to the Hillsboro County Commissioners that the task force be made responsible to the Board of Health. Currently, no changes are anticipated.

The state contributes 50 percent of the Medicaid program and has indicated that, given anticipated Medicaid cost increases, it will either raise taxes statewide or require counties to contribute 10 to 25 percent of the Medicaid expenditures in their county. Under one of these plans, the state Medicaid program would pay 80 percent of allowable charges on the statewide fee schedule and the county would pay the remaining 20 percent. According to Snow, such a plan would bankrupt public health and prevent it from fulfilling its mission.

In keeping with its population growth, the Town of Jasper continues to expand its municipal water and sewage systems. Fifteen years ago, town water and sewer systems covered 12 percent of the property in Jasper. Today, these systems cover 54 percent. The town estimates that 88 percent of the households in Jasper will be serviced with town water and sewer systems within six years. However, Jasper recently declared a moratorium on adding fluoridation to town water effective in July 2020. In 2019, the Jasper Town Council received an against-fluoridation petition with 6,100 signatures. This led to the council's continued position against fluoridation. Two members of the council—Jennifer Kip and Alan Simpson—have continued to vote against fluoridation.

Nationally, the number of cases of community-acquired MRSA (methicillin-resistant Staphylococcus aureus) has attracted local concern. Snow has asked the senior staff for policy recommendations on this issue.

More statistics about HCHD and its programs can be found in the tables 9.1 through 9.14.

On the web at ache.org/books/ Middleboro2

	2019	2014	2009
Annual Licensed Food Establishments	712	745	523
Routine Inspections Conducted	1,258	956	1,320
Reinspections Conducted	101	177	237
Complaint Investigations Conducted	153	167	163
Temporary Food Stand Inspections	228	312	102
Food Certification Classes	14	23	9
Potable Water Supply			
Water Well Permits Issued	68	56	45
Water Wells Installed	43	32	15
New Water Wells Inspected	42	28	20
Complaint Investigations Conducted	2	18	12
Private On-Site Wastewater Disposal			
Systems Permits Issued	187	177	152
Systems Installed	169	101	98
Systems Inspected	197	130	164
Complaint Investigations Conducted	24	14	21
Lead Hazards Removal			
Environmental Assessments	146	77	60
Homes Mitigated	174	85	15
Other			
Indoor Tanning Establishment Inspections	27	24	15
Body Art Establishment Inspections	7	5	4
Camp (Summer) Inspections	40	58	59
Health Facility Inspections	19	18	12
Public Swimming Pool Inspections	11	11	10
Rabies Control Investigations	16	8	5
Radon Control Inspections	13	14	12
Vector Control Public Contacts	225	201	245
Vector Control Inspections	157	133	80

	2019	2014	2009
Adult Health Program			
Health Clinics Conducted	20	18	21
Clients Seen	1,177	1,466	1,405
Vision Screening Clients	544	689	459
Hearing Screening Clients	801	818	857
Substance Abuse Pamphlets Distributed	14,000	1,400	1,350
Health Promotion Presentations			
Community Programs Given	99	80	34
Community Program Attendees	1,277	1,326	978
School Health Program Presentations	201	156	159
School Health Program Attendees	4,106	3,648	3,948
Health Fairs Attendees	16	14	16
Osteoporosis Prevention and Screening			
Women Screened	190	203	224
Tobacco-Free Community Programs			
Smoking Cessation Program Enrollees	180	167	112
Program Classes	27	36	14
Smoke-Free Complaints	44	81	64
Smoke-Free Inspections	6	3	5
Smoke-Free Fines Assessed	5	3	8

Table 9.2
HCHD Community Health and Health Promotion Statistics

Table 9.3		2019	2014	2009
Communicable Diseases Reported				
Giardiasis		6	9	5
Lyme Disease		15	9	22
Meningitis (Viral)		0	1	0
Salmonellosis		13	14	9
Shigellosis		3	11	5
Tuberculosis		0	3	1
Case Investigations (Includes STD)		11	6	9
Dental Health Program				
Examinations		2,145	2,503	3,277
Sealants		565	503	509
Other Dental Services		4,423	4,129	3,715
Family Planning				
Clinics Held		8	5	4
Immunizations				
Adult Immunization, Doses Administered		3,718	3,823	3,512
Adult Immunization, Clients Served		2,247	2,156	2,546
Childhood Immunization, Doses Administered		8,560	8,934	9,213
Childhood Immunization, Clients Served		3,369	3,312	3,068
H1N1 Vaccine, Doses Administered		1,422	1,201	823
Influenza Immunization, Adult Doses		827	623	434
Influenza Immunization, Infant/Child Doses		801	602	338
Sexually Transmitted Disease (STD)				
Clinic Patient Encounters		2,178	2,099	1,856
HIV Counseling and Testing at Clinics		1,002	757	892
Chlamydia Cases Reported		1,268	1,130	956
Gonorrhea Cases Reported		406	386	402
Syphilis Cases Reported		1	1	0
Women, Infants, and Children (WIC) Program				
Clients Certified		6,835	6,022	5,103
Clients Attending Nutrition Classes		3,821	3,156	3,046
Breastfeeding Peer-Counseling Contracts		203	187	N/A
High-Risk Infant Visits		202	134	87
Children with Elevated Blood Lead Levels		44	51	69
Women's Health				
Clients Seen		2,544	2,014	2,056

Table 9.3
HCHD Disease
Prevention
Statistics

	2019	2018	2017
Revenues			
County Appropriation/Tax Levy	2,421,165	2,553,000	2,870,525
Federal Grants			
CDC—Environmental Health Tracking	8,450	8,450	8,200
EPA—Asthma	37,566	35,688	33,903
Oral Health	21,705	24,340	27,393
Rural Healthcare Development	194,204	212,440	215,383
Rural Poverty and Homelessness	103,440	90,450	85,303
State Grants			
County Health Department Development	215,400	200,000	200,000
EMS Assistance	121,000	110,000	110,000
EMS Preparedness	45,000	45,000	45,000
HIV Control and Prevention	55,000	55,000	55,000
Immunization	68,445	50,000	50,000
Lead Control Program	15,787	15,000	12,450
Medicaid Oral Health	118,407	94,818	56,282
Primary Health Care—Demo	234,040	212,494	0
STD Control and Prevention	83,817	85,000	85,000
Tobacco Use	56,818	72,404	86,249
WIC—Administration	85,000	85,000	85,000
WIC—Services	357,202	325,493	365,292
Private Foundations			
Breast Cancer Awareness	40,000	30,000	0
Obesity Control and Prevention	2,175	0	0
Subtotal External Grants and Contracts	**1,863,456**	**1,751,577**	**1,520,455**
Licenses and Permits			
Food Services	6,219	5,740	5,952
Campgrounds	1,250	1,433	1,340
Tanning Facilities	450	560	0
Special Fees and Fines	2,430	3,145	3,767
Overhead Recovery+*	100,113	125,000	150,300
Other—Miscellaneous	204	612	120
Subtotal Noncounty Tax Revenue	**1,974,122**	**1,888,067**	**1,681,934**
Total Revenue	**4,395,287**	**4,441,067**	**4,552,459**

Table 9.4
HCHD Statement of Revenues and Expenses

On the web at ache.org/books/Middleboro2

continued

Table 9.4
HCHD
Statement
of Revenues
and Expenses
(continued)

*On the web at
ache.org/books/
Middleboro2*

	2019	2018	2017
Expenses			
Office of the Director			
Salaries and Wages	262,969	257,710	249,978
Benefits	73,631	79,890	77,493
Supplies	18,540	21,500	20,340
Equipment	24,660	24,302	12,560
Utilities*	2,422	2,200	2,030
Marketing and Promotion	4,000	4,000	5,000
Staff Development	500	4,000	4,000
Miscellaneous	2,366	596	856
Grants to Local Agencies	4,800	6,800	6,800
Subtotal	**393,888**	**400,998**	**379,057**
Administrative Services Division			
Salaries and Wages	523,420	500,200	553,486
Benefits	157,026	155,062	171,581
Supplies	84,284	94,563	99,363
Equipment	4,803	5,234	4,109
Utilities*	28,383	26,440	28,304
Marketing and Promotion	450	500	500
Staff Development	1,000	1,500	2,000
Miscellaneous	200	140	167
Grants to Local Agencies	0	0	0
Subtotal	**799,566**	**783,639**	**859,510**
Environmental Health Division			
Salaries and Wages	452,320	456,675	446,905
Benefits	135,696	141,569	138,541
Supplies	6,579	6,500	5,356
Equipment	1,039	2,546	2,946
Utilities*	37,669	36,122	35,476
Marketing and Promotion	3,825	4,024	6,034
Staff Development	500	4,000	4,000
Miscellaneous—Lab Contracts	4,375	3,760	3,700
Miscellaneous	243	201	103
Grants to Local Agencies	0	0	0
Subtotal	**642,246**	**655,397**	**643,061**

continued

	2019	2018	2017
Community Health and Health Promotion Division			
Salaries and Wages	765,744	762,971	735,923
Benefits	222,066	236,521	228,136
Supplies	98,161	103,453	117,506
Equipment	39,445	23,450	12,404
Utilities*	22,341	23,460	24,354
Marketing and Promotion	4,512	5,500	5,500
Staff Development	355	5,000	5,000
Miscellaneous	456	402	450
Grants to Local Agencies	124,565	135,400	150,220
Subtotal	**1,277,645**	**1,296,157**	**1,279,493**
Disease Prevention Division			
Salaries and Wages	765,957	780,156	847,233
Benefits	237,447	241,848	262,642
Supplies	103,288	110,393	114,506
Equipment	23,693	12,000	4,500
Utilities*	34,552	34,595	30,282
Marketing and Promotion	2,300	2,500	2,500
Staff Development	1,800	4,800	4,800
Miscellaneous	356	221	498
Grants to Local Agencies	112,445	118,340	124,303
Subtotal	**1,281,838**	**1,304,853**	**1,391,264**
Total Expenses	**4,395,183**	**4,441,045**	**4,552,385**
Excess Revenue**	104	22	75

Table 9.4
HCHD
Statement
of Revenues
and Expenses
(continued)

*On the web at
ache.org/books/
Middleboro2*

Notes: (1) *Total charges for utilities allocated on the basis of square feet occupied. (2) +*The amount included in grants to cover overhead; used to reduce expenses. (3) ** Excess revenue is returned to the general fund at the end of the fiscal year. (4) Years Ending December 31. (5) Numbers are in US dollars. (6) CDC: Centers for Disease Control and Prevention; EMS: emergency medical services; EPA: Environmental Protection Agency; STD: sexually transmitted disease; WIC: women, infants, and children.

Table 9.5
HCHD Budget
by Source of
Funds

*On the web at
ache.org/books/
Middleboro2*

	Office of the Director	Administrative Services	Environmental Health	Community Health	Disease Prevention	Total
Federal Grants						
CDC—Environmental Health Tracking			8,450			8,450
EPA Asthma			37,566			37,566
Oral Health					21,705	21,705
Rural Healthcare Development	21,000	50,000	80,060	43,144		194,204
Rural Poverty and Homelessness	18,000			74,800	10,640	103,440
State Grants						
County Health Department Development	118,450	950	32,000	32,000	32,000	215,400
EMS Assistance				121,000		121,000
EMS Preparedness				45,000		45,000
HIV Control and Prevention				30,000	25,000	55,000
Immunization					68,445	68,445
Lead Control Program			15,787			15,787
Medicaid Oral Health					118,407	118,407
Primary Healthcare—Demo			9,475	224,565		234,040
STD Control and Prevention					83,817	83,817
Tobacco Use				56,818		56,818
WIC—Administration	25,500	15,600			43,900	85,000
WIC—Services					357,202	357,202
Private Foundations						
Breast Cancer Awareness				40,000		40,000
Obesity Control and Prevention				2,175		2,175
Total Grants and Contract	**182,950**	**66,550**	**183,338**	**669,502**	**761,116**	**1,863,456**

continued

	Office of the Director	Administrative Services	Environmental Health	Community Health	Disease Prevention	Total
Other Revenue	10,553					10,553
Overhead Recovery		100,113				100,113
Total Noncounty Revenue	193,503	166,663	183,338	669,502	761,116	1,974,122
County Tax Appropriation	200,385	632,903	458,908	608,143	520,722	2,421,061
Total Budget By Division	393,888	799,566	642,246	1,277,645	1,281,838	4,395,183
% Total Budget–County Funds	50.9	79.2	71.5	47.6	40.6	55.1

Table 9.5
HCHD Budget by Source of Funds *(continued)*

On the web at ache.org/books/ Middleboro2

Notes: (1) For calendar year 2019. (2) Numbers are in US dollars, except where indicated. (3) CDC: Centers for Disease Control and Prevention; EMS: emergency medical services; EPA: Environmental Protection Agency; STD: sexually transmitted disease; WIC: women, infants, and children.

Table 9.6
HCHD Staffing
Budget

*On the web at
ache.org/books/
Middleboro2*

	2019		2018		2017	
	FTE	Budgeted Salary	FTE	Budgeted Salary	FTE	Budgeted Salary
Office of the Director						
Director	1.0	140,174	1.0	137,447	1.0	130,174
Administrative Assistant III	1.0	39,262	1.0	38,477	1.0	37,322
Administrative Assistant II	0.5	31,348	0.5	30,721	0.5	29,799
Health Info Tech	0.5	44,560	0.5	43,669	0.5	42,359
Intern	0.2	7,625	0.4	10,000	0.5	16,754
Subtotal	**3.2**	**262,969**	**3.4**	**260,314**	**3.5**	**256,408**
Administrative Services Division						
Director, Administration	1.0	92,330	1.0	90,483	1.0	88,674
Health Officer/Medical Examiner	0.5	98,517	0.5	98,517	0.5	98,517
Business Services Officer	1.2	90,315	1.0	73,787	**1.0**	72,340
Customer Services Rep II	1.0	53,315	1.0	52,249	1.0	51,204
Administrative Services Manager	1.0	51,230	2.0	50,205	2.0	49,201
Administrative Assistant II	1.0	31,348	1.0	30,721	1.0	30,107
Custodian	2.5	106,365	3.0	104,238	4.0	163,444
Subtotal	**8.2**	**523,420**	**9.5**	**500,200**	**10.5**	**553,487**
Environmental Health Division						
Director, Environmental Health	1.0	103,233	1.0	101,168	1.0	101,168
Environ Health Specialist IV	1.0	54,223	1.0	53,139	1.0	53,139
Environ Health Specialist II	4.0	135,056	4.0	132,408	4.0	129,812
Public Health Specialist II	2.0	128,460	2.0	125,891	2.0	119,598
Administrative Assistant II	1.0	31,348	1.0	30,721	1.0	30,107
Administrative Assistant I	0.0	0	0.5	13,348	0.5	13,081
Subtotal	**9.0**	**452,320**	**9.5**	**456,675**	**9.5**	**446,905**
Community Health and Health Promotion Division						
Director, Community Health	1.0	93,274	1.0	88,610	1.0	86,838
Community Health Nurse	6.0	379,260	6.0	367,882	6.0	360,525
Public Health Specialist II	3.0	192,960	3.0	183,312	3.0	179,646
Public Health Preparedness Admin	1.0	86,200	1.3	109,819	1.0	82,752
Administrative Assistant I	0.5	14,050	0.5	13,348	1.0	26,163
Subtotal	**11.5**	**765,744**	**11.8**	**762,971**	**12.0**	**735,924**

continued

	2019		2018		2017	
	FTE	Budgeted Salary	FTE	Budgeted Salary	FTE	Budgeted Salary
Disease Prevention Division						
Director, Personal Health	1.0	104,330	1.0	99,114	1.0	97,131
Public Health Specialist III	2.0	120,068	2.0	114,065	3.0	111,783
Program Director, Women's Health	1.0	84,670	1.0	80,437	1.0	78,828
Public Health Nurse	5.0	332,115	5.0	315,509	5.0	247,360
Case Control Investigators	1.0	84,550	1.4	86,173	2.0	162,336
Community Services Assistant	0.5	24,550	1.5	69,968	2.0	91,425
Administrative Assistant II	0.5	15,674	1.0	14,890	2.0	58,370
Subtotal	**11.0**	**765,957**	**12.9**	**780,156**	**16.0**	**847,233**
Total	**42.9**	**2,770,410**	**47.1**	**2,760,316**	**51.5**	**2,839,957**

Table 9.6
HCHD Staffing Budget *(continued)*

On the web at ache.org/books/ Middleboro2

Notes: (1) Numbers are in US dollars, except where indicated. (2) FTE: full-time equivalent.

Table 9.7
HCHD Special
Study: Oral
Health and
Fluoridation

City/Town	Percentage of Households in Hillsboro County Served by Municipal Water System		
	2019	2014	2009
Boalsburg	0	0	0
Carterville	12	12	10
Harris City	8	4	5
Jasper	54	50	44
Middleboro	74	73	70
Mifflenville	22	24	30
Minortown	5	10	12
Statesville	18	20	9

City/Town	Percentage of Households in Hillsboro County Served by Flouridated Water System		
	2019	2014	2009
Boalsburg	0	0	0
Carterville	4	4	4
Harris City	0	0	0
Jasper	54	50	44
Middleboro	54	58	56
Mifflenville	22	24	0
Minortown	0	0	0
Statesville	0	10	12

City/Town	Percentage of 3rd-Grade Students with	
	Tooth Decay	Untreated Tooth Decay
Boalsburg	43.6	12.9
Carterville	19.3	14.3
Harris City	28.2	13.2
Jasper	23.5	8.1
Middleboro	24.9	10.7
Mifflenville	32.9	15.2
Minortown	31.4	23.7
Statesville	29.7	11.4

continued

City/Town	Time Since Last Cleaning by Dentist or Hygienist		
	2 Years	5 Years	6 Years or More*
Boalsburg	60	15	25
Carterville	56	10	34
Harris City	62	17	21
Jasper	79	10	11
Middleboro	70	14	16
Mifflenville	64	14	22
Minortown	77	10	13
Statesville	56	12	32

Table 9.7
HCHD Special Study: Oral Health and Fluoridation *(continued)*

Note: * "Never" or "Did not know" included.

Table 9.8
HCHD Special
Study: HIV and
AIDS Prevalence

	AIDS Cases per 100,000 Population, All Ages			
Location	2019	2014	2009	2004
Hillsboro County	3.1	3.4	3.6	3.9
Capital City	4.1	4.2	4.7	5.6
Statewide	5.3	6.2	6.7	7.2

	AIDS Cases per 100,000 Population, Adults and Adolescents			
Location	2019	2014	2009	2004
Hillsboro County	3.5	3.5	3.7	4.1
Capital City	4.3	4.3	4.8	5.7
Statewide	8.2	7.6	8.0	9.3
By Sex, Hillsboro County				
Male	10.7	10.4	12.7	8.6
Female	3.0	3.2	4.0	2.7
By Sex, Capital City				
Male	12.3	11.5	12.0	10.6
Female	3.8	3.8	3.8	3.9
By Sex, Statewide				
Male	10.2	11.5	23.2	15.1
Female	3.5	3.7	3.5	3.7

	HIV Infections per 100,000 Population			
Location	2019	2014	2009	2004
Hillsboro County	10.1	11.4	10.7	12.2
Capital City	17.5	17.3	18.4	19.8
Statewide	23.8	25.8	24.2	25.6

	2019	2014
Total Population with Asthma		
Hillsboro County	12.4	10.0
Statewide	11.8	10.5
Males with Asthma		
Hillsboro County	13.2	10.1
Statewide	12.4	10.3
Females with Asthma		
Hillsboro County	14	13.5
Statewide	17.5	14.3
By Age, Hillsboro County		
18–34	12.4	11.7
35–64	10.9	10.8
65+	7.0	7.6
By Household Income, Hillsboro County		
<$25,000	16.3	15.8
$25,000+	8.5	9.3
By Education, Hillsboro County		
Less Than High School	19.4	18.3
At Least High School/GED	10.3	10.0
By Employment Status, Hillsboro County		
Employed	9	9.4
Unemployed	14.5	12.7
Unable to Work	28.7	27.5
Homemaker/Student	12.3	14.0
Retired	7.4	7.9
Statewide	23.8	25.8

Table 9.9
HCHD Special Study: Asthma Prevalence

Notes: (1) All data, except total population, are percentage of population aged 18 years or older. (2) GED: general educational development.

Table 9.10
HCHD Special Study: Child Health

	2019	2014
Percentage of Low Birthweight Births		
Hillsboro County—All	8.0	7.5
White	7.0	5.9
Black	9.3	9.4
Hispanic	7.0	7.4
Capital City—All	9.0	8.8
White	6.0	6.1
Black	12.0	13.0
Hispanic	8.0	9.0
Percentage of Preterm Births		
Hillsboro County—All	11.0	13.0
White	10.4	11.2
Black	15.0	14.6
Hispanic	11.2	11.4
Capital City–All	13.3	15.3
White	8.0	8.2
Black	17.0	17.4
Hispanic	12.9	9.3
Percentage of Overweight or Obese Children (Aged 10–17 Years)		
Hillsboro County—All	31.5	33.0
White	24.5	28.2
Black	36.3	38.4
Hispanic	33.5	31.2
Capital City—All	35.0	36.1
White	29.0	30.1
Black	37.2	34.8
Hispanic	32.4	33.8
Percentage of Children (Aged 0–17 Years) Who Had Medical and Dental Visits in Past 12 Months		
Hillsboro County—All	69.3	62.4
White	74.0	68.2
Black	61.0	58.9
Hispanic	60.1	52.3
Capital City—All	76.8	62.3
White	77.9	70.2
Black	65.9	60.3
Hispanic	70.2	63.2

continued

	2019	2014
Percentage of Children (Aged 1–17 Years) with Oral Health Problems		
Hillsboro County—All	17.3	17.0
White	16.2	15.3
Black	18.9	18.3
Hispanic	17.4	17.0
Capital City–All	18.6	19.4
White	16.0	15.9
Black	17.5	17.5
Hispanic	17.1	16.8
Percentage of Children (Aged 2–17 Years) with Emotional, Developmental, or Behavioral Problems Who Received Mental Healthcare		
Hillsboro County—All	58.2	53.5
White	63.4	62.5
Black	45.2	40.3
Hispanic	49.2	49.3
Capital City—All	58.9	52.5
White	66.2	60.2
Black	43.4	40.8
Hispanic	45.3	40.2
Percentage of Children (Aged 19–35 Months) Who Are Immunized*		
Hillsboro County—All	68.5	63.2
White	74.9	72.4
Black	66.5	60.2
Hispanic	74.6	70.4
Capital City—All	65.5	64.9
White	72.0	71.4
Black	60.7	59.4
Hispanic	70.3	70.9

Table 9.10
HCHD Special Study: Child Health *(continued)*

Note: * Includes DTaP1, poliovirus, measles, Hib, HepB, varicella, and PCV vaccines.

Table 9.11
HCHD Special
Study: Sexually
Transmitted
Diseases

	2019
Chlamydia	
Reported Cases in Hillsboro County	690
Percentage, Male	28.1
Percentage, Female	71.9
Reported Cases in Capital City	828
Percentage, Male	25.0
Percentage, Female	75.0
Gonorrhea	
Reported Cases in Hillsboro County	184
Percentage, Male	47.5
Percentage, Female	52.5
Reported Cases in Capital City	267
Percentage, Male	46.2
Percentage, Female	53.8
Syphilis	
Reported Cases in Hillsboro County	10
Percentage, Male	94.1
Percentage, Female	5.9
Reported Cases in Capital City	34
Percentage, Male	95.3
Percentage, Female	4.7

	2019	2014
Cervical Cancer Deaths in Hillsboro County		
Rate per 100,000 Women		
All Hillsboro County	2.7	2.6
White	7.4	7.8
Black	7.7	8.1
Hispanic	6.5	6.9
Incidence Rate per 100,000		
All Hillsboro County	7.5	7.4
White	7.4	7.1
Black	7.7	8.3
Hispanic	N/A	N/A
Breast Cancer Prevalence in Hillsboro County		
Rate per 100,000 Women		
All Hillsboro County	21.7	23.1
White	20.9	20.1
Black	33.8	34.6
Hispanic	N/A	N/A
Incidence Rate per 100,000		
All Hillsboro County	118.6	115.4
White	113.6	113.7
Black	126.2	125.2
Hispanic	88.8	93.6
Legal Abortions in Hillsboro County		
Rate per 1,000 Women (Aged 15–44)		
All Hillsboro County	5.1	6.8
Percentage by Age		
Up to 19	14	16
20–29	58	545
30–39	25	26
40+	3	4
Percentage by Race		
White	80	83
Black	16	
Other	4	3

Table 9.12
HCHD Special Study: Women's Health

Table 9.13
Behavioral
Risk Factor
Surveillance
System Data:
Hillsboro
County vs.
Capital City

	Hillsboro County (%)	Capital City (%)
Alcohol Consumption		
Adults who have had at least one drink of alcohol within the past 30 days	38.2	58.5
Heavy drinkers (adult men having more than two drinks per day; adult women having more than one drink per day)	2.5	5.1
Binge drinkers (adults having five or more drinks on one occasion)	8.4	14.2
Arthritis		
Adults who have been told they have arthritis (Yes)	29.3	24.0
Asthma		
Adults who have been told they currently have asthma (Yes)	10.5	9.0
Adults who have ever been told they have asthma (Yes)	13.8	13.2
Cardiovascular Disease		
Adults who have ever been told they had a heart attack (myocardial infarction)	4.3	4.3
Adults who have ever been told they had angina or coronary heart disease	5.3	4.7
Adults who have ever been told they had a stroke	3.3	2.7
Cholesterol Awareness		
Adults who have had their blood cholesterol checked within the past five years (Yes)	65.3	71.2
Adults who have ever had their blood cholesterol checked (Yes)	82.4	73.2
Adults who have had their blood cholesterol checked and have been told it was high (Yes)	56.6	40.4
Colorectal Cancer		
Adults aged 50+ who have had a blood stool test within the past two years	15.6	21.3
Adults aged 50+ who have had a sigmoidoscopy or colonoscopy	51.0	68.0
Diabetes		
Have you ever been told by a doctor that you have diabetes? (No)	93.5	83.4
Disability		
Adults with health problems that require the use of special equipment (Yes)	8.3	21.2
Adults who are limited in any activities because of physical, mental, or emotional problems (Yes)	12.3	17.4
Exercise		
Adults who participated in any physical activities during the past month (Yes)	80.3	70.2
Fruits and Vegetables		
Adults who have consumed fruits and vegetables five or more times per day (Yes)	29.4	19.4
Healthcare Access/Coverage		
Adults who have any kind of healthcare coverage (Yes)	78.2	72.3

continued

	Hillsboro County (%)	Capital City (%)
Health Status		
Excellent	22.2	23.4
Very Good	25.5	37.6
Good	27.0	30.5
Fair	14.5	6.3
Poor	10.8	2.2
Hypertension Awareness		
Adults who have been told they have high blood pressure (Yes)	34.5	26.3
Immunization Status		
Adults aged 65+ who had a flu shot within the past year (Yes)	43.4	54.2
Adults aged 65+ who have ever had a pneumonia vaccination (Yes)	23.5	43.4
Oral Health		
Adults aged 65+ who have had all their natural teeth extracted	18.9	13.4
Adults who have had any permanent teeth extracted	64.2	58.3
Adults who have visited the dentist or dental clinic within the past year for any reason	61.3	70.8
Physical Activity		
Adults with 30+ minutes of moderate physical activity five or more days per week, or vigorous physical activity for 20+ minutes three or more days per week (Yes)	52.2	40.4
Adults with 20+ minutes of vigorous physical activity three or more days per week (Yes)	30.4	28.9
Prostate Cancer		
Men aged 40+ who have had a PSA test within the past two years	59.3	53.3
Women's Health		
Women aged 50+ who have had a mammogram within the past two years	77.1	82.4
Women aged 18+ who have had a Pap test within the past three years	77.5	82.8
Women aged 40+ who have had a mammogram with the past two years	65.8	70.3
Tobacco Use		
Four-level smoking status		
Smokes every day	24.5	21.4
Some days	7.5	6.7
Former smoker	14.0	20.2
Never smoked	54.0	51.7
Adults who are current smokers	32.0	28.1
Demographics: Age (Years)		
18–24	9.0	12.5
25–34	19.5	16.5
35–44	20.4	21.5
35–44	20.4	21.5

Table 9.13
Behavioral Risk Factor Surveillance System Data: Hillsboro County vs. Capital City *(continued)*

continued

Table 9.13
Behavioral
Risk Factor
Surveillance
System Data:
Hillsboro
County vs.
Capital City
(continued)

	Hillsboro County (%)	Capital City (%)
45–54	23.5	19.5
55–64	8.8	14.0
65+	18.8	16.0
Demographics: Race/Ethnicity		
White	84.0	78.0
Black	10.0	12.5
Hispanic	4.0	5.5
Other	1.0	2.0
Multiracial	1.0	2.0
Demographic: Marital Status		
Married	73.0	65.0
Divorced	6.0	10.3
Widowed	8.8	7.3
Separated	1.3	1.0
Never Married	10.5	14.2
Partnered	0.4	2.2
Demographic: Children in Household		
None	50.1	63.2
One	16.9	17.2
Two	22.5	15.2
Three	5.5	3.1
Four	3.2	1.0
Five or More	1.8	0.3
Demographics: Highest Grade in School		
Less than High School	10.2	11.3
High School or GED	44.5	34.5
Some College	18.2	28.3
College+	27.1	25.9
Demographic: Employment		
Employed	54.3	48.2
Self-Employed	10.5	7.5
No Work >Year	0.4	2.3
No Work <Year	1.2	2.9
Homemaker	9.3	6.9
Student	4.0	4.8
Retired	17.3	22.2
Unable to Work	3.0	5.2

continued

	Hillsboro County (%)	Capital City (%)
Demographics: Household Income (US Dollars)		
Less than $15,000	12.4	14.8
$15,000–24,999	18.3	11.3
$25,000–34,999	10.2	10.8
$35,000–49,999	18.9	11.8
$50,000+	40.2	51.3
Demographics: Gender	100.0	100.0
Male	49.5	46.3
Female	51.5	53.7
Demographics: Weight Classification		
Neither Overweight nor Obese (BMI below 24.8)	33.2	29.0
Overweight (BMI 25.0–29.9)	38.8	39.0
Obese (BMI 30.0–99.8)	28.0	32.0
Sample Size (Number)	860	1,245

Table 9.13 Behavioral Risk Factor Surveillance System Data: Hillsboro County vs. Capital City *(continued)*

Notes: (1) Sample study conducted in 2018. (2) Reported percentages are based on cell sizes >50. (3) BMI: body-mass index; GED: general educational development; PSA: prostate-specific antigen.

Table 9.14
Healthy People
2020 National
Goals and
Recent State
Statistics

	Note	National Goals (2020)	Statewide (2019)
Access to Health Services			
Percentage of adults aged 18–64 with specific source of ongoing care		89.0	72.0
Percentage of adults aged 65+ with specific source of ongoing care		100.0	74.0
Arthritis, Osteoporosis, and Chronic Back Condition			
Percentage of adults with doctor-diagnosed arthritis whose usual activities are limited in any way by arthritis		35.5	26.0
Percentage of adults aged 18–64 diagnosed with arthritis who are unemployed or unable to work		31.5	22.0
Hospitalization rate for hip fracture among females aged 65+	1	741.2	819.2
Hospitalization rate for hip fracture among males aged 65+	1	418.4	490.5
Cancer			
Lung cancer death rate	1	48.5	52.4
Breast cancer death rate	1	20.6	25.0
Cervical cancer death rate	1	2.2	2.6
Colorectal cancer death rate	1	14.5	19.4
Oropharyngeal cancer death rate	1	2.3	2.2
Prostate cancer death rate	1	21.2	27.1
Melanoma (skin) cancer death rate	1	2.4	2.7
Percentage of women aged 21–65 who have received cervical cancer screening based on the most recent guidelines		93.0	81.2
Percentage of adults aged 50+ who received a fecal occult blood test (FOBT) for colorectal cancer within the past 2 years	1	17.0	17.0
Percentage of adults aged 50 who ever received a sigmoidoscopy for colorectal cancer	1	72.0	68.0
Percentage of women aged 50–74 with a mammogram in last 2 years	1	81.1	70.0
Chronic Kidney Disease			
End-stage renal disease incidence rate	2	318.5	358.6
Diabetes			
Percentage of adults with diabetes who have an annual foot examination	1	74.8	66.1
Percentage of adults with diabetes who have an annual dilated eye examination	1	58.7	68.3
Percentage of adults with diabetes who have a glycosylated hemo-globin measurement at least twice a year	1	71.7	66.4
Percentage of adults with diabetes who perform self-blood-glucose monitoring at least once daily	1	70.4	55.8
Percentage of adults diagnosed with diabetes who have attended class in managing diabetes	1	62.5	60.0

continued

	Note	National Goals (2020)	Statewide (2019)
Environmental Health			
Number of days the air quality index (AQI) exceeds 100		10.0	26.0
Percentage of persons receiving safe drinking water from community water systems		91.0	90.0
Waterborne disease outbreaks from community water systems		0.0	0.0
State monitors environmentally related diseases		Yes	Yes
Family Planning			
Pregnancy rate among adolescent females aged 15–17	3	36.2	23.6
Food Safety			
Campylobacter species incidence	4	8.5	12.8
Shiga toxin–producing *E. coli*	4	0.6	1.2
Salmonella incidence rate	4	11.4	13.7
Outbreaks of infections associated with beef		0.0	0.0
Hearing and Other Sensory or Communication Disorder			
Percentage of infants (with possible hearing loss) who receive audiologic evaluation by age 3 months		72.6	70.9
Heart Disease and Stroke			
Coronary heart disease death rate	1	100.8	153.1
Stroke death rate	1	33.8	47.9
Percentage of adults aged 20 or older who have ever been told their blood pressure was high		10% less	29.0
Percentage of adults who had their blood cholesterol checked within the past 5 years		82.1	75.0
Hospitalization rate for heart failure as the principal diagnosis (aged 65–74)	5	8.8	12.4
Hospitalization rate for heart failure as the principal diagnosis (aged 75–84)	5	20.2	30.1
Hospitalization rate for heart failure as the principal diagnosis (aged 85+)	5	38.6	67.2
HIV			
AIDS incidence rate (persons aged 13+)	6	13.0	14.2
Number of new AIDS cases among men aged 13+ who have sex with men		10% less	438.0
Number of new AIDS cases among persons aged 13+ who inject drugs		10% less	353.0
Number of new cases of perinatally acquired AIDS		10% less	4.0
HIV disease death rate	1	3.3	2.9
Percentage of persons aged 25–44 with tuberculosis who have been tested for HIV		71.5	79.0

Table 9.14
Healthy People 2020 National Goals and Recent State Statistics *(continued)*

continued

Table 9.14
Healthy People
2020 National
Goals and
Recent State
Statistics
(continued)

	Note	National Goals (2020)	Statewide (2019)
Percentage of unmarried sexually active women (aged 18–44) who use condoms (to prevent pregnancy)		38.0	21.5
Percentage of unmarried sexually active men (aged 18–44) who use condoms (to prevent pregnancy)		60.7	NA
Immunization and Infectious Disease			
Number of new reported cases of vaccine-preventable diseases: Pertussis (under aged 1)		Reduce	82.0
Number of new reported cases of vaccine-preventable diseases: Pertussis (aged 11–18)		Reduce	140.0
Number of new reported cases of vaccine-preventable diseases: Varicella or chicken pox (under aged 18)		Reduce	4,869.0
Meningococcal disease incidence rate	1	0.3	0.5
Percentage of vaccination coverage levels of 4 doses diphtheria-tetanus-acellular pertussis (DTaP) (children aged 19–35 months)		90.0	87.8
Percentage of vaccination coverage levels for 3 doses Haemophilus influenza type b (Hib) (children aged 19–35 months)		90.0	95.0
Percentage of vaccination coverage levels for 3 doses hepatitis B (hep B) (children aged 19–35 months)		90.0	92.4
Percentage of vaccination coverage levels for 1 dose measles-mumps-rubella (MMR) (children aged 19–35 months)		90.0	94.0
Percentage of vaccination coverage levels for 3 doses polio (children aged 19–35 months)		90.0	93.9
Percentage of vaccination coverage levels for 1 dose varicella (children aged 19–35 months)		90.0	88.9
Percentage of vaccination coverage levels for 4 doses pneumococcal conjugate (children aged 19–35 months)		90.0	75.8
Percentage of fully immunized children (children aged 19–35 months)		80.0	68.3
Percentage of adults aged 18–64 with flu shot in past year		80.0	31.2
Percentage of adults aged 65+ with flu shot in past year		90.0	72.2
Percentage of adults aged 65+ ever vaccinated against pneumococcal disease		90.0	69.0
Percentage of adults aged 18–64 ever had vaccination against pneumococcal disease		10% more	15.2
Percentage of public health providers who had vaccination coverage levels among children in their practice population measured within the past year		50.0	80.0
Percentage of children under aged 6 who participate in population-based immunization registries		10% more	17.0
Hepatitis A incidence rate	1	0.3	0.5
Hepatitis B incidence rate (persons aged 19+)	1	1.5	1.1

continued

	Note	National Goals (2020)	Statewide (2019)
Hepatitis C incidence rate	1	0.2	0.4
Tuberculosis incidence rate	1	1.0	2.7
Percentage of tuberculosis patients who complete curative therapy within 12 months		93.0	74.0
Percentage of persons with latent tuberculosis infection who complete a course of treatment		79.0	41.0
Injury and Violence Prevention			
Hospitalization rate for nonfatal traumatic brain injuries	1	10% less	39.6
Hospitalization rate for nonfatal spinal cord injuries	1	3.2	5.8
State-level child fatality review of external causes for children aged 17 or under		Yes	Yes
Statewide emergency department surveillance system that collects data on external causes of injury		Yes	No
State collects data on external causes of injury through hospital discharge data systems		Yes	Yes
Poisoning death rate	1	13.1	15.3
Unintentional injury death rate	1	36.0	39.4
Motor vehicle crash death rate per 100,000 population	1	12.4	12.2
Motor vehicle crash death rate per 100 million miles traveled	1	1.2	1.5
Percentage of adults using safety belts		92.4	75.1
Pedestrian death rate	1	1.3	1.4
State law requiring bicycle helmets for riders under age 18		Yes	No
Accidental falls death rate	1	7.0	6.5
Unintentional suffocation death rate	1	1.7	2.3
Drowning death rate	1	1.1	0.9
Residential fire death rate	1	0.9	1.2
Homicide rate	1	5.5	6.3
Firearm-related death rate	1	9.2	10.8
Weapon possession among adolescents on school property	8	10% less	1.8
Child maltreatment fatality rate	9	2.2	1.1
Maltreatment of children under age 18	9	8.5	8.0
Maternal, Infant, and Child Health			
Fetal mortality rate (20+ weeks of gestation)	10	5.6	6.0
Perinatal mortality rate (fetal and infant mortality rate during perinatal period)	10	5.9	7.1
Infant mortality rate (under age 1)	10	6.0	7.2
Neonatal mortality rate (aged 0–27 days)	10	4.1	5.1

Table 9.14
Healthy People
2020 National
Goals and
Recent State
Statistics
(continued)

continued

	Note	National Goals (2020)	Statewide (2019)
Postneonatal mortality rate (aged 28–364 days)	10	2.0	2.1
Infant mortality rate for birth defects	10	1.3	1.3
Infant mortality rate for congenital heart defects	10	0.3	0.4
Infant mortality rate for sudden infant death syndrome (SIDS)	10	0.5	0.4
Child death rate for ages 1–4	11	25.7	26.1
Child death rate for ages 5–9	11	12.3	13.1
Adolescent death rate for ages 10–14	11	15.2	16.6
Adolescent death rate for ages 15–19	11	55.7	57.4
Young adult death rate for ages 20–24	11	88.5	103.5
Maternal mortality rate	10	11.4	10.3
Rate of maternal complications during hospitalized labor and delivery	12	28.0	35.1
Percentage of low-risk, first-time mothers giving birth by cesarean		23.9	27.5
Percentage of low-risk women giving birth by cesarean with a prior cesarean birth		81.7	86.0
Percentage of infants born at low birthweight (LBW)		7.8	8.5
Percentage of infants born at very low birthweight (VLBW)		1.4	1.6
Percentage of preterm live births		11.4	10.2
Percentage of live births at 34–36 weeks of gestation		8.1	7.3
Percentage of live births at 32–33 weeks of gestation		1.4	1.3
Percentage of live births at less than 32 weeks of gestation		1.8	1.8
Percentage of births to mothers beginning prenatal care in first trimester		77.9	71.5
Percentage of live births to mothers who received early and adequate prenatal care		77.6	66.3
Percentage of live births to mothers who did not smoke during pregnancy		98.6	82.4
Percentage of mothers who breastfeed their babies		81.9	64.6
All newborns screened at birth for conditions as mandated by state programs		Yes	Yes
Percentage of very low birthweight infants born at Level III hospitals		83.7	83.7
Mental Health and Mental Disorder			
Suicide rate	1	10.2	10.7
Nutrition and Weight Status			
Percentage of healthy weight adults (aged 20+)		33.9	34.2
Percentage of obese adults (aged 20+)		30.6	29.2
Percentage of children grades K–6 who are obese		15.7	17.3
Percentage of students grades 7–12 who are obese		16.1	17.2

continued

	Note	National Goals (2020)	Statewide (2019)
Occupational Safety and Health			
Work-related injury death rate for all industries (aged 16+)	13	3.6	3.2
Work-related injury death rate for construction industry (aged 16+)	13	9.7	7.9
Work-related injury death rate for transportation and warehousing industry (aged 16+)	13	14.8	10.7
Number of pneumoconiosis deaths (aged 15+)		10% less	329.0
Work-related homicides (aged 16+)		10% less	29.0
Oral Health			
Percentage of adults aged 45–64 who ever had a permanent tooth extracted due to dental caries or periodontal disease		68.8	55.5
Percentage of oral and pharyngeal cancers detected at the earliest stage		35.8	31.7
Percentage of adults who have visited a dentist in the past year, aged 18+ and aged 65+		10% more	70.2 and 65.3
Percentage of population served by optimally fluoridated community water systems		79.6	46.0
State has a system for referring infants/children with cleft lips, cleft palates, and other craniofacial anomalies to rehabilitative teams		Yes	Yes
State has an oral and craniofacial state-based surveillance system		Yes	No
State has an effective public dental health program directed by a dental professional with public health training		Yes	Yes
Physical Activity			
Percentage of adults who engage in no leisure-time physical activity		32.6	23.2
Percentage of adults who engage in vigorous or moderate physical activity		10% more	51.2
Respiratory Disease			
Asthma death rate (persons under age 35)	14	10% less	4.5
Asthma death rate (persons aged 35–64)	14	6.0	12.6
Asthma death rate (persons aged 65+)	14	22.9	37.8
Hospitalization rate for asthma (children under age 5)	15	18.1	47.1
Hospitalization rate for asthma (persons aged 5–64)	15	8.6	14.9
Hospitalization rate for asthma (persons aged 65+)	15	20.3	28.2
Death rate due to chronic obstructive pulmonary disease (COPD) among adults aged 45+	1	98.5	109.7
Death rate due to chronic obstructive pulmonary disease (COPD) among adults aged 45+	1	98.5	109.7

Table 9.14
Healthy People 2020 National Goals and Recent State Statistics *(continued)*

continued

	Note	National Goals (2020)	Statewide (2019)
Sexually Transmitted Disease			
Gonorrhea incidence rate among females aged 14–44	1	257.0	225.4
Gonorrhea incidence rate among males aged 15–44	1	198.0	164.2
Incidence rate of primary and secondary syphilis among females	1	1.4	0.5
Incidence rate of primary and secondary syphilis among males	1	6.8	3.8
Substance Abuse			
Percentage of high school seniors who never used any alcoholic beverages		30.5	17.3
Percentage of 8th graders who disapprove of drinking alcohol regularly		86.4	87.2
Percentage of 10th graders who disapprove of drinking alcohol regularly		85.4	61.3
Percentage of 12th graders who disapprove of drinking alcohol regularly		77.6	48.2
Percentage of 8th graders who said they would never use marijuana		82.8	84.2
Percentage of 10th graders who said they would never use marijuana		66.1	65.4
Percentage of 12th graders who said they would never use marijuana		60.3	50.5
Cirrhosis death rate	1	8.2	7.2
Drug-induced death rate	1	11.3	14.6
Percentage of high school seniors who engaged in binge drinking in the past two weeks		22.7	34.4
Tobacco Use			
Percentage of adults who smoke cigarettes		12.0	22.2
Percentage of adults who use smokeless (spit) tobacco		0.3	3.1
Percentage of adults who smoke cigars		0.2	7.1
Percentage of students in grades 9–12 who used tobacco products in past month		21.0	25.3
Percentage of students in grades 9–12 who smoked cigarettes in past month		16.0	17.3
Percentage of students in grades 9–12 who used smokeless (spit) tobacco in past month		6.9	6.2
Percentage of students in grades 9–12 who used cigars in past month		8.0	10.2

continued

	Note	National Goals (2020)	Statewide (2019)
Percentage of adult smokers who attempted to quit smoking		80.0	57.4
Percentage of smoke cessation during first trimester of pregnancy		30.0	24.8
Percentage of students in grades 9–12 who tried to quit smoking		64.0	66.8
State has smoke-free indoor air laws that prohibit smoking		Yes	Mixed

Table 9.14
Healthy People 2020 National Goals and Recent State Statistics *(continued)*

Notes:

1. per 100,000
2. per 1,000,000
3. per 1,000 women aged 15–17
4. Cases per 100,000
5. per 1,000 by age group
6. per 100,000 aged 13+
7. per million miles traveled
8. per 1,000 students
9. per 100,000 children under age 18
10. per 1,000 live births
11. per 100,000 in age group
12. per 100 deliveries
13. per 100,000 workers aged 16+
14. per 10,000

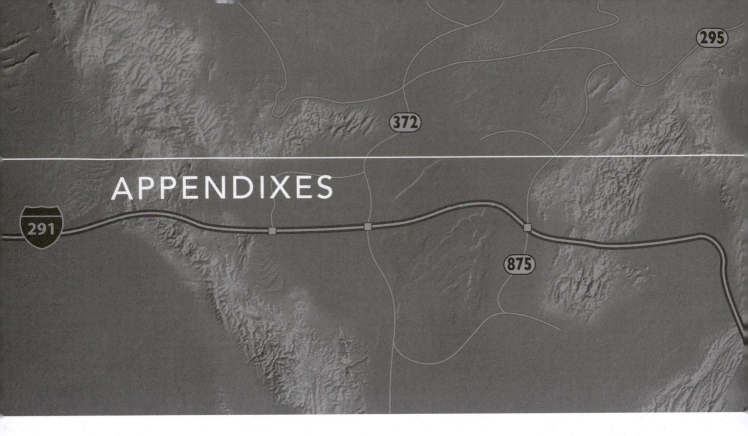

APPENDIXES

Appendixes include supplemental information on Capital City. Although not located in Hillsboro County, Capital City is near Jasper. As stated in case 8, Jasper is slowly becoming a commuter town for Capital City, as an increasing number of Jasper residents work in Capital City. The opening of the new interstate highway will significantly reduce the travel time between Jasper and Capital City. Capital City also remains the medical referral center for Hillsboro County.

The following tables are included here. An asterisk (*) indicates that an Excel version of the table is available on the web at *ache.org/books/Middleboro2*.

	2019	2014	2009	2004	1999
All Races					
Ward I	40,293	41,250	40,320	41,249	39,339
Ward II	50,392	52,395	50,395	47,502	46,503
Ward III	35,202	31,595	31,370	29,720	21,340
Ward IV	51,673	38,200	38,145	36,869	13,268
Total	**177,560**	**163,440**	**160,230**	**155,340**	**120,450**
White					
Ward I	19,241	25,949	26,646	28,272	31,898
Ward II	38,668	44,057	42,599	39,815	38,987
Ward III	27,212	25,350	25,971	24,590	17,088
Ward IV	48,936	35,387	37,123	35,867	12,603
Total	**134,057**	**130,743**	**132,339**	**128,544**	**100,576**
Black					
Ward I	19,202	13,612	12,096	11,627	6,506
Ward II	10,294	7,218	6,826	6,927	6,927
Ward III	7,067	5,365	4,516	4,368	3,820
Ward IV	1,612	1,590	597	379	212
Total	**38,175**	**27,785**	**24,035**	**23,301**	**17,465**
Other					
Ward I	1,850	1,689	1,578	1,350	935
Ward II	1,430	1,120	970	760	589
Ward III	923	880	883	762	432
Ward IV	1,125	1,223	425	623	453
Total	**5,328**	**4,912**	**3,856**	**3,495**	**2,409**

Table A.1
Capital City Population by Race

*On the web at
ache.org/books/
Middleboro2*

Table A.2
Capital City Age Profile by Sex

	2019 Total	Under 5	5–14	15–24	25–44	45–64	65–74	75+
Ward I	40,293	2,759	5,698	5,317	12,001	8,660	3,497	2,361
Male	19,938	1,396	2,991	2,692	5,284	4,446	2,133	997
Female	20,355	1,364	2,707	2,626	6,717	4,213	1,364	1,364
Ward II	50,392	3,450	7,122	6,649	15,024	10,826	4,364	2,957
Male	24,692	1,728	3,704	3,333	6,543	5,506	2,642	1,235
Female	25,700	1,722	3,418	3,315	8,481	5,320	1,722	1,722
Ward III	35,202	2,408	4,962	4,640	10,545	7,551	3,018	2,078
Male	16,489	1,154	2,473	2,226	4,370	3,677	1,764	824
Female	18,713	1,254	2,489	2,414	6,175	3,874	1,254	1,254
Ward IV	51,673	3,537	7,294	6,815	15,440	11,093	4,454	3,040
Male	24,803	1,736	3,720	3,348	6,573	5,531	2,654	1,240
Female	26,870	1,800	3,574	3,466	8,867	5,562	1,800	1,800
Total	**177,560**	**12,154**	**25,076**	**23,421**	**53,010**	**38,130**	**15,333**	**10,436**
Male	**85,922**	**6,014**	**12,888**	**11,599**	**22,770**	**19,161**	**9,193**	**4,296**
Female	**91,638**	**6,140**	**12,188**	**11,821**	**30,240**	**18,969**	**6,140**	**6,140**
% Male	**48.4**	**49.5**	**51.4**	**49.5**	**43.0**	**50.3**	**60.0**	**41.2**
% Female	**51.6**	**50.5**	**48.6**	**50.5**	**57.0**	**49.7**	**40.0**	**58.8**

Table A.3
Capital City Vital Statistics

	2019	2014	2009	2004	1999
Live Births	2,556	2,257	2,163	2,051	1,723
Death (Except Fetal)	1,456	1,379	1,362	1,398	1,145
Infant Deaths*	18	19	21	22	24
Neonatal Deaths+*	11	12	14	14	15
Postneonatal**	7	7	7	8	9
Maternal Deaths	2	1	3	2	0
Out-of-Wedlock Births	890	689	565	315	245
Marriages	1,367	1,358	1,433	1,325	1,325

Notes: *Under 1 year; +*Under 28 days; **28 days–11 months.

Cause of Death	ICD-10 Codes	2019	2014	2009	2004	1999	1994
Diseases of the Heart	I00–I09, I11, I13, 120-151	418	376	361	365	295	268
Malignant Neoplasms	C00–C97	340	300	298	296	267	210
Cerebrovascular Diseases	I60–I69	96	85	80	84	78	68
All Accidents	V01–X59, Y85–Y86	67	60	50	58	56	60
Chronic Lower Respiratory Disease	J40–J47	77	69	60	67	58	49
Influenza and Pneumonia	J10–J18	40	30	41	38	39	38
Diabetes Mellitus	E10–E14	45	34	31	40	30	34
Alzheimer's Disease	G30	39	30	18	39	16	12
Intentional Self-Harm	U03, X60–X84, Y87.0	19	17	15	21	35	22
Nephritis, Nephrotic Syndrome, and Nephrosis	N00–N07, N17–N19, N25–N27	25	20	20	28	19	25
Septicemia	A40–A41	20	20	12	12	18	10
Total Leading Causes		1,186	1,041	986	1,048	911	796
All Deaths		1,456	1,340	1,378	1,398	1,152	1,049

Table A.4
Capital City Resident Deaths by Cause of Death

Table A.5
Capital City
Causes of
Resident Death
by Age Group

Cause of Death	Total	>1	1–4	5–14	15–24	25–44	45–64	65–74	75+
Diseases of the Heart									
2019	418	0	0	0	0	11	50	139	218
2014	376	0	0	0	0	9	40	101	226
Malignant Neoplasms									
2019	340	0	0	2	4	9	15	145	165
2014	300	0	3	4	6	24	41	94	128
Cerebrovascular Diseases									
2019	96	0	0	0	0	2	14	33	47
2014	85	0	0	0	0	5	17	26	37
All Accidents									
2019	67	3	3	4	16	15	12	5	9
2014	60	6	1	2	13	16	8	3	11
Chronic Lower Respiratory Disease									
2019	77	0	0	0	0	0	21	29	27
2014	69	0	0	0	4	9	18	24	14
Influenza and Pneumonia									
2019	40	3	2	0	0	0	2	8	25
2014	40	0	1	0	0	4	4	9	22
Diabetes Mellitus									
2019	45	0	0	0	0	4	20	12	9
2014	34	0	0	0	0	5	12	12	5
Alzheimer's Disease									
2019	39	0	0	0	0	0	1	10	28
2014	30	0	0	0	0	0	4	9	17
Intentional Self-Harm									
2019	19	0	1	6	3	3	3	2	1
2014	17	0	0	3	2	3	6	1	2
Nephritis, Nephrotic Syndrome, and Nephrosis									
2019	25	1	0	4	2	4	6	2	6
2014	20	0	1	5	3	1	2	2	6
Septicemia									
2019	20	2	0	0	0	0	6	5	7
2014	20	1	0	2	0	5	4	4	4
Total Listed Causes									
2019	1,186	9	6	16	25	48	150	390	542
2014	1,041	7	6	16	28	81	146	285	472
Total All Deaths									
2019	1,456	18	36	35	48	79	193	438	609
2014	1,379	19	20	23	45	95	188	300	589

Category	CMS Core Measure	Benchmark	CCG	OMC
Timely and Effective Heart Attack Care	Average number of minutes before outpatients with chest pain or possible heart attack who needed specialized care were transferred to another hospital	58 min	82 min	61 min
Timely and Effective Heart Attack Care	Average number of minutes before outpatients with chest pain or possible heart attack got an ECG (electrocardiogram)	7 min	7 min	7 min
Timely and Effective Heart Attack Care	Percentage of outpatients with chest pain or possible heart attack who got drugs to break up blood clots within 30 minutes of arrival	59%	78%	79%
Timely and Effective Heart Attack Care	Percentage of outpatients with chest pain who received aspirin within 24 hours of arrival or before transferring from the emergency department	97%	96%	97%
Timely and Effective Heart Attack Care	Percentage of heart attack patients who got drugs to break up blood clots within 30 minutes of arrival	60%	65%	57%
Timely and Effective Heart Attack Care	Percentage of heart attack patients given a procedure to open blocked blood vessels within 90 minutes of arrival	96%	77%	83%
Effective Heart Failure Care	Percentage of heart failure patients given an evaluation of LVS (left ventricular systolic) function	99%	100%	100%
Effective Pneumonia Care	Percentage of pneumonia patients given the most appropriate initial antibiotic(s)	96%	97%	95%
Timely Surgical Care	Percentage of surgery patients who were given an antibiotic at the right time (within 1 hour of surgery) to help prevent infection	99%	98%	99%
Timely Surgical Care	Percentage of surgery patients whose preventive antibiotics were stopped at the right time (within 2 hours after surgery)	98%	99%	98%
Timely Surgical Care	Percentage of patients who got treatment at the right time (within 24 hours before or after surgery) to help prevent blood clots after certain types of surgery	100%	99%	100%
Effective Surgical Care	Percentage of surgery patients taking heart drugs called beta blockers before coming to the hospital who were kept on the beta blockers during the period just before and after surgery	98%	99%	99%
Effective Surgical Care	Percentage of surgery patients who were given the right kind of antibiotic to help prevent infection	99%	100%	100%
Effective Surgical Care	Percentage of surgery patients whose urinary catheters were removed on the first or second day after surgery	98%	99%	99%
Timely Emergency Dept. Care	Average time patients who came to the emergency department with broken bones had to wait before getting pain medication	54 min	42 min	45 min
Timely Emergency Dept. Care	Percentage of patients who left the emergency department before being seen	2%	3%	3%
Timely Emergency Dept. Care	Percentage of patients who came to the emergency department with stroke symptoms who received brain scan results within 45 minutes of arrival	66%	71%	69%

Table A.6
Performance Against CMS Core Measures: Capital City General Hospital (CCG) vs. Osteopathic Medical Center (OMC)

continued

Category	CMS Core Measure	Benchmark	CCG	OMC
Timely Emergency Dept. Care	Average median time patients spent in the emergency department before they were admitted to the hospital as an inpatient	260 min	325 min	303 min
Timely Emergency Dept. Care	Average (median) time patients spent in the emergency department before leaving from the visit	89 min	154 min	132 min
Timely Emergency Dept. Care	Average time patients spent in the emergency department before leaving from the visit	142 min	163 min	154 min
Timely Emergency Dept. Care	Average time patients spent in the emergency department before they were seen by a healthcare professional	26 min	33 min	31 min
Preventive Care	Percentage of patients assessed and given influenza vaccination	94%	97%	85%
Preventive Care	Percentage of healthcare workers given influenza vaccination	84%	94%	94%
Effective Children's Asthma Care	Percentage of children and their caregivers who received home management plan-of-care documents while hospitalized for asthma	90%	N/A	N/A
Effective Stroke Care	Percentage of ischemic stroke patients who got medicine to break up a blood clot within 3 hours after symptoms started	81%	85%	82%
Effective Stroke Care	Percentage of ischemic stroke patients who received medicine known to prevent complications caused by blood clots within 2 days of hospital admission	98%	94%	97%
Effective Stroke Care	Percentage of ischemic or hemorrhagic stroke patients who received treatment to keep blood clots from forming anywhere in the body within 2 days of hospital admission	97%	95%	95%
Effective Stroke Care	Percentage of ischemic stroke patients who received a prescription for medicine known to prevent complications caused by blood clots at discharge	99%	99%	98%
Effective Stroke Care	Percentage of ischemic stroke patients with a type of irregular heartbeat who were given a prescription for a blood thinner at discharge	97%	96%	95%
Effective Stroke Care	Percentage of ischemic stroke patients needing medicine to lower bad cholesterol who were given a prescription for this medicine at discharge	97%	93%	97%
Effective Stroke Care	Percentage of ischemic or hemorrhagic stroke patients or caregivers who received written educational material about stroke care and prevention during the hospital stay	94%	94%	93%
Blood Clot Prevention	Percentage of patients who got treatment to prevent blood clots on the day of or day after hospital admission or surgery	93%	91%	92%
Blood Clot Prevention	Percentage of patients who got treatment to prevent blood clots on the day of or the day after being admitted to the ICU (intensive care unit)	96%	97%	90%
Blood Clot Prevention	Percentage of patients who developed a blood clot while in the hospital who did not get treatment that could have prevented it	5%	3%	3%

continued

Category	CMS Core Measure	Benchmark	CCG	OMC
Blood Clot Treatment	Percentage of patients with blood clots who got recommended treatment, which includes using two different blood thinner medicines at the same time	95%	94%	95%
Blood Clot Treatment	Percentage of patients with blood clots who were treated with an intravenous blood thinner and then were checked to determine if the blood thinner caused unplanned complications	99%	98%	98%
Blood Clot Treatment	Percentage of patients with blood clots who were discharged on a blood thinner medicine and received written instructions about that medicine	90%	88%	84%
Pregnancy and Delivery Care	Percentage of mothers whose deliveries were scheduled too early (1–2 weeks early) when a scheduled delivery was not medically necessary	3%	3%	4%
Use of Medical Imaging	Percentage of outpatients with low back pain who had a magnetic resonance imaging (MRI) scan without trying recommended treatments first, such as physical therapy	40%	31%	53%
Use of Medical Imaging	Percentage of outpatients who had a mammogram, an ultrasound, or an MRI of the breast within 45 days after a screening mammogram	9%	8%	8%
Use of Medical Imaging	Percentage of outpatients who had CT (computed tomography) scans of the chest that were "combination" (double) scans	2%	8%	10%
Use of Medical Imaging	Percentage of outpatient CT scans of the abdomen that were "combination" scans	9%	3%	5%
Use of Medical Imaging	Percentage of outpatients who got cardiac imaging stress tests before low-risk outpatient surgery	5%	8%	7%
Use of Medical Imaging	Percentage of outpatients with brain CT scans who got a sinus CT scan at the same time	3%	5%	5%
Surgical Complications	Rate of complications for hip/knee replacement patients	3%	2%	2%
Surgical Complications	Rate of serious complications (from AHRQ)	<1%	No Difference from National Rate	No Difference from National Rate
Surgical Complications	Death rate among patients with serious treatable complications after surgery	117.5 per 1,000 dis.	No Difference from National Rate	No Difference from National Rate
Healthcare-Associated Infections	Rate of central line–associated bloodstream infections (CLABSIs) in ICUs and selected wards	N/A	No Difference from National Rate	No Difference from National Rate
Healthcare-Associated Infections	Rate of CLABSIs in ICUs only	N/A	No Difference from National Rate	No Difference from National Rate

Table A.6
Performance Against CMS Core Measures: Capital City General Hospital (CCG) vs. Osteopathic Medical Center (OMC) *(continued)*

continued

Category	CMS Core Measure	Benchmark	CCG	OMC
Healthcare-Associated Infections	Rate of catheter-associated urinary tract infections (CAUTIs) in ICUs and selected wards	N/A	No Difference from National Rate	No Difference from National Rate
Healthcare-Associated Infections	Rate of CAUTIs in ICUs only	N/A	No Difference from National Rate	No Difference from National Rate
Healthcare-Associated Infections	Rate of surgical-site infections from abdominal hysterectomy	N/A	No Difference from National Rate	No Difference from National Rate
Healthcare-Associated Infections	Rate of MRSA (Methicillin-resistant Staphylococcus aureus) blood laboratory identified events (bloodstream infections)	N/A	No Difference from National Rate	No Difference from National Rate
Healthcare-Associated Infections	Rate of C. diff (Clostridium difficile) laboratory identified events (intestinal infections)	N/A	No Difference from National Rate	No Difference from National Rate
Readmissions and Deaths	Rate of unplanned readmission for COPD (chronic obstructive pulmonary disease) patients	20%	No Difference from National Rate	Higher than National Rate
Readmissions and Deaths	Death rate for COPD patients	8%	No Difference from National Rate	No Difference from National Rate
Readmissions and Deaths	Rate of unplanned readmission for heart attack patients	22%	No Difference from National Rate	No Difference from National Rate
Readmissions and Deaths	Death rate for heart attack patients	12%	No Difference from National Rate	No Difference from National Rate
Readmissions and Deaths	Rate of unplanned readmission for heart failure patients	22%	No Difference from National Rate	No Difference from National Rate
Readmissions and Deaths	Death rate for heart failure patients	11%	No Difference from National Rate	No Difference from National Rate
Readmissions and Deaths	Rate of unplanned readmission for pneumonia patients	17%	No Difference from National Rate	No Difference from National Rate
Readmissions and Deaths	Death rate for pneumonia patients	11%	No Difference from National Rate	No Difference from National Rate

continued

Category	CMS Core Measure	Benchmark	CCG	OMC
Readmissions and Deaths	Rate of unplanned readmission for stroke patients	13%	No Difference from National Rate	No Difference from National Rate
Readmissions and Deaths	Death rate for stroke patients	15%	No Difference from National Rate	No Difference from National Rate
Readmissions and Deaths	Rate of unplanned readmission for coronary artery bypass graft (CABG) surgery patients	15%	No Difference from National Rate	No Difference from National Rate
Readmissions and Deaths	Death rate for CABG surgery patients	3%	No Difference from National Rate	No Difference from National Rate
Readmissions and Deaths	Rate of unplanned readmission after hip/knee surgery	5%	No Difference from National Rate	No Difference from National Rate
Readmissions and Deaths	Rate of unplanned readmission after discharge from hospital (hospitalwide)	15%	Better than National Rate	No Difference from National Rate
Payment and Value of Care	Payment for heart attack patients	N/A	More than National Average	No Difference from National Rate
Payment and Value of Care	Payment for heart failure patients	N/A	More than National Average	No Difference from National Rate
Payment and Value of Care	Payment for pneumonia patients	N/A	More than National Average	No Difference from National Rate
Payment and Value of Care	Death rate for heart attack patients	N/A	No Difference from National Rate	No Difference from National Rate
Payment and Value of Care	Payment for heart attack patients	N/A	More than National Average	No Difference from National Rate
Payment and Value of Care	Death rate for heart failure patients	N/A	More than National Average	More than National Average
Payment and Value of Care	Payment for heart failure patients	N/A	More than National Average	More than National Average

Table A.6
Performance Against CMS Core Measures: Capital City General Hospital (CCG) vs. Osteopathic Medical Center (OMC) *(continued)*

continued

Table A.6
Performance
Against CMS
Core Measures:
Capital City
General
Hospital (CCG)
vs. Osteopathic
Medical
Center (OMC)
(continued)

Category	CMS Core Measure	Benchmark	CCG	OMC
Payment and Value of Care	Death rate for pneumonia patients	N/A	No Difference from National Rate	No Difference from National Rate
Payment and Value of Care	Payment for pneumonia patients	N/A	No Difference from National Rate	No Difference from National Rate
Patient Survey	Percentage of patients who reported that their nurses "always" communicated well	80%	86%	80%
Patient Survey	Percentage of patients who reported that their doctors "always" communicated well	82%	91%	80%
Patient Survey	Percentage of patients who reported that they "always" received help as soon as they wanted	68%	78%	70%
Patient Survey	Percentage of patients who reported that their pain was "always" well controlled	71%	78%	61%
Patient Survey	Percentage of patients who reported that staff "always" explained the medication before giving it to them	65%	83%	66%
Patient Survey	Percentage of patients who reported that their room and bathroom were "always" cleaned	74%	91%	76%

Notes: (1) N/A means not applicable and either the data are not available or the number of cases is too small for a legitimate conclusion. (2) "Better" means better than national average. (3) "No difference" means no statistical difference exists between the hospital and the national average. (4) AHRQ: Agency for Healthcare Research and Quality; CMS: Centers for Medicare & Medicaid Services.

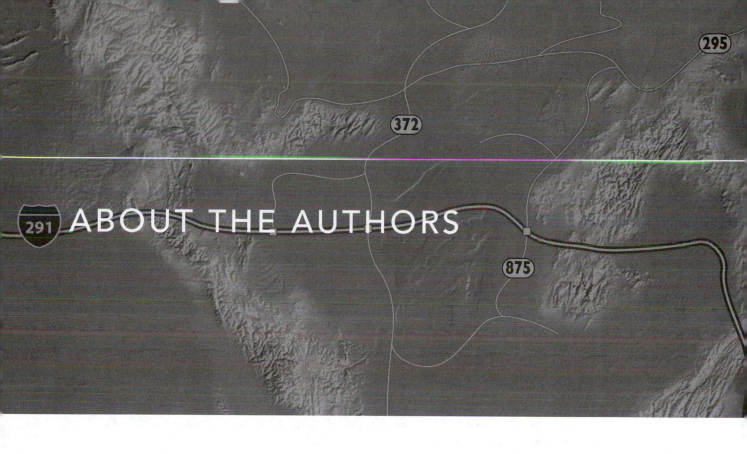

ABOUT THE AUTHORS

Lee F. Seidel, PhD, is professor emeritus of health management and policy at the University of New Hampshire (UNH) and visiting professor in the executive MBA in health administration program at the University of Colorado, Denver. He teaches capstone courses in both settings and courses in financial management and healthcare systems at UNH. He is the founding director of the UNH Center for Excellence in Teaching & Learning, and he managed the center for 15 years. The center is a recipient of a national Theodore M. Hesburgh Award.

UNH awarded Dr. Seidel the Jean Brierley Award, its highest honor for effective teaching. He is the first Association of University Programs in Health Administration (AUPHA) board chair from a baccalaureate program. In addition, he has authored four books and numerous articles on health administration, health administration education, and effective college teaching. His work has been supported by numerous sources, including the W.K. Kellogg Foundation and the Fund for the Improvement of Postsecondary Education of the US Department of Education.

Prior to his academic career, he worked with Arthur Andersen and Company and for the Office of the Mayor, City of New York. Dr. Seidel holds an MPA and PhD in community systems planning and development with emphasis in health administration from the Pennsylvania State University.

James B. Lewis, ScD, is associate professor of health management and policy at the University of New Hampshire (UNH). At UNH, he has taught baccalaureate- and graduate-level courses in health finance, health marketing, social marketing, strategic planning, strategic management, health reimbursement, managed care, and introduction to the healthcare system. He has also directed the university's undergraduate and graduate programs in health management and public health and served as department chair for several years.

Dr. Lewis holds an MBA from Northwestern University and an ScD from the Johns Hopkins School of Hygiene and Public Health. Prior to his academic appointment, he was a healthcare management consultant specializing in strategy and strategic planning, having been a principal with the firm of William M. Mercer and the national manager of healthcare strategic planning for Coopers & Lybrand. In these positions, he provided advice to dozens of healthcare organizations, insurance companies, and purchasers of healthcare services.

Dr. Lewis has coauthored three books and approximately 20 journal articles and case studies. He has served on the editorial boards and reviewed manuscripts for several healthcare journals. He is a member of AUPHA and has been a program reviewer at both the undergraduate and graduate levels.